REFERENCE EDITION

ESAP™ 2020

Endocrine Society's
Endocrine Self-Assessment Program
Questions, Answers, and Discussions

Lisa R. Tannock, MD, Program Chair
Professor of Medicine
Chief, Division of Endocrinology
and Molecular Medicine
University of Kentucky and
Department of Veterans Affairs

Barbara Gisella Carranza Leon, MD
Assistant Professor of Medicine
Division of Diabetes, Endocrinology,
and Metabolism
Vanderbilt University Medical Center

Alice Y. Chang, MD, MSc
Assistant Professor
Division of Endocrinology,
Diabetes, and Nutrition
Mayo Clinic

Stephen Clement, MD
Medical Director, Endocrine Services
Inova Fairfax Hospital

Dima Lutfi Diab, MD
Associate Professor of Clinical Medicine
University of Cincinnati

Nazanene H. Esfandiari, MD
Associate Professor
University of Michigan

Mathis Grossmann, MD, PhD, FRACP
Professor of Medicine
University of Melbourne
Austin Health

**Mark Gurnell, MBBS, MA
(Med Ed), PhD, FRCP**
Professor of Clinical Endocrinology
& Clinical SubDean
University of Cambridge,
Wellcome Trust-MRC Institute
of Metabolic Science &
School of Clinical Medicine

Jacqueline Jonklaas, MD, PhD
Professor
Division of Endocrinology
and Metabolism
Georgetown University

Steven B. Magill, MD, PhD
Associate Clinical Professor of Medicine
Endocrinology, Diabetes, and Metabolism
Medical College of Wisconsin

Deepika Reddy, MD
Assistant Professor
Division of Diabetes, Endocrinology,
and Metabolism
University of Utah Healthcare

Roberto Salvatori, MD
Professor of Medicine
Medical Director,
Johns Hopkins Pituitary Center
Johns Hopkins University

Aniket Sidhaye, MD
Assistant Professor of Medicine
Johns Hopkins University

Savitha Subramanian, MD
Associate Professor of Medicine
University of Washington

Anand Vaidya, MD, MMSC
Associate Professor of Medicine
Brigham and Women's Hospital
Harvard Medical School

Thomas J. Weber, MD
Associate Professor of Medicine
Division of Endocrinology,
Metabolism, and Nutrition
Duke University Medical Center

Abbie L. Young, MS, CGC, ELS(D)
Medical Editor

Endocrine Society
2055 L Street NW, Suite 600, Washington, DC 20036
1-888-ENDOCRINE • www.endocrine.org

ENDOCRINE
SOCIETY

Hormone Science to Health

ENDOCRINE
SOCIETY
Hormone Science to Health

The Endocrine Society is the world's largest, oldest, and most active organization working to advance the clinical practice of endocrinology and hormone research. Founded in 1916, the Society now has more than 18,000 global members across a range of disciplines. The Society has earned an international reputation for excellence in the quality of its peer-reviewed journals, educational resources, meetings, and programs that improve public health through the practice and science of endocrinology.

Visit us at:
education.endocrine.org
endocrine.org

Other Publications:
https://www.endocrine.org/publications

ISBN: 978-1-879225-72-5

Library of Congress Control Number: 2019951669

On the Cover: © Shutterstock. Doctor or medical student concentrating on textbook for medical research, close up (By TippaPatt).

OVERVIEW

The Endocrine Self-Assessment Program (ESAP™) is a self-study curriculum aimed at physicians wanting a self-assessment and a broad review of endocrinology. The ESAP Reference Edition consists of 120 brand-new multiple-choice questions in all areas of endocrinology, diabetes, and metabolism. There is extensive discussion of each correct answer, a comprehensive syllabus, and references. ESAP is updated annually with new questions.

The ESAP reference book is intended primarily for consultation and self-assessment of knowledge relating to endocrinology. As a reference book, educational credits are not available upon completion of the multiple-choice questions included. For information on educational products that include educational credit, please visit endocrine.org/store.

LEARNING OBJECTIVES

ESAP 2020 will allow learners to assess their knowledge of all aspects of endocrinology, diabetes, and metabolism.

Completion of this educational activity enables learners to accomplish key objectives:

- Recognize clinical manifestations of endocrine and metabolic disorders and select among current options for diagnosis, management, and therapy.
- Identify risk factors for endocrine and metabolic disorders and develop strategies for prevention.
- Evaluate endocrine and metabolic manifestations of systemic disorders.
- Use existing resources pertaining to clinical guidelines and treatment recommendations for endocrine and related metabolic disorders to guide diagnosis and treatment.

TARGET AUDIENCE

ESAP is a self-study curriculum aimed at physicians seeking initial certification or recertification in endocrinology, program directors interested in a testing and training instrument, and clinicians simply wanting a self-assessment and a broad review of endocrinology.

STATEMENT OF INDEPENDENCE

The Endocrine Society has a policy of ensuring that the content and quality of this educational activity are balanced, independent, objective, and scientifically rigorous. The scientific content of this activity was developed under the supervision of the Endocrine Society's ESAP Faculty Working Group.

DISCLOSURE POLICY

The faculty, committee members, and staff who are in position to control the content of this activity are required to disclose to the Endocrine Society and to learners any relevant financial relationship(s) of the individual or spouse/partner that have occurred within the last 12 months with any commercial interest(s) whose products or services are related to the content. Financial relationships are defined by remuneration in any amount from the commercial interest(s) in the form of grants; research support; consulting fees; salary; ownership interest (e.g., stocks, stock options, or ownership interest excluding diversified mutual funds); honoraria or other payments for participation in speakers' bureaus, advisory boards, or boards of directors; or other financial benefits. The intent of this disclosure is not to prevent planners with relevant financial relationships from planning or delivering content, but rather to provide learners with information that allows them to make their own judgments of whether these financial relationships may have influenced the educational activity with regard to exposition or conclusion. The Endocrine Society has reviewed all disclosures and resolved or managed all identified conflicts of interest, as applicable.

The following faculty reported relevant financial relationship(s): **Alice Y. Chang, MD, MSc**, is a site investigator and on the advisory board for clinical trial for Millendo Therapeutics. She is also on the national advisory board for Corcept Therapeutics. **Roberto Salvatori, MD**, receives grant funds from Roche, and he is on the advisory board of Pfizer and NovoNordisk. He serves as a clinical trial investigator for Novartis, Chiasma, OPKO, Strongbridge Biopharma, Corcept Therapeutics, and Crinetics Pharmaceuticals. **Savitha Subramanian, MD**, serves on the advisory board for Sanofi. **Anand Vaidya, MD, MMSC**, is a consultant for Selenity Therapeutics, HRA Pharma, and Orphagen Pharmaceuticals. **Thomas J. Weber, MD**, is a consultant for Ultragenyx Pharmaceutical and Pharmacosmos, He is also a primary investigator for Ultragenyx Pharmaceutical. His spouse is an editor for Nivalis Therapeutics and a primary investigator for AstraZeneca.

The following committee members reported no relevant financial relationships: **Lisa R. Tannock, MD**; **Barbara Gisella Carranza Leon, MD**; **Stephen Clement, MD**; **Dima Lutfi Diab, MD**; **Nazanene H. Esfandiari, MD**; **Mathis Grossmann, MD, PhD, FRCP**; **Mark Gurnell, MBBS, MA (Med Ed), PhD, FRCP**; **Jacqueline Jonklaas, MD, PhD**; **Steven B. Magill, MD, PhD**; **Deepika Reddy, MD**; **Aniket Sidhaye, MD**.

The medical editor for this program, **Abbie L. Young, MS, CGC, ELS(D)**, reported no relevant financial relationships.

The Endocrine Society staff associated with the development of content for this activity reported no relevant financial relationships.

DISCLAIMERS

The information presented in this activity represents the opinion of the faculty and is not necessarily the official position of the Endocrine Society.

USE OF PROFESSIONAL JUDGMENT:

The educational content in this self-assessment test relates to basic principles of diagnosis and therapy and does not substitute for individual patient assessment based on the health care provider's examination of the patient and consideration of laboratory data and other factors unique to the patient. Standards in medicine change as new data become available.

DRUGS AND DOSAGES:

When prescribing medications, the physician is advised to check the product information sheet accompanying each drug to verify conditions of use and to identify any changes in drug dosage schedule or contraindications.

POLICY ON UNLABELED/OFF-LABEL USE

The Endocrine Society has determined that disclosure of unlabeled/off-label or investigational use of commercial product(s) is informative for audiences and therefore requires this information to be disclosed to the learners at the beginning of the presentation. Uses of specific therapeutic agents, devices, and other products discussed in this educational activity may not be the same as those indicated in product labeling approved by the Food and Drug Administration (FDA). The Endocrine Society requires that any discussions of such "off-label" use be based on scientific research that conforms to generally accepted standards of experimental design, data collection, and data analysis. Before recommending or prescribing any therapeutic agent or device, learners should review the complete prescribing information, including indications, contraindications, warnings, precautions, and adverse events.

ACKNOWLEDGMENT OF COMMERCIAL SUPPORT

This activity is not supported by educational grant(s) or other funds from any commercial supporter.

PUBLICATION DATE: February 2020

Laboratory Reference Ranges

Reference ranges vary among laboratories. The listed reference ranges should be used when interpreting laboratory values presented in ESAP™. Conventional units are listed first with SI units in parentheses.

Lipid Values

High-density lipoprotein (HDL) cholesterol

    Optimal ----------------------------- >60 mg/dL (>1.55 mmol/L)

    Normal ------------------------ 40-60 mg/dL (1.04-1.55 mmol/L)

    Low ------------------------------------- <40 mg/dL (<1.04 mmol/L)

Low-density lipoprotein (LDL) cholesterol

    Optimal -----------------------------------<100 mg/dL (<2.59 mmol/L)

    Low ---------------------------------100-129 mg/dL (2.59-3.34 mmol/L)

    Borderline-high --------------130-159 mg/dL (3.37-4.12 mmol/L)

    High -----------------------160-189 mg/dL (4.14-4.90 mmol/L)

    Very high --------------------------≥190 mg/dL (≥4.92 mmol/L)

Non-HDL cholesterol

    Optimal -----------------------------------<130 mg/dL (<3.37 mmol/L)

    Borderline-high --------------130-159 mg/dL (3.37-4.12 mmol/L)

    High --------------------------------≥240 mg/dL (≥6.22 mmol/L)

Total cholesterol

    Optimal -----------------------------<200 mg/dL (<5.18 mmol/L)

    Borderline-high --------------200-239 mg/dL (5.18-6.19 mmol/L)

    High -----------------------------------≥240 mg/dL (≥6.22 mmol/L)

Triglycerides

    Optimal ----------------------------<150 mg/dL (<1.70 mmol/L)

    Borderline-high --------------150-199 mg/dL (1.70-2.25 mmol/L)

    High -----------------------200-499 mg/dL (2.26-5.64 mmol/L)

    Very high --------------------------≥500 mg/dL (≥5.65 mmol/L)

Lipoprotein (a) ----------------------------≤30 mg/dL (≤1.07 μmol/L)

Apolipoprotein B ------------------------ 50-110 mg/dL (0.5-1.1 g/L)

Hematologic Values

Erythrocyte sedimentation rate -------------------------- 0-20 mm/h

Haptoglobin ------------------------ 30-200 mg/dL (300-2000 mg/L)

Hematocrit----------------------------- 41%-50% (0.41-0.51) (male);

    35%-45% (0.35-0.45) (female)

Hemoglobin A_{1c}----------------------- 4.0%-5.6% (20-38 mmol/mol)

Hemoglobin ------------------- 13.8-17.2 g/dL (138-172 g/L) (male);

    12.1-15.1 g/dL (121-151 g/L) (female)

International normalized ratio ----------------------------------0.8-1.2

Mean corpuscular volume (MCV)-----------80-100 μm³ (80-100 fL)

Platelet count-------------------- 150-450 × 10³/μL (150-450 × 10⁹/L)

Protein (total) ---------------------------------6.3-7.9 g/dL (63-79 g/L)

Reticulocyte count-------0.5%-1.5% of red blood cells (0.005-0.015)

White blood cell count------------4500-11,000/μL (4.5-11.0 × 10⁹/L)

Thyroid Values

Thyroglobulin ------------ 3-42 ng/mL (3-42 μg/L) (after surgery and

    radioactive iodine treatment: <1.0 ng/mL [<1.0 μg/L])

Thyroglobulin antibodies --------------------- ≤4.0 IU/mL (≤4.0 kIU/L)

Thyrotropin (TSH) ------------------------------------0.5-5.0 mIU/L

Thyrotropin-receptor antibodies (TRAb) ------------------ ≤1.75 IU/L

Thyroid-stimulating immunoglobulin-------- ≤120% of basal activity

Thyroperoxidase (TPO) antibodies ----------- <2.0 IU/mL (<2.0 kIU/L)

Thyroxine (T_4) (free) ------------- 0.8-1.8 ng/dL (10.30-23.17 pmol/L)

Thyroxine (T_4) (total) --------- 5.5-12.5 μg/dL (94.02-213.68 nmol/L)

Free thyroxine (T_4) index ------------------------------------- 4-12

Triiodothyronine (T_3) (free)--------- 2.3-4.2 pg/mL (3.53-6.45 pmol/L)

Triiodothyronine (T_3) (total) ------- 70-200 ng/dL (1.08-3.08 nmol/L)

Triiodothyronine (T_3), reverse -------- 10-24 ng/dL (0.15-0.37 nmol/L)

Triiodothyronine uptake, resin -----------------------------25%-38%

Radioactive iodine uptake -- 3%-16% (6 hours); 15%-30% (24 hours)

Endocrine Values

Serum

Aldosterone----------------------- 4-21 ng/dL (111.0-582.5 pmol/L)

Alkaline phosphatase ---------------- 50-120 U/L (0.84-2.00 μkat/L)

Alkaline phosphatase (bone-specific) --------≤20 μg/L (adult male);

    ≤14 μg/L (premenopausal female); ≤22 μg/L (postmenopausal

    female)

Androstenedione ---- 65-210 ng/dL (2.27-7.33 nmol/L) (adult male);

    30-200 ng/dL (1.05-6.98 nmol/L) (adult female)

Antimullerian hormone -----------0.7-19.0 ng/mL (5.0-135.7 pmol/L)

    (male, >12 years);

    0.9-9.5 ng/mL (6.4-67.9 pmol/L) (female, 13-45 years);

    <1.0 ng/mL (<7.1 pmol/L) (female, >45 years)

Calcitonin ------------------<16 pg/mL (<4.67 pmol/L) (basal, male);

    <8 pg/mL (<2.34 pmol/L) (basal, female);

    ≤130 pg/mL (≤37.96 pmol/L) (peak calcium infusion, male);

    ≤90 pg/mL (≤26.28 pmol/L) (peak calcium infusion, female)

Carcinoembryonic antigen ------------------- <2.5 ng/mL (<2.5 μg/L)

Chromogranin A------------------------------ <93 ng/mL (<93 μg/L)

Corticosterone ------ 53-1560 ng/dL (1.53-45.08 nmol/L) (>18 years)

Corticotropin (ACTH) ---------------- 10-60 pg/mL (2.2-13.2 pmol/L)

Cortisol (8 AM) -------------------- 5-25 μg/dL (137.9-689.7 nmol/L)

Cortisol (4 PM)-----------------------2-14 μg/dL (55.2-386.2 nmol/L)

C-peptide ------------------------- 0.9-4.3 ng/mL (0.30-1.42 nmol/L)

C-reactive protein ----------------0.8-3.1 mg/L (7.62-29.52 nmol/L)

Cross-linked N-telopeptide of type 1 collagen ----------------------

    5.4-24.2 nmol BCE/mmol creat (male);

    6.2-19.0 nmol BCE/mmol creat (female)

Dehydroepiandrosterone sulfate (DHEA-S)

Patient Age	Female	Male
18-29 years	44-332 μg/dL	89-457 μg/dL
	(1.19-9.00 μmol/L)	(2.41-12.38 μmol/L)
30-39 years	31-228 μg/dL	65-334 μg/dL
	(0.84-6.78 μmol/L)	(1.76-9.05 μmol/L)

Patient Age	Female	Male
40-49 years	18-244 µg/dL	48-244 µg/dL
	(0.49-6.61 µmol/L)	(1.30-6.61 µmol/L)
50-59 years	15-200 µg/dL	35-179 µg/dL
	(0.41-5.42 µmol/L)	(0.95-4.85 µmol/L)
≥60 years	15-157 µg/dL	25-131 µg/dL
	(0.41-4.25 µmol/L)	(0.68-3.55 µmol/L)

Deoxycorticosterone ----------<10 ng/dL (<0.30 nmol/L) (>18 years)

1,25-Dihydroxyvitamin D_3---------16-65 pg/mL (41.6-169.0 pmol/L)

Estradiol -------------------- 10-40 pg/mL (36.7-146.8 pmol/L) (male);

    10-180 pg/mL (36.7-660.8 pmol/L) (follicular, female);

    100-300 pg/mL (367.1-1101.3 pmol/L) (midcycle, female);

    40-200 pg/mL (146.8-734.2 pmol/L) (luteal, female);

    <20 pg/mL (<73.4 pmol/L) (postmenopausal, female)

Estrone -------------------- 10-60 pg/mL (37.0-221.9 pmol/L) (male);

    17-200 pg/mL (62.9-739.6 pmol/L) (premenopausal female);

    7-40 pg/mL (25.9-147.9 pmol/L) (postmenopausal female)

α-Fetoprotein ----------------------------------- <6 ng/mL (<6 µg/L)

Follicle-stimulating hormone (FSH) ----------------------------------

    1.0-13.0 mIU/mL (1.0-13.0 IU/L) (male);

    <3.0 mIU/mL (<3.0 IU/L) (prepuberty, female);

    2.0-12.0 mIU/mL (2.0-12.0 IU/L) (follicular, female);

    4.0-36.0 mIU/mL (4.0-36.0 IU/L) (midcycle, female);

    1.0-9.0 mIU/mL (1.0-9.0 IU/L) (luteal, female);

    >30 mIU/mL (>30 IU/L) (postmenopausal, female)

Free fatty acids -------------------- 10.6-18.0 mg/dL (0.4-0.7 nmol/L)

Gastrin----------------------------------- <100 pg/mL (<100 ng/L)

Growth hormone (GH)----- 0.01-0.97 ng/mL (0.01-0.97 µg/L) (male);

    0.01-3.61 ng/mL (0.01-3.61 µg/L) (female)

Homocysteine ----------------------------- ≤1.76 mg/L (≤13 µmol/L)

β-Human chorionic gonadotropin (β-hCG) ----------------------------

    <3.0 mIU/mL (<3.0 IU/L) (nonpregnant female);

    >25 mIU/mL ------- (>25 IU/L) indicates a positive pregnancy test

β-Hydroxybutyrate ----------------------<3.0 mg/dL (<288.2 µmol/L)

17-Hydroxypregnenolone --------- 29-189 ng/dL (0.87-5.69 nmol/L)

17α-Hydroxyprogesterone - <220 ng/dL (<6.67 nmol/L) (adult male);

    <80 ng/dL (<2.42 nmol/L) (follicular, female);

    <285 ng/dL (<8.64 nmol/L) (luteal, female);

    <51 ng/dL (<1.55 nmol/L) (postmenopausal, female)

25-Hydroxyvitamin D ------- <20 ng/mL (<49.9 nmol/L) (deficiency);

    21-29 ng/mL (52.4-72.4 nmol/L) (insufficiency);

    30-80 ng/mL (74.9-199.7 nmol/L) (optimal levels);

    >80 ng/mL (>199.7 nmol/L) (toxicity possible)

Inhibin B -----------------------------15-300 pg/mL (15-300 ng/L)

Insulinlike growth factor 1 (IGF-1)

Patient Age	Female	Male
18 years	162-541 ng/mL	170-640 ng/mL
	(21.2-70.9 nmol/L)	(22.3-83.8 nmol/L)
19 years	138-442 ng/mL	147-527 ng/mL
	(18.1-57.9 nmol/L)	(19.3-69.0 nmol/L)
20 years	122-384 ng/mL	132-457 ng/mL
	(16.0-50.3 nmol/L)	(17.3-59.9 nmol/L)

Patient Age	Female	Male
21-25 years	116-341 ng/mL	116-341 ng/mL
	(15.2-44.7 nmol/L)	(15.2-44.7 nmol/L)
26-30 years	117-321 ng/mL	117-321 ng/mL
	(15.3-42.1 nmol/L)	(15.3-42.1 nmol/L)
31-35 years	113-297 ng/mL	113-297 ng/mL
	(14.8-38.9 nmol/L)	(14.8-38.9 nmol/L)
36-40 years	106-277 ng/mL	106-277 ng/mL
	(13.9-36.3 nmol/L)	(13.9-36.3 nmol/L)
41-45 years	98-261 ng/mL	98-261 ng/mL
	(12.8-34.2 nmol/L)	(12.8-34.2 nmol/L)
46-50 years	91-246 ng/mL	91-246 ng/mL
	(11.9-32.2 nmol/L)	(11.9-32.2 nmol/L)
51-55 years	84-233 ng/mL	84-233 ng/mL
	(11.0-30.5 nmol/L)	(11.0-30.5 nmol/L)
56-60 years	78-220 ng/mL	78-220 ng/mL
	(10.2-28.8 nmol/L)	(10.2-28.8 nmol/L)
61-65 years	72-207 ng/mL	72-207 ng/mL
	(9.4-27.1 nmol/L)	(9.4-27.1 nmol/L)
66-70 years	67-195 ng/mL	67-195 ng/mL
	(8.8-25.5 nmol/L)	(8.8-25.5 nmol/L)
71-75 years	62-184 ng/mL	62-184 ng/mL
	(8.1-24.1 nmol/L)	(8.1-24.1 nmol/L)
76-80 years	57-172 ng/mL	57-172 ng/mL
	(7.5-22.5 nmol/L)	(7.5-22.5 nmol/L)
>80 years	53-162 ng/mL	53-162 ng/mL
	(6.9-21.2 nmol/L)	(6.9-21.2 nmol/L)

Insulinlike growth factor binding protein 3 --------------2.5-4.8 mg/L

Insulin---------------------------- 1.4-14.0 µIU/mL (9.7-97.2 pmol/L)

Islet-cell antibody assay------- 0 Juvenile Diabetes Foundation units

Luteinizing hormone (LH)------ 1.0-9.0 mIU/mL (1.0-9.0 IU/L) (male);

    <1.0 mIU/mL (<1.0 IU/L) (prepuberty, female);

    1.0-18.0 mIU/mL (1.0-18.0 IU/L) (follicular, female);

    20.0-80.0 mIU/mL (20.0-80.0 IU/L) (midcycle, female);

    0.5-18.0 mIU/mL (0.5-18.0 IU/L) (luteal, female);

    >30 mIU/mL (>30 IU/L) (postmenopausal, female)

Metanephrines (plasma fractionated)

    Metanephrine ------------------------<99 pg/mL (<0.50 nmol/L)

    Normetanephrine -------------------- <165 pg/mL (<0.90 nmol/L)

75-g oral glucose tolerance test blood glucose values---------------

    60-100 mg/dL (3.3-5.6 mmol/L) (fasting);

    <200 mg/dL (<11.1 mmol/L) (1 hour);

    <140 mg/dL (<7.8 mmol/L) (2 hour); between 140-200 mg/dL

    (7.8-11.1 mmol/L) is considered impaired glucose tolerance or

    prediabetes. Greater than 200 mg/dL (11.1 mmol/L) is a sign of

    diabetes mellitus.

50-g oral glucose tolerance test for gestational diabetes -----------

    <140 mg/dL (<7.8 mmol/L) (1 hour)

100-g oral glucose tolerance test for gestational diabetes ----------

    <95 mg/dL (<5.3 mmol/L) (fasting);

    <180 mg/dL (<10.0 mmol/L) (1 hour);

    <155 mg/dL (<8.6 mmol/L) (2 hour);

    <140 mg/dL (<7.8 mmol/L) (3 hour)

Osteocalcin --------------------------9.0-42.0 ng/mL (9.0-42.0 µg/L)

Parathyroid hormone, intact (PTH) ------- 10-65 pg/mL (10-65 ng/L)

Parathyroid hormone–related protein (PTHrP) -----------<2.0 pmol/L

Progesterone ----------------------≤1.2 ng/mL (≤3.8 nmol/L) (male);

    ≤1.0 ng/mL (≤3.2 nmol/L) (follicular, female);

    2.0-20.0 ng/mL (6.4-63.6 nmol/L) (luteal, female);

    ≤1.1 ng/mL (≤3.5 nmol/L) (postmenopausal, female);

    >10.0 ng/mL (>31.8 nmol/L) (evidence of ovulatory adequacy)

Proinsulin ----------------------- 26.5-176.4 pg/mL (3.0-20.0 pmol/L)

Prolactin ----------------------4-23 ng/mL (0.17-1.00 nmol/L) (male);

    4-30 ng/mL (0.17-1.30 nmol/L) (nonlactating female);

    10-200 ng/mL (0.43-8.70 nmol/L) (lactating female)

Prostate-specific antigen (PSA) - <2.0 ng/mL (<2.0 µg/L) (≤40 years);

    <2.8 ng/mL (<2.8 µg/L) (≤50 years);

    <3.8 ng/mL (<3.8 µg/L) (≤60 years);

    <5.3 ng/mL (<5.3 µg/L) (≤70 years);

    <7.0 ng/mL (<7.0 µg/L) (≤79 years);

    <7.2 ng/mL (<7.2 µg/L) (≥80 years)

Renin activity, plasma, sodium replete, ambulatory -- 0.6-4.3 ng/mL per h

Renin, direct concentration ------------- 4-44 pg/mL (0.1-1.0 pmol/L)

Sex hormone–binding globulin (SHBG) --------------- 1.1-6.7 µg/mL

    (10-60 nmol/L) (male);

    2.2-14.6 µg/mL (20-130 nmol/L) (female)

α-Subunit of pituitary glycoprotein hormones - <1.2 ng/mL (<1.2 µg/L)

Testosterone (bioavailable)---------0.8-4.0 ng/dL (0.03-0.14 nmol/L)

    (20-50 years, female on oral estrogen);

    0.8-10.0 ng/dL (0.03-0.35 nmol/L)

    (20-50 years, female not on oral estrogen);

    83.0-257.0 ng/dL (2.88-8.92 nmol/L) (male 20-29 years);

    72.0-235.0 ng/dL (2.50-8.15 nmol/L) (male 30-39 years);

    61.0-213.0 ng/dL (2.12-7.39 nmol/L) (male 40-49 years);

    50.0-190.0 ng/dL (1.74-6.59 nmol/L) (male 50-59 years);

    40.0-168.0 ng/dL (1.39-5.83 nmol/L) (male 60-69 years)

Testosterone (free)-------- 9.0-30.0 ng/dL (0.31-1.04 nmol/L) (male);

    0.3-1.9 ng/dL (0.01-0.07 nmol/L) (female)

Testosterone (total) ------- 300-900 ng/dL (10.4-31.2 nmol/L) (male);

    8-60 ng/dL (0.3-2.1 nmol/L) (female)

Vitamin B_{12} ----------------------- 180-914 pg/mL (133-674 pmol/L)

Chemistry Values

Alanine aminotransferase ------------- 10-40 U/L (0.17-0.67 µkat/L)

Albumin------------------------------------3.5-5.0 g/dL (35-50 g/L)

Amylase --------------------------- 26-102 U/L (0.43-1.70 µkat/L)

Aspartate aminotransferase ---------- 20-48 U/L (0.33-0.80 µkat/L)

Bicarbonate ------------------------- 21-28 mEq/L (21-28 mmol/L)

Bilirubin (total) ---------------------- 0.3-1.2 mg/dL (5.1-20.5 µmol/L)

Blood gases

    Po_2, arterial blood ----------------80-100 mm Hg (10.6-13.3 kPa)

    Pco_2, arterial blood ------------------35-45 mm Hg (4.7-6.0 kPa)

Blood pH--7.35-7.45

Calcium ---------------------------8.2-10.2 mg/dL (2.1-2.6 mmol/L)

Calcium (ionized) ---------------- 4.60-5.08 mg/dL (1.2-1.3 mmol/L)

Carbon dioxide ---------------------- 22-28 mEq/L (22-28 mmol/L)

CD_4 cell count------------------------500-1400/µL (0.5-1.4 × 109/L)

Chloride---------------------------- 96-106 mEq/L (96-106 mmol/L)

Creatine kinase ----------------------- 50-200 U/L (0.84-3.34 µkat/L)

Creatinine----------------0.7-1.3 mg/dL (61.9-114.9 µmol/L) (male);

    0.6-1.1 mg/dL (53.0-97.2 µmol/L) (female)

Ferritin ------------------------- 15-200 ng/mL (33.7-449.4 pmol/L)

Folate ------------------------------------- ≥4.0 ng/mL (≥4.0 µg/L)

Glucose ----------------------------- 70-99 mg/dL (3.9-5.5 mmol/L)

γ-Glutamyltransferase ----------------- 2-30 U/L (0.03-0.50 µkat/L)

Iron ------------------------50-150 µg/dL (9.0-26.8 µmol/L) (male);

    35-145 µg/dL (6.3-26.0 µmol/L) (female)

Lactate dehydrogenase --------------- 100-200 U/L (1.7-3.3 µkat/L)

Lactic acid --------------------------5.4-20.7 mg/dL (0.6-2.3 mmol/L)

Lipase ------------------------------- 10-73 U/L (0.17-1.22 µkat/L)

Magnesium ------------------------- 1.5-2.3 mg/dL (0.6-0.9 mmol/L)

Osmolality --------------------275-295 mOsm/kg (275-295 mmol/kg)

Phosphate -------------------------- 2.3-4.7 mg/dL (0.7-1.5 mmol/L)

Potassium -------------------------- 3.5-5.0 mEq/L (3.5-5.0 mmol/L)

Prothrombin time --------------------------------------- 8.3-10.8 s

Serum urea nitrogen--------------------8-23 mg/dL (2.9-8.2 mmol/L)

Sodium --------------------------136-142 mEq/L (136-142 mmol/L)

Transferrin saturation -------------------------------------14%-50%

Troponin I ----------------------------------- <0.6 ng/mL (<0.6 µg/L)

Tryptase --------------------------------- <11.5 ng/mL (<11.5 µg/L)

Uric acid ------------------------ 3.5-7.0 mg/dL (208.2-416.4 µmol/L)

Urine

Albumin-----------------30-300 µg/mg creat (3.4-33.9 µg/mol creat)

Albumin-to-creatinine ratio ------------------------- <30 mg/g creat

Aldosterone------------------------ 3-20 µg/24 h (8.3-55.4 nmol/d)

    (should be <12 µg/24 h [<33.2 nmol/d] with oral sodium

    loading—confirmed with 24-hour urinary sodium >200 mEq)

Calcium ------------------------ 100-300 mg/24 h (2.5-7.5 mmol/d)

Catecholamine fractionation

    Normotensive normal ranges:

        Dopamine ----------------------- <400 µg/24 h (<2610 nmol/d)

        Epinephrine -----------------------<21 µg/24 h (<115 nmol/d)

        Norepinephrine --------------------<80 µg/24 h (<473 nmol/d)

Citrate ----------------------- 320-1240 mg/24 h (16.7-64.5 mmol/d)

Cortisol ----------------------------- 4-50 µg/24 h (11-138 nmol/d)

Cortisol following dexamethasone suppression test (low-dose:

    2 day, 2 mg daily) -------------------- <10 µg/24 h (<27.6 nmol/d)

Creatinine------------------------ 1.0-2.0 g/24 h (8.8-17.7 mmol/d)

Glomerular filtration rate (estimated) ------ >60 mL/min per 1.73 m2

5-Hydroxyindole acetic acid---------2-9 mg/24 h (10.5-47.1 µmol/d)

Iodine (random)--- >100 µg/L

17-Ketosteroids ------- 6.0-21.0 mg/24 h (20.8-72.9 µmol/d) (male);

    4.0-17.0 mg/24 h (13.9-59.0 µmol/d) (female)

Metanephrine fractionation

    Normotensive normal ranges:

        Metanephrine ----------- <261 µg/24 h (<1323 nmol/d) (male);

        <180 µg/24 h (<913 nmol/d) (female)

Normetanephrine -------------------- age and sex dependent

Total metanephrine ------------------- age and sex dependent

Osmolality ---------------- 150-1150 mOsm/kg (150-1150 mmol/kg)

Oxalate -------------------------------- <40 mg/24 h (<456 mmol/d)

Phosphate ---------------------- 0.9-1.3 g/24 h (29.1-42.0 mmol/d)

Potassium ------------------------17-77 mEq/24 h (17-77 mmol/d)

Sodium ------------------------40-217 mEq/24 h (40-217 mmol/d)

Uric acid ------------------------------<800 mg/24 h (<4.7 mmol/d)

Saliva

Cortisol (salivary), midnight --------------- <0.13 µg/dL (<3.6 nmol/L)

Semen

Semen analysis ---------------- >20 million sperm/mL; >50% motility

Abbreviations

ACTH ---corticotropin

ACE inhibitor--------------- angiotensin-converting enzyme inhibitor

ALT --------------------------------------- alanine aminotransferase

AST --------------------------------------- aspartate aminotransferase

BMI --- body mass index

CNS--- central nervous system

CT---computed tomography

DHEA -------------------------------------- dehydroepiandrosterone

DHEA-S---------------------------- dehydroepiandrosterone sulfate

DNA --- deoxyribonucleic acid

DPP-4 inhibitor ----------------------dipeptidyl-peptidase 4 inhibitor

DXA------------------------------dual-energy x-ray absorptiometry

FDA---------------------------------Food and Drug Administration

FGF-23 ---------------------------------- fibroblast growth factor 23

FNA--fine-needle aspiration

FSH --------------------------------------- follicle-stimulating hormone

GH -- growth hormone

GHRH------------------------- growth hormone–releasing hormone

GLP-1 receptor agonist----- glucagonlike peptide 1 receptor agonist

GnRH -----------------------------gonadotropin-releasing hormone

hCG --------------------------------- human chorionic gonadotropin

HDL--high-density lipoprotein

HIV----------------------------------- human immunodeficiency virus

HMG-CoA reductase inhibitor---------- 3-hydroxy-3-methylglutaryl
coenzyme A reductase inhibitor

IGF-1------------------------------------- insulinlike growth factor 1

LDL --low-density lipoprotein

LH --- luteinizing hormone

MCV --mean corpuscular volume

MIBG------------------------------------ meta-iodobenzylguanidine

MRI ---------------------------------- magnetic resonance imaging

NPH insulin --------------------- neutral protamine Hagedorn insulin

PCSK9 inhibitor ---- proprotein convertase subtilisin/kexin 9 inhibitor

PET ---------------------------------------positron emission tomography

PSA --------------------------------------- prostate-specific antigen

PTH ---parathyroid hormone

PTHrP-----------------------------parathyroid hormone–related protein

SGLT-2 inhibitor ----------sodium-glucose cotransporter 2 inhibitor

SHBG --------------------------------- sex hormone–binding globulin

T$_3$ -- triiodothyronine

T$_4$ -- thyroxine

TPO antibodies ------------------------- thyroperoxidase antibodies

TRH---------------------------------- thyrotropin-releasing hormone

TRAb -------------------------------thyrotropin-receptor antibodies

TSH --- thyrotropin

VLDL----------------------------------- very low-density lipoprotein

ENDOCRINE SELF-ASSESSMENT PROGRAM 2020

Part I

1 A 58-year-old woman with vitamin D deficiency and end-stage hepatitis C sustains a fracture of her right hip after falling. DXA scan reveals T-scores of –4.5 (Z-score, –3.2) in the spine and –3.0 (Z-score, –2.1) in the left total hip. She went through natural menopause at age 40 years and has not taken estrogen. She has esophageal varices with history of upper gastrointestinal bleeding. Liver transplant is currently being considered. She has no history of kidney stones, parathyroid disease, or thyroid disease. She smokes cigarettes and is planning to have multiple teeth extracted in the near future.

Her dietary calcium intake is limited and she does not take any calcium supplements, but she does take over-the-counter cholecalciferol, 2000 IU daily.

Her physical examination reveals poor oral hygiene and ascites.

Laboratory test results (6 months after hip fracture):
Serum calcium = 8.6 mg/dL (8.2-10.2 mg/dL) (SI: 2.2 mmol/L [2.1-2.6 mmol/L])
Serum phosphate = 3.0 mg/dL (2.3-4.7 mg/dL) (SI: 1.0 mmol/L [0.7-1.5 mmol/L])
Serum creatinine = 0.6 mg/dL (0.6-1.1 mg/dL) (SI: 53.0 μmol/L [53.0-97.2 μmol/L])
Glomerular filtration rate (estimated) = 72 mL/min per 1.73 m^2 (>60 mL/min per 1.73 m^2)
Serum intact PTH = 30 pg/mL (10-65 pg/mL) (SI: 30 ng/L [10-65 ng/L])
Serum 25-hydroxyvitamin D = 26 ng/mL (30-80 ng/mL [optimal]) (SI: 64.9 nmol/L [74.9-199.7 nmol/L])
Serum albumin = 3.4 g/dL (3.5-5.0 g/dL) (SI: 34 g/L [35-50 g/L])
Serum alkaline phosphatase = 110 U/L (50-120 U/L) (SI: 1.84 μkat/L [0.84-2.00 μkat/L])

Which of the following should be recommended in addition to adequate calcium and vitamin D supplementation?
A. Alendronate
B. Zoledronic acid
C. Denosumab
D. Teriparatide
E. Raloxifene

2 A 35-year-old woman is admitted to the hospital for workup of hypoglycemia. About 6 months ago, she started having episodes of hunger and sweating in the early morning hours. Symptoms would resolve after eating. Subsequently, she started having postprandial symptoms later in the day associated with dizziness and irritability. She was brought to the emergency department on 2 occasions over the last 4 months for these symptoms. She briefly lost consciousness during one of the episodes, and emergency medical technicians were called to her house. On both occasions, she was treated conservatively with intravenous fluids and sent home. She was previously healthy and takes no medications.

While in the emergency department, a random cortisol concentration was documented to be 21 μg/dL (579.3 nmol/L). Her glucose concentration was 32 mg/dL (1.8 mmol/L), and intravenous dextrose was administered with resolution of symptoms. She is now admitted to the hospital for a supervised 72-hour fast. The fast is terminated at 18 hours and the following laboratory values are obtained:

Glucose = 53 mg/dL (SI: 2.9 mmol/L)
Insulin = 4.3 μIU/mL (SI: 29.9 pmol/L)
C-peptide = 2.08 ng/mL (SI: 0.69 nmol/L)

The patient is given glucagon intravenously at 7:30 AM. The plasma glucose concentration at 7:50 AM is 91 mg/dL (5.1 mmol/L). Imaging studies are pursued on the basis of the clinical presentation and test results. Magnetic resonance cholangiopancreatography and endoscopic ultrasonography are performed and neither identifies a discrete adenoma.

Which of the following is the best next step in this patient's management?
  A.   Intraarterial calcium stimulation with a selective hepatic venous sampling test
  B.   Surgical pancreatic exploration
  C. ^{111}In pentetreotide scanning
  D.   Oral diazoxide
  E.   Small frequent meals

3 A 57 year-old woman with a history of goiter and hypothyroidism is found to have a thyroid nodule. Recent ultrasonography shows a left thyroid lobe that measures 1.5 (anteroposterior) × 1.5 (transverse) × 5.3 (longitudinal) cm with a 0.61 × 0.72 × 1.02-cm thyroid nodule and a right thyroid lobe that measures 1.1 × 1.5 × 5.8 cm (*see image*). The isthmus is 0.24 cm. She is referred to you for evaluation of her left thyroid nodule. She currently takes levothyroxine, 100 mcg daily. She has no history of radiation therapy to her head and neck. Her mother has a history of thyroid cancer.

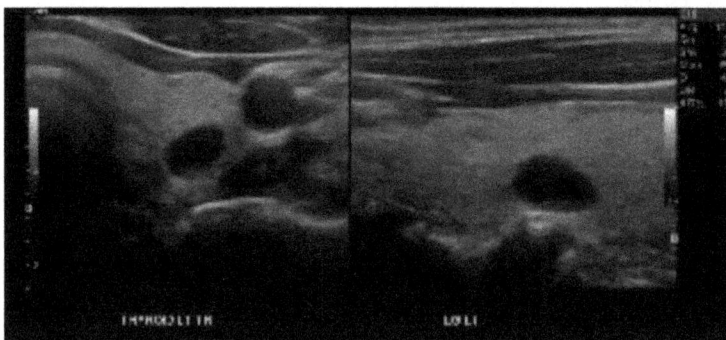

On physical examination, her blood pressure is 120/60 mm Hg and pulse rate is 74 beats/min. Her height is 65 in (165 cm) and weight is 125 lb (56.8 kg) (BMI = 20.8 kg/m^2). Her thyroid gland is 40 g with no palpable nodules or cervical lymphadenopathy. The rest of the examination findings are unremarkable.

Laboratory test results:
  TSH = 1.2 mIU/L (0.5-5.0 mIU/L)
  Free T$_4$ = 1.1 ng/dL (0.8-1.8 ng/dL) (SI: 14.2 pmol/L [10.30-23.17 pmol/L])
  Calcium = 8.9 mg/dL (8.2-10.2 mg/dL) (SI: 2.2 mmol/L [2.1-2.6 mmol/L])

Which of the following is the best next step in this patient's management?
  A.   Thyroid scan
  B.   FNA biopsy of the thyroid nodule
  C.   Left hemithyroidectomy
  D.   Neck ultrasonography in 2 years to monitor thyroid nodule size
  E.   An increase in the levothyroxine dosage to maintain her TSH <0.1 mIU/L

4 A 35-year-old woman is admitted to the hospital with severe abdominal pain, nausea, and vomiting. The pain radiates to her back. She has no history of diabetes mellitus.

On physical examination, her blood pressure is 110/60 mm Hg and pulse rate is 100 beats/min. Her temperature is 99.5°F (37.5°C). Her height is 60.5 in (153.7 cm), and weight is 198 lb (90 kg) (BMI = 38 kg/m^2). She has truncal obesity and acanthosis nigricans at the base of the neck and in the axillae bilaterally. On abdominal examination, there is tenderness to deep palpation below the xiphoid process in the midline. There are minimal bowel sounds.

Laboratory tests results (sample drawn at admission):

Serum sodium = 132 mEq/L (136-142 mEq/L) (SI: 132 mmol/L [136-142 mmol/L])

Serum glucose = 480 mg/dL (70-99 mg/dL) (SI: 26.6 mmol/L [3.9-5.5 mmol/L])

Bicarbonate = 15 mEq/L (21-28 mEq/L) (SI: 15 mmol/L [21-28 mmol/L])

Potassium = 5.5 mEq/L (3.5-5.0 mEq/L) (SI: 5.5 mmol/L [3.5-5.0 mmol/L])

Phosphate = 3.5 mEq/L (2.3-4.7 mg/dL) (SI: 1.1 mmol/L [0.7-1.5 mmol/L])

Arterial blood pH = 7.20 (7.35-7.45)

Anion gap = 22

Lipase = 450 U/L (10-73 U/L) (SI: 7.52 μkat/L [0.17-1.22 μkat/L])

Hemoglobin A$_{1c}$ = 12.0% (4.0%-5.6%) (108 mmol/mol [20-38 mmol/mol])

Qualitative hCG, negative

CT of the abdomen shows stranding around the pancreas and no fluid collection.

The patient is currently being treated with intravenous insulin and fluids. On hospital day 2, her anion gap is starting to close and her serum glucose value is 280 mg/dL (15.4 mmol/L). Her pain is controlled by intravenous narcotics. Diet is restricted to nothing-by-mouth.

Which of the following is the best next step in this patient's care?

A. Measure glutamic acid decarboxylase antibodies and C-peptide

B. Refer for endoscopic retrograde cholangiopancreatography (or endoscopic ultrasonography)

C. Order a lipid panel

D. Perform abdominal ultrasonography

E. Measure serum and ionized calcium

5 A 34-year-old woman is referred for evaluation of amenorrhea and rising DHEA-S. Menarche was at age 13 years, and she initially had regular menses, occurring every 30 to 35 days. She initiated combined oral contraceptive birth control at age 17 years and switched to the etonogestrel/ethinyl estradiol vaginal ring 3 years ago. With this form of birth control, she developed elevated blood pressure, so she discontinued its use. However, the hypertension has persisted. Within a few months of discontinuing birth control, she developed acne and irregular menses occurring every other month. Polycystic ovary syndrome was diagnosed 2 years ago on the basis of symptoms of acne, irregular menses, and the following laboratory test results:

TSH = 0.5 mIU/L (0.5-5.0 mIU/L)

Total testosterone = 30 ng/dL (8-60 ng/dL) (SI: 1.0 nmol/L [0.3-2.1 nmol/L])

Prolactin = 11 ng/mL (4-30 ng/mL) (SI: 0.48 nmol/L [0.17-1.30 nmol/L])

LH = 2.8 mIU/mL (0.5-18.0 mIU/mL [luteal]) (SI: 2.8 IU/L [0.5-18.0 IU/L])

Day 21 progesterone = 1.2 ng/mL (2.0-20.0 ng/mL [luteal]) (SI: 3.8 nmol/L [6.4-63.6 nmol/L])

FSH = 4.5 mIU/mL (1.0-9.0 mIU/mL [luteal]) (SI: 4.5 IU/L [1.0-9.0 IU/L])

Androstenedione = 376 ng/dL (30-200 ng/dL) (SI: 13.1 nmol/L [1.05-6.98 nmol/L])

DHEA-S = 418 μg/dL (31-228 μg/dL) (SI: 11.33 μmol/L [0.84-6.78 μmol/L])

Estradiol = 29 pg/mL (40-200 pg/mL [luteal]) (SI: 106.5 pmol/L [146.8-734.2 pmol/L])

17-Hydroxyprogesterone = 320 ng/dL (<285 ng/dL [luteal]) (SI: 9.70 nmol/L [<8.64 nmol/L])

She reports a 20-lb (9.1-kg) weight gain over the past several years. She has not had any menses in the past 6 months. Her DHEA-S concentration is currently 578 μg/dL (15.67 μmol/L).

On physical examination, her height is 66 in (167.6 cm) and weight is 149.5 lb (68 kg) (BMI = 24.1 kg/m²). Her blood pressure is 156/96 mm Hg. She has facial plethora and supraclavicular fat pads. There is mild papular acne. No violaceous striae or ecchymoses are observed. Terminal hair growth is present only on the upper lip and upper arms. She is able to rise and walk without difficulty.

Which of the following is the best next step in this patient's management?
  A. Perform a 250-mcg cosyntropin-stimulation test
  B. Perform abdominal CT
  C. Perform a 1-mg dexamethasone suppression test
  D. Initiate spironolactone
  E. Restart a combined oral contraceptive

6 A 67-year-old woman is found to have a 2-cm left adrenal mass on abdominal CT performed for evaluation of left loin pain and suspected renal colic. The mass has a density of 35 Hounsfield units after intravenous contrast. She has a 10-year history of type 2 diabetes mellitus and hypertension and had an inferior myocardial infarction 2 years ago. Her current medications are aspirin, atenolol, atorvastatin, indapamide, metformin, and ramipril.

On physical examination, she is obese in a predominantly centripetal distribution. Her height is 64 in (162.6 cm) and weight is 225 lb (102.3 kg) (BMI = 38.6 kg/m²). Her blood pressure is 145/90 mm Hg, and pulse rate is 60 beats/min and regular. Fundoscopic examination reveals grade 2 hypertensive retinopathy and background diabetic retinopathy. No other specific endocrine stigmata are observed.

Laboratory test results:
  Serum potassium = 3.4 mEq/L (3.5-5.0 mEq/L) (SI: 3.4 mmol/L [3.5-5.0 mmol/L])
  Plasma renin activity = 0.8 ng/mL per h (0.6-4.3 ng/mL per h)
  Serum aldosterone = 6.2 ng/dL (4-21 ng/dL) (SI: 172 pmol/L [111.0-582.5 pmol/L])
  Cortisol following 1-mg dexamethasone suppression test = 2.0 μg/dL (SI: 55.2 nmol/L)
  Plasma metanephrine = 82 pg/mL (<99 pg/mL) (SI: 0.42 nmol/L [<0.50 nmol/L])
  Plasma normetanephrine = 185 pg/mL (<165 pg/mL) (SI: 1.01 nmol/L [<0.90 nmol/L])

Which of the following is the most likely cause of her hypertension?
  A. Cushing syndrome
  B. Essential hypertension (primary hypertension)
  C. Pheochromocytoma or paraganglioma
  D. Primary aldosteronism
  E. Renovascular disease

7 A 47-year-old male research scientist presents for management of cardiovascular risk. One year ago, he developed chest pain and underwent an extensive cardiac workup, which was unrevealing for cardiac ischemia. Statin therapy was offered, but he declined treatment. Symptoms resolved with use of an H2 receptor blocker. He does not smoke cigarettes and drinks 1 alcoholic beverage per week. He is an avid runner and continues to train for marathons without problems. His family history is negative for premature atherosclerotic cardiovascular disease, and both of his parents are alive and well in their 70s. He currently takes no medication and would prefer to avoid medication unless there is a clear indication.

On physical examination, his blood pressure is 124/72 mm Hg and pulse rate is 72 beats/min. His height is 75 in (190.5 cm), and weight is 195 lb (88.6 kg) (BMI = 24.4 kg/m²). No hepatosplenomegaly or xanthomas are noted on examination.

Laboratory test results (sample drawn while fasting):
  Total cholesterol = 175 mg/dL (<200 mg/dL [optimal]) (SI: 4.53 mmol/L [<5.18 mmol/L])
  Triglycerides = 49 mg/dL (<150 mg/dL [optimal]) (SI: 0.55 mmol/L [<1.70 mmol/L])
  HDL cholesterol = 43 mg/dL (>60 mg/dL [optimal]) (SI: 1.11 mmol/L [>1.55 mmol/L])
  LDL cholesterol = 122 mg/dL (<100 mg/dL [optimal]) (SI: 3.16 mmol/L [<2.59 mmol/L])
  Non-HDL cholesterol = 132 mg/dL (<130 mg/dL [optimal]) (SI: 3.42 mmol/L [<3.37 mmol/L])
  Hemoglobin A₁c = 5.4% (4.0%-5.6%) (36 mmol/mol [20-38 mmol/mol])
  TSH = 1.28 mIU/L (0.5-5.0 mIU/L)
  Fasting plasma glucose = 91 mg/dL (70-99 mg/dL) (SI: 5.05 mmol/L [3.9-5.5 mmol/L])

His 10-year atherosclerotic cardiovascular disease risk is 2.3% based on the American College of Cardiology/American Heart Association cardiovascular risk calculator. Despite these numbers, he is concerned about his cardiovascular risk and inquires about advanced lipid testing.

Which of the following is the best next step in this patient's management?
   A. No further testing needed now
   B. Measure direct LDL cholesterol
   C. Measure apolipoprotein B
   D. Measure high-sensitivity C-reactive protein
   E. Obtain lipoprotein analysis by nuclear magnetic resonance spectroscopy

8 A 72-year-old woman comes to your office for advice regarding management of osteoporosis. She has a known history of osteoporosis based on a recent DXA scan, which revealed lumbar spine, right femoral neck, and total hip T-scores of –3.2, –2.2, and –1.8, respectively. She had previously taken alendronate, which she did not tolerate because of significant musculoskeletal pain. She also has a history of 2 moderate and 1 severe compression fractures that were identified through a recent lateral chest x-ray and which occurred in the absence of major trauma or injury. Aside from menopausal status, she has no additional risk factors for osteoporosis, including no family history of hip fracture. Her medical history is notable for atrial fibrillation, for which she takes a β-adrenergic blocker and aspirin.

On physical examination, her height is 64.5 in (163.8 cm), which is 2.5 in (~6 cm) below her adult maximum height. Pulse is irregularly irregular. She has moderate lower thoracic kyphosis without palpable vertebral tenderness. Rib to pelvis distance is diminished at one-half fingerbreadth. The rest of her examination findings are normal.

Laboratory evaluation reveals normal chemistries, including calcium, creatinine, TSH, and 25-hydroxyvitamin D.

On the basis of her clinical presentation, which of the following is the best recommendation to manage her osteoporosis?
   A. Raloxifene
   B. Risedronate
   C. Teriparatide
   D. Zoledronic acid
   E. Calcium and vitamin D

9 A 32-year-old man presents with a 12-month history of increasing fatigue, reduced libido, and reduced exercise tolerance, which he attributes to declining muscle strength. He is an avid weekend hiker, and he feels less motivated to maintain his hiking activities and has gained 4.4 lb (2 kg) over the last 6 months. He has had no headaches or vision disturbances. He reports no history of head trauma or significant medical or family history. He takes no prescribed or illicit drugs. He has a normal sense of smell, and he underwent normal puberty.

On physical examination, his blood pressure is 122/63 mm Hg, and pulse rate is 68 beats/min. His height is 72 in (183 cm), and weight is 200 lb (90.9 kg) (BMI = 27.1 kg/m²). Visual fields are full to confrontation, and he has a full range of eye movements. Body hair is mildly reduced. There is no muscle wasting, gynecomastia, facial plethora, or purple striae. Testes are 20 mL bilaterally.

Laboratory test results (sample drawn at 8 AM while fasting):
   Total testosterone = 150 ng/dL (300-900 ng/dL) (SI: 5.2 nmol/L [10.4-31.2 nmol/L]) (repeated measurement = 140 ng/dL (SI: 4.9 nmol/L))
   LH = 2.0 mIU/mL (1.0-9.0 mIU/mL) (SI: 2.0 IU/L [1.0-9.0 IU/L])
   FSH = 2.5 mIU/mL (1.0-13.0 mIU/mL) (SI: 2.5 IU/L [1.0-13.0 IU/L])
   Hemoglobin = 12.8 g/dL (13.8-17.2 g/dL) (SI: 128 g/L [138-172 g/L])
   Complete blood cell count, otherwise normal
   Renal function, normal
   Liver function, normal
   Thyroid function, normal

Which of the following is the best next step in this patient's evaluation?
  A. Serum prolactin measurement
  B. Serum free testosterone measurement
  C. 1-mg dexamethasone-suppression test
  D. Urinary anabolic steroid screen
  E. Pituitary-directed MRI

10 A 32-year-old pregnant woman is being seen in the clinic for treatment of type 1 diabetes mellitus. She is currently at 9 weeks' gestation with her second pregnancy. Diabetes was diagnosed at age 16 years. She has background retinopathy and mild peripheral neuropathy. She has a history of hypoglycemia unawareness. Recent glycemic control has been reasonable, and her hemoglobin A_{1c} level has been in the range of 6.6% to 7.4% (49-57 mmol/mol) over the past 3 years. She does not smoke cigarettes or drink alcohol. She has had mild morning sickness and occasional nausea and has not gained any weight during the pregnancy thus far. She has occasional mild hypoglycemia in the evening.

She started insulin pump therapy during her first pregnancy at age 26 years to optimize glucose control and reduce the risk of hypoglycemia. Her baby girl was born via cesarean delivery at 37 weeks' gestation with a birth weight of 8 lb 2 oz (3685 g). The baby had mild jaundice as the only complication.

She uses insulin lispro in the pump. She uses an insulin-to-carbohydrate ratio of 1 unit per 7 g of carbohydrate before meals and boluses insulin 10 to 15 minutes before each meal. The total insulin amount per day is 48 units. The bolus and correctional insulin, on average, is 31.3 units per day.

The basal insulin rates are as follows:
Midnight to 4 AM	0.80 units per hour
4 AM to 7 AM	1.00 units per hour
7 AM to 5 PM	0.65 units per hour
5 PM to midnight	0.80 units per hour

On physical examination, her height is 67 in (170 cm) and weight is 194 lb (88.2 kg) (BMI = 30.4 kg/m²). Her blood pressure is 102/72 mm Hg, and pulse rate is 72 beats/min. Examination findings are normal except for mildly reduced sensation to monofilament touch and vibrational sense in each foot.

Laboratory test results:
  Hemoglobin A_{1c} = 6.8% (4.0%-5.6%) (51 mmol/mol [20-38 mmol/mol])
  Creatinine = 1.0 mg/dL (0.6-1.1 mg/dL) (SI: 88.4 μmol/L [53.0-97.2 μmol/L])
  TSH = 1.8 mIU/L (0.5-5.0 mIU/L)
  Urinary albumin-to-creatinine ratio = 6 mg/g creat (<30 mg/g creat)

Continuous glucose sensor data are shown (*see image*). Blue arrows indicate meal times.

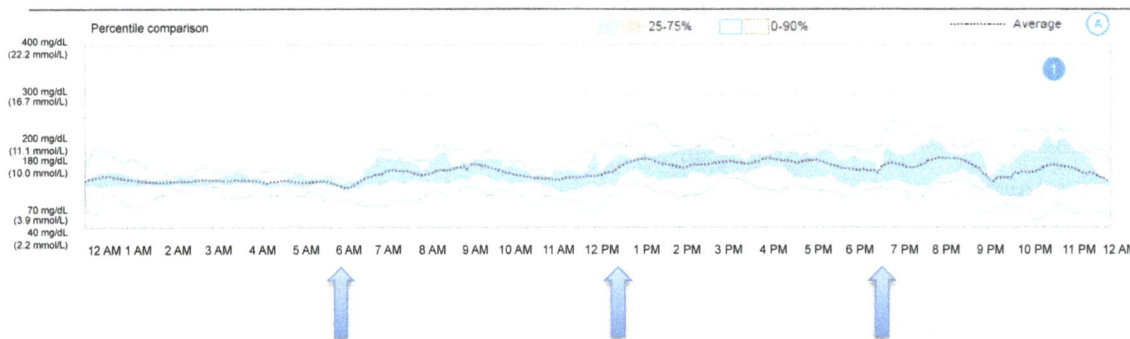

In addition to referring the patient for review of carbohydrate counting, which of the following is the best approach to manage her diabetes?
   A. Change the insulin-to-carbohydrate ratio to 1 unit per 6 g before lunch and dinner
   B. Change the insulin-to-carbohydrate ratio to 1 unit per 6 g before each meal
   C. Increase the basal insulin rate at midnight, 4 AM, and 7 AM
   D. Decrease the basal insulin rate at midnight and increase the basal rate at 7 AM and 5 PM
   E. Increase the basal insulin rate at 7 AM and change the insulin-to-carbohydrate ratio to 1 unit per 8 g before each meal

11 A 74-year-old woman with metastatic papillary cancer is being prepared for treatment with radioactive iodine. She underwent thyroidectomy 5 weeks ago and is suspected to have lung metastases based on the findings observed on chest CT. MRI of the brain was unrevealing. Her treating endocrinologist felt that it was best to prepare her for radioiodine therapy using a protocol involving treatment in the hypothyroid state. Therefore, levothyroxine was not initiated after thyroidectomy. In addition, she is following a low-iodine diet, which she started 2 weeks before the week of her intended radioactive iodine treatment. During the second week of her low-iodine diet, she started to feel nauseated. After receiving a 3-mCi diagnostic dose of ^{123}I, the patient experiences a headache and worsening nausea. These symptoms do not remit and, in fact, the patient progresses into confusion. She is taken to the emergency department from the nuclear medicine facility.

On physical examination, she is no longer oriented to place or time. Her blood pressure is 130/80 mm Hg, and pulse rate is 58 beats/min. She has facial and extremity edema, cool skin, and a delayed relaxation phase of her deep tendon reflexes.

Laboratory test results:
   TSH = 76 mIU/L (0.5-5.0 mIU/L)
   Free T$_4$ = 0.1 ng/dL (0.8-1.8 ng/dL) (SI: 1.3 pmol/L [10.30-23.17 pmol/L])

Which of the following is the most likely direct cause of this patient's symptoms?
   A. Brain metastases from thyroid cancer
   B. Azotemia
   C. Hyponatremia
   D. Iodine allergy
   E. Adrenal insufficiency

12 A 48-year-old woman is referred for elevated estradiol in the context of menometrorrhagia. She has a several-year history of heavy menses and intermenstrual irregular bleeding. Her evaluation thus far has not revealed any uterine abnormalities, and she has had several significantly elevated estradiol measurements in the range of 900 to 1300 pg/mL (3304-4772 pmol/L). These measurements were performed with chemiluminescence assays. Total testosterone concentrations have been normal (by tandem mass spectrometry).

Before she had her 3 children, she had irregular periods that were shorter in cycle length, but she never skipped periods. Menses were also accompanied by cramping. She had no difficulty conceiving. At age 40 years, her periods became heavier and more frequent. She underwent endometrial ablation 5 years ago, but she still has bleeding almost daily despite taking progesterone, 200 mg twice daily. Most recently, her gynecologist prescribed a GnRH analogue without any effect. She has no history of hirsutism or acne.

A year ago, she underwent a pituitary evaluation, and the following laboratory test results were documented:

   Prolactin = 13 ng/mL (4-30 ng/mL) (SI: 0.57 nmol/L [0.17-1.30 nmol/L])
   GH = 0.19 ng/mL (0.01-3.61 ng/mL) (SI: 0.19 µg/L [0.01-3.61 µg/L])
   IGF-1 = 139 ng/mL (91-246 ng/mL) (SI: 18.2 nmol/L [11.9-32.2 nmol/L])
   FSH = 6.0 mIU/mL (2.0-12.0 mIU/mL [follicular]) (SI: 6.0 IU/L [2.0-12.0 IU/L])
   α-Subunit = 0.9 ng/mL (<1.2 ng/mL) (SI: 0.9 µg/L [<1.2 µg/L])
   hCG = <3.0 mIU/mL (<3.0 mIU/mL) (SI: <3.0 IU/L [<3.0 IU/L])

She is referred to you for a second opinion regarding the elevated estradiol.

On physical examination, her height is 66.5 in (169 cm) and weight is 336 lb (152.7 kg) (BMI = 53.4 kg/m²). Her blood pressure is 115/72 mm Hg. Examination findings are otherwise unremarkable.

Laboratory test results now:

TSH = 1.4 mIU/L (0.5-5.0 mIU/L)

Prolactin = 18.7 ng/mL (4-30 ng/mL) (SI: 0.81 nmol/L [0.17-1.30 nmol/L])

FSH = 4.7 mIU/mL (2.0-12.0 mIU/mL [follicular]) (SI: 4.7 IU/L [2.0-12.0 IU/L])

Estradiol (by liquid chromatography/tandem mass spectrometry) = 403 pg/mL (40-200 pg/mL [luteal]) (SI: 1479.4 pmol/L [146.8-734.2 pmol/L])

Progesterone = 5.7 ng/mL (2.0-20.0 ng/mL [luteal]) (SI: 18.1 nmol/L [6.4-63.6 nmol/L])

Pelvic ultrasonography documents an endometrium measuring 9 mm in greatest diameter. Evaluation is somewhat limited due to previous endometrial ablation. Both ovaries are visualized in limited views transabdominally and have no masses.

Gynecology is consulted but does not recommend hysterectomy or oophorectomy without further evidence of an ovarian or uterine source.

Which of the following is the best next step in this patient's management?

A. Perform pelvic CT

B. Start tamoxifen

C. Start letrozole

D. Perform ovarian venous sampling

E. Initiate an oral contraceptive

13 A 31-year-old woman (G1, P0) with type 1 diabetes mellitus since age 5 years presents for a follow-up visit. She is currently 32 weeks' gestation. She self-manages her diabetes with insulin pump therapy. After her last visit 1 week ago, she had sudden onset of frequent hypoglycemia during both day and night, prompting a reduction in her basal rates by 15%. Three days ago, she was still having mild hypoglycemic reactions during the night and between meals, prompting a further reduction in her evening basal rates and a change in her insulin-to-carbohydrate ratio from 1:10 to 1:15. She exercises by walking 10,000 steps daily.

On physical examination, her blood pressure is 117/75 mm Hg. Her weight is 135 lb (61.4 kg) (she has gained 26 lb [11.8 kg] during this pregnancy). Her abdomen is gravid. Neurologic examination demonstrates reduced sensation in both feet to monofilament testing. She has no lower-extremity edema.

Laboratory test results:

Hemoglobin A₁c = 6.5% (4.0%-5.6%) (48 mmol/mol [20-38 mmol/mol])

TSH = 0.5 mIU/L (0.5-5.0 mIU/L)

Total T₄ = 16.0 μg/dL (5.5-12.5 μg/dL) (SI: 205.92 nmol/L [94.02-213.68 nmol/L])

Serum sodium = 139 mEq/L (136-142 mEq/L) (SI: 139 mmol/L [136-142 mmol/L])

Serum potassium = 4.0 mEq/L (3.5-5.0 mEq/L) (SI: 4.0 mmol/L [3.5-5.0 mmol/L])

Serum creatinine = 0.8 mg/dL (0.6-1.1 mg/dL) (SI: 70.7 μmol/L [53.0-97.2 μmol/L])

Urinalysis, moderately positive for protein

Which of the following is the best next step in this patient's management?

A. Recommend increasing her carbohydrate intake at the evening meal and adding a bedtime snack

B. Perform a cosyntropin-stimulation test

C. Counsel her to reduce her daily exercise to 5000 steps

D. Call her obstetrician and recommend that she be seen immediately

E. Start methimazole, 10 mg daily

14 A 75-year-old woman with hypertension presents for evaluation of osteoporosis after sustaining a left femur fracture. This occurred spontaneously while walking down some steps. She subsequently underwent an intramedullary nail placement in her left femur. DXA scan revealed T-scores of −2.4 in the spine and −3.3 in the left one-third radius. She takes calcium and vitamin D supplements but has never taken osteoporosis medications. She has no history of long-term glucocorticoid exposure. She underwent surgical menopause at age 47 years. She has no history of kidney stones, parathyroid disease, or thyroid disease. She has hypertension treated with hydrochlorothiazide.

Her physical examination findings are unremarkable.

Laboratory test results:

Serum calcium = 10.0 mg/dL (8.2-10.2 mg/dL) (SI: 2.5 mmol/L [2.1-2.6 mmol/L])

Serum phosphate = 3.7 mg/dL (2.3-4.7 mg/dL) (SI: 1.2 mmol/L [0.7-1.5 mmol/L])

Serum creatinine = 1.1 mg/dL (0.6-1.1 mg/dL) (SI: 97.2 μmol/L [53.0-97.2 μmol/L])

Glomerular filtration rate (estimated) = 52 mL/min per 1.73 m^2 (>60 mL/min per 1.73 m^2)

Serum 25-hydroxyvitamin D = 51 ng/mL (30-80 ng/mL [optimal]) (SI: 127.3 nmol/L [74.9-199.7 nmol/L])

Serum albumin = 4.7 g/dL (3.5-5.0 g/dL) (SI: 47 g/L [35-50 g/L])

Serum alkaline phosphatase = 130 U/L (50-120 U/L) (SI: 2.17 μkat/L [0.84-2.00 μkat/L])

Her imaging results are shown (*see images*).

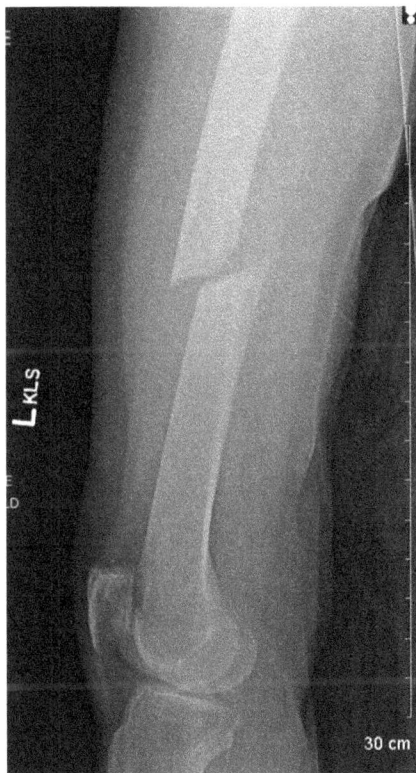

Plain x-ray of the left femur (status post intramedullary nailing).

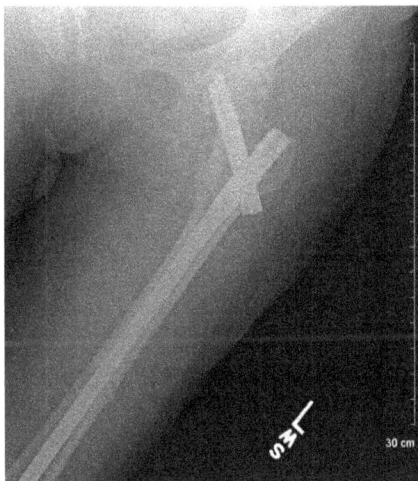

Plain x-ray of the left femur.

Which of the following should be recommended as the best next step regarding this patient's bone health?

A. Measure serum protein electrophoresis

B. Measure serum intact PTH

C. Measure 24-hour urinary calcium

D. Obtain whole-body bone scan

E. Obtain a radiograph of the right femur

15 A 34-year-old man presents for evaluation of generalized muscle weakness and low libido. He recalls that he was diagnosed with congenital adrenal hyperplasia shortly after birth; however, all of his medical care was at another facility and the records to confirm his diagnosis and treatment are not available. He had normal male genitalia at birth and was treated with dexamethasone and fludrocortisone during childhood, and then prednisone and fludrocortisone from his teenage years to the present. He recalls going through pubertal changes, such as deepening of the voice and facial hair growth, at the same time as other boys in his class. However, he has never had much facial or body hair. He is not aware of any impairment in his linear growth or development of secondary sexual characteristics, but he does think his testes are small. He has never fathered a child, but has never tried to do so either.

On physical examination, his blood pressure is 131/65 mm Hg, and pulse rate is 67 beats/min. He is well developed without any obvious features of Cushing syndrome. His genital examination is notable for no palpable testicular masses and a testicular size of 7 mL bilaterally.

A biochemical assessment, before and after cosyntropin stimulation, is performed in the morning, 24 hours after his last doses of prednisone and fludrocortisone (*see table*).

Measurement	8 AM	→ → → → →	9 AM
Cortisol	<0.2 μg/dL (SI: <5.5 nmol/L) (reference range, 5-25 μg/dL [SI: 137.9-689.7 nmol/L])		<0.2 μg/dL (SI: <5.5 nmol/L)
ACTH	1998 pg/mL (SI: 439.6 pmol/L) (reference range, 10-60 pg/mL [SI: 2.2-13.2 pmol/L])		...
Aldosterone	<4.0 ng/dL (SI: <111.0 pmol/L) (reference range, 4-21 ng/dL [SI: 111.0-582.5 pmol/L])		<4.0 ng/dL (SI: <111.0 pmol/L)
Plasma renin activity	3.7 ng/mL per h (reference range, 0.6-4.3 ng/mL per h)		...
17-Hydroxyprogesterone	85 ng/dL (SI: 2.6 nmol/L) (reference range, <220 ng/dL [SI: <6.67 nmol/L])		113 ng/dL (SI: 3.4 nmol/L)
11-Deoxycortisol	<5.0 ng/dL (SI: <0.14 nmol/L) (reference range, 10-79 ng/dL [SI: 0.29-2.28 nmol/L])	→ → → → →	<5.0 ng/dL (SI: <0.14 nmol/L)
11-Deoxycorticosterone	<5.0 ng/dL (SI: <0.15 nmol/L) (reference range, <10 ng/dL [SI: <0.30 nmol/L])	Administration of intravenous bolus of cosyntropin, 250 mcg	<5.0 ng/dL (SI: <0.15 nmol/L)
DHEA-S	8 μg/dL (SI: 0.22 μmol/L) (reference range, 65-334 μg/dL [SI: 1.76-9.05 μmol/L])		...
Total testosterone	176 ng/dL (SI: 6.1 nmol/L) (reference range, 300-900 ng/dL [SI: 10.4-31.2 nmol/L])		...
Free testosterone	4.54 ng/dL (0.16 nmol/L) (reference range, 4.85-19.0 ng/dL [SI: 0.17-0.66 nmol/L])		...
SHBG	9.4 μg/mL (SI: 84 nmol/L) (reference range, 1.1-6.7 μg/mL [SI: 10-60 nmol/L])		...
LH	2.7 mIU/mL (SI: 2.7 IU/L) (reference range, 1.0-9.0 mIU/mL [SI: 1.0-9.0 IU/L])		...
Prolactin	9.6 ng/mL (SI: 0.42 nmol/L) (reference range, 4-23 ng/mL [SI: 0.17-1.00 nmol/L])		...

Which of the following genes is most likely to harbor a pathogenic variant?

A. *CYP17A1* (resulting in 17-hydroxylase/17,20-lyase deficiency)

B. *CYP21A2* (resulting in 21-hydroxylase deficiency)

C. *CYP11B1* (resulting in 11-hydroxylase deficiency)

D. *HSD3B2* (resulting in 3β-hydroxysteroid dehydrogenase deficiency)

E. *NR0B1* (also known as *DAX1*) (resulting in adrenal hypoplasia congenita)

16 A 58-year-old woman presents with a 6-week history of retro-orbital headaches and deteriorating vision. She has no relevant medical history. She finds coping with her busy job increasingly difficult.

On physical examination, her height is 63 in (160 cm) and weight is 161 lb (73.2 kg) (BMI = 28.5 kg/m²). Her resting pulse rate is 56 beats/min and regular, and blood pressure is 105/75 mm Hg. Visual acuity is 20/80 (6/24) in the right eye and 20/40 (6/12) in the left eye.

Laboratory test results:

Prolactin = 85 ng/mL (4-30 ng/mL) (SI: 3.70 nmol/L [0.17-1.30 nmol/L])

TSH = 1.4 mIU/L (0.5-5.0 mIU/L)

Free T$_4$ = 0.75 ng/dL (0.8-1.8 ng/dL) (SI: 9.65 pmol/L [10.30-23.17 pmol/L])

Serum cortisol (9 AM) = 6.5 µg/dL (5-25 µg/dL) (SI: 179.3 nmol/L [137.9-689.7 nmol/L])

IGF-1 = 88 ng/mL (78-220 ng/mL) (SI: 11.5 nmol/L [10.2-28.8 nmol/L])

FSH = 7.2 mIU/mL (>30 mIU/mL [postmenopausal]) (SI: 7.2 IU/L [>30 IU/L])

LH = 8.0 mIU/mL (>30 mIU/mL [postmenopausal]) (SI: 8.0 IU/L [>30 IU/L])

The results of formal visual field assessment are shown (*see image*).

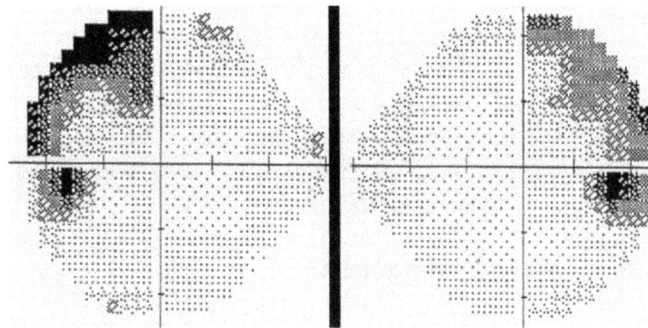

MRI of the sella (T1 noncontrast) is shown (*see images*).

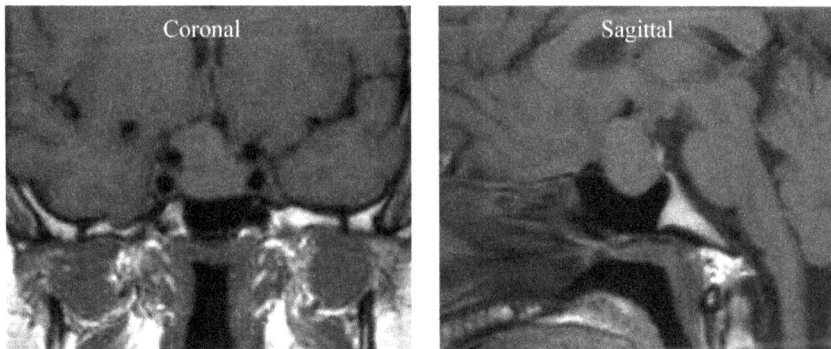

Which of the following is this patient's most likely diagnosis?

A. Autoimmune hypophysitis

B. Craniopharyngioma

C. Gonadotropinoma

D. Prolactinoma

E. Rathke cleft cyst

17 A 60-year-old woman presents with a chief concern of difficulty with hand movements. Her medical history is notable for type 2 diabetes mellitus diagnosed 8 years ago, although she had prediabetes for 5 to 7 years before diagnosis. She reports no complications except for background diabetic retinopathy. She felt well until 3 years ago when she developed right thumb "trigger finger." One year after symptom onset, she underwent right thumb trigger release and a right flexor pollicis longus tendon repair and her symptoms improved. However, she subsequently developed stiffness and swelling of the first and second digits on her right hand that spread to her other fingers on both hands. She cannot identify a particular joint that is more affected and notes that her overriding symptom is tightness of the palms. Her shoe size has not changed. She does not have an underbite or overbite and has had no headaches or vision changes.

Workup to date has included serologic studies documenting normal values of rheumatoid factor, cyclic citrullinated peptide antibodies, and antinuclear antibodies. Her hemoglobin A_{1c} level has ranged between 6.8% and 7.2% (51-55 mmol/mol) over the last 2 years, although it was less well controlled in previous years. Serum protein electrophoresis, urine protein electrophoresis, kappa-to-lambda ratio, and fat-pad biopsy are negative. Hand x-ray shows mild degenerative changes. The urinary albumin-to-creatine ratio is 21 mg/g creat (<30 mg/g creat).

She does not use tobacco or illicit drugs and does not drink alcohol. Her family history is notable for type 2 diabetes in multiple maternal relatives. There is no history of rheumatologic disease. Medications include glipizide, metformin, atorvastatin, multivitamins, and a nonsteroidal antiinflammatory drug.

On physical examination, her blood pressure is 138/78 mm Hg and pulse rate is 82 beats/min. Her height is 63 in (160 cm), and weight is 160 lb (72.7 kg) (BMI = 28.3 kg/m²). There is no evidence of synovitis in the small joints of the hands, wrists, shoulders, elbows, hips, knees, or ankles. She has flexion contractures, and all fingers of both hands have lost range of motion. She cannot place her palms flat against each other in opposition. She has impaired active range of motion of her left shoulder. Both knees are cool to touch without effusions. There is no ankle effusion or synovitis of her metatarsophalangeal joints.

Which of the following is the most likely diagnosis?
   A. Reflex sympathetic dystrophy
   B. Dupuytren contracture
   C. Limited joint mobility syndrome
   D. Rheumatoid arthritis
   E. Stiff-person syndrome

18 A 2.4-cm right thyroid nodule is identified in a 39-year-old woman. Thyroid ultrasonography shows a hypoechoic nodule with several echogenic foci. The left thyroid lobe is homogeneous without nodules. She undergoes FNA biopsy of the right thyroid nodule and the pathology report describes a follicular lesion of undetermined significance. She undergoes total thyroidectomy. The final pathology confirms a 2.0-cm tumor in the right thyroid lobe. The pathology slides are shown (*see images*). The surgical report mentions no capsular or vascular invasion. No lymph nodes are removed. She is prescribed levothyroxine, 100 mcg daily, after thyroidectomy.

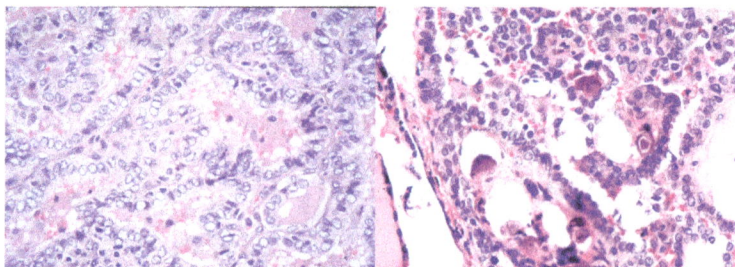

You see the patient 12 weeks after thyroidectomy. On physical examination, her blood pressure is 120/70 mm Hg and pulse rate is 65 beats/min. Her height is 64 in (162.6 cm), and weight is 134 lb (60.9 kg) (BMI = 23 kg/m²). There is a well-healed scar at the base of her neck, and there are no palpable cervical lymph nodes. The rest of the examination findings are normal.

Laboratory test results:
TSH = 3.5 mIU/L (0.5-5.0 mIU/L)
Thyroglobulin = 0.2 ng/mL (3-42 ng/mL) (0.2 µg/L [3-42 µg/L])

Which of the following is the best next step in this patient's management?
A. Continue levothyroxine, 100 mcg daily
B. Increase the levothyroxine dosage to maintain TSH between 0.5 and 2.0 mIU/L
C. Increase the levothyroxine dosage to maintain TSH around 0.1 mIU/L
D. Proceed with radioiodine treatment after thyroid hormone withdrawal
E. Proceed with radioiodine treatment after recombinant human TSH injection

19 A 65-year-old woman is referred to you for evaluation following abnormal results from a recent bone mineral density study. She underwent DXA scanning for routine menopausal health management and was found to be osteopenic based on femoral neck and total T-scores of –1.6 and –1.4, respectively, with normal bone mineral density at the lumbar spine (T-score, –0.8). Lumbar spine DXA images do not show apparent degenerative changes. She has no history of low-trauma fractures.

She underwent menopause at age 52 years and has never taken hormone therapy. Further review of secondary osteoporosis risk factors is unrevealing. There is no family history of osteoporosis or hip fracture. She has a 10-year history of type 2 diabetes mellitus, which has primarily been controlled with diet, exercise, and metformin, although her glycemic control has worsened recently based on a hemoglobin A_{1c} measurement of 7.7% (61 mmol/mol). Review of her home blood glucose values shows a fairly homogeneous increase in values through the day (fasting and 2-hour postprandial) compared with previous measurements. She does have proteinuria, but she has no history of other microvascular or macrovascular complications. The patient expresses an unwillingness to initiate insulin therapy.

Current medications include metformin, benazepril, metoprolol, atorvastatin, calcium with vitamin D_3, and aspirin.

On physical examination, her blood pressure is 110/65 mm Hg and pulse rate is 70 beats/min. Her height is 63 in (160 cm), and weight is 140 lb (63.6 kg) (BMI = 24.8 kg/m²). Self-reported maximum height is 64 in (162.6 cm). She has normal spinal curvature with preserved rib-to-pelvis distance of 2 fingerbreadths. The rest of the examination findings are normal, with no peripheral edema and normal 5.07 g monofilament testing of the feet bilaterally.

Laboratory investigations reveal normal chemistries, including normal creatinine, calcium corrected for albumin, TSH, serum 25-hydroxyvitamin D, and 24-hour urinary calcium and creatinine. Fasting lipid profile is within normal limits. Spot urine albumin is 140 µg/g creat (30-300 µg/mg creat) (SI: 15.8 µg/mol creat [3.4-33.9 µg/mol creat]).

The patient's 10-year risks of hip and major osteoporotic fracture by FRAX are 1.1% and 9.1%, respectively.

On the basis of her clinical history, which of the following is the best approach to her endocrine clinical management?
A. No changes are indicated
B. Start sitagliptin
C. Start rosiglitazone
D. Start canagliflozin
E. Start alendronate

20 A 24-year-old man is referred for management of dyslipidemia. One year ago, nephrotic syndrome was diagnosed after he developed abdominal pain and bilateral lower-extremity swelling. Severe hyperlipidemia was noted on initial presentation, and atorvastatin was initiated at a dosage of 20 mg daily. His clinical course was complicated by pulmonary embolism and poor response to steroids and tacrolimus. His nephrologist tells you that the patient has treatment-resistant nephrotic syndrome. Lipid levels remained persistently high, and the atorvastatin dosage was increased to 80 mg daily, and ezetimibe, 10 mg daily, was added. He does not smoke cigarettes or drink alcoholic beverages. His other medications include torsemide, 100 mg daily;

lisinopril, 40 mg daily; amlodipine, 5 mg daily; warfarin, 5 mg daily; and cholecalciferol, 1000 units daily. He is adherent to his medication regimen.

On physical examination, he is an anxious-appearing man. His blood pressure is 146/88 mm Hg. His height is 72 in (183 cm), and weight is 167 lb (76 kg) (BMI = 22.2 kg/m^2). There are no xanthomas. Bilateral pedal edema (1+) is present.

Laboratory test results (sample drawn while fasting, on atorvastatin, 80 mg daily, and ezetimibe, 10 mg daily):
  Total cholesterol = 464 mg/dL (<200 mg/dL [optimal]) (SI: 12.02 mmol/L [<5.18 mmol/L])
  Triglycerides = 196 mg/dL (<150 mg/dL [optimal]) (SI: 2.21 mmol/L [<1.70 mmol/L])
  HDL cholesterol = 46 mg/dL (>60 mg/dL [optimal]) (SI: 1.19 mmol/L [>1.55 mmol/L])
  LDL cholesterol = 379 mg/dL (<100 mg/dL [optimal]) (SI: 9.82 mmol/L [<2.59 mmol/L])
  Non-HDL cholesterol = 418 mg/dL (<130 mg/dL [optimal]) (SI: 10.83 mmol/L [<3.37 mmol/L])
  Apolipoprotein B = 350 mg/dL (50-110 mg/dL) (SI: 3.5 g/dL [0.5-1.1 g/dL])
  Lipoprotein (a) = 342 mg/dL (≤30 mg/dL) (>95th percentile) (SI: 12.2 μmol/L [≤1.07 μmol/L])
  Hemoglobin A$_{1c}$ = 5.5% (4.0%-5.6%) (37 mmol/mol [20-38 mmol/mol])
  Creatinine = 2.2 mg/dL (0.7-1.3 mg/dL) (SI: 194.5 μmol/L [61.9-114.9 μmol/L])
  Albumin = 0.9 mg/dL (3.5-5.0 g/dL) (SI: 9 g/L [35-50 g/L])
  TSH = 3.23 mIU/L (0.5-5.0 mIU/L)
  Fasting plasma glucose = 78 mg/dL (70-99 mg/dL) (SI: 7.3 mmol/L [3.9-5.5 mmol/L])

Which of the following is the best next therapy to manage this patient's hyperlipidemia?
  A. Switch to rosuvastatin, 40 mg daily
  B. Start fenofibrate
  C. Start marine omega-3 fatty acids
  D. Start a PCSK9 inhibitor
  E. Perform LDL apheresis

21 A 26-year-old amateur runner presents with fatigue and declining race performance. Over the last 4 months, he scaled up his training program in preparation for a marathon. He reports an intentional weight loss of 15.5 lb (7.0 kg), fatigue, and reduced libido. He describes longstanding intermittent and minor abdominal bloating attributed to lactose intolerance. He underwent normal puberty. He is unsure about fertility, as he has not attempted to achieve fatherhood. He does not use prescribed or illicit drugs, except for infrequent use of nonsteroidal antiinflammatory drugs. There is no history of head trauma.

On physical examination, his height is 70 in (177.8 cm) and weight is 148 lb (67.3 kg) (BMI = 21.2 kg/m^2). Blood pressure is 110/68 mm Hg, and resting pulse rate is 50 beats/min. There is no clinical visual field defect, and he has full range of eye movements. Muscle bulk appears normal, and testes are 25 mL bilaterally.

Laboratory test results (sample drawn at 8 AM while fasting):
  Total testosterone = 55 ng/dL (300-900 ng/dL) (SI: 1.9 nmol/L [10.4-31.2 nmol/L]) (repeat measurement = 66 ng/dL [SI: 2.3 nmol/L])
  SHBG = 8.9 μg/mL (1.1-6.7 μg/mL) (SI: 79.2 nmol/L [10-60 nmol/L])
  LH = 0.2 mIU/mL (1.0-9.0 mIU/mL) (SI: 0.2 IU/L [1.0-9.0 IU/L])
  FSH = 0.7 mIU/mL (1.0-13.0 mIU/mL) (SI: 0.7 IU/L [1.0-13.0 IU/L])
  Hemoglobin = 12.6 g/dL (13.8-17.2 g/dL) (SI: 126 g/L [138-172 g/L])
  Prolactin = 20 ng/mL (4-23 ng/mL) (SI: 0.87 nmol/L [0.17-1.00 nmol/L])
  Ferritin = 220 ng/mL (15-200 ng/mL) (SI: 494.3 pmol/L [33.7-449.4 pmol/L])
  Transferrin saturation = 35% (14%-50%)
  TSH = 1.24 mIU/L (0.5-5.0 mIU/L)
  Free T$_4$ = 0.87 ng/dL (0.8-1.8 ng/dL) (SI: 11.2 pmol/L [10.30-23.17 pmol/L])
  Free T$_3$ = 2.1 pg/mL (2.3-4.2 pg/mL) (SI: 3.22 pmol/L [3.53-6.45 pmol/L])

Which of the following is the most likely diagnosis?
  A. Covert anabolic steroid use
  B. Pituitary adenoma
  C. Hemochromatosis
  D. Functional hypogonadotropic hypogonadism
  E. Celiac disease

22 An 84-year-old woman with a history of anemia, hypertension, hypothyroidism, end-stage renal disease, paroxysmal atrial fibrillation, chronic diastolic congestive heart failure, and peripheral artery disease presents to the emergency department with hypoglycemia. She was at a dialysis appointment when she became tremulous and clammy. Her fingerstick glucose value was 23 mg/dL (1.3 mmol/L), and 1 ampule of dextrose 50% was administered. Three hours later, she was still clammy and became confused. A repeated blood glucose measurement was "too low to read" and she was given another ampule of dextrose 50%. At that time, her blood pressure was 90/40 mm Hg. She was sent to the emergency department for further evaluation.

The patient is a resident at a local nursing home. She does not have diabetes mellitus and does not take insulin or any diabetes medication. She had consumed 2 eggs and bacon in the morning, but did not eat lunch before her dialysis appointment. The patient's daughter states that she has been having no difficulty with eating and her weight has been stable. The patient has no history of hypoglycemia.

In the emergency department, her glucose concentration is documented to be 19 mg/dL (1.1 mmol/L). An infusion of dextrose 10% is started at a rate of 50 cc/h.

Medications listed on the transfer note are acetaminophen as needed for pain, alprazolam, amiodarone, amlodipine, atorvastatin, famotidine, fluticasone ACT nasal spray, furosemide, gabapentin, hydralazine, levetiracetam, levothyroxine, loperamide as needed for diarrhea, loratadine, metoprolol, midodrine, sertraline, sevelamer, and warfarin.

Physical examination findings are unremarkable. Her height is 64 in (162.6 cm), and weight is 154 lb (70 kg) (BMI = 26.4 kg/m²).

In addition to screening for hypoglycemic agents and measuring insulin and C-peptide, which of the following is the best next step?
  A. Call the head nurse at the nursing home to review the patient's medications
  B. Stop the β-adrenergic blocker
  C. Perform a cosyntropin-stimulation test
  D. Perform a 48-hour fast
  E. Stop loperamide

23 A 28-year-old woman with minimal medical history is 28 weeks pregnant. Gestational diabetes and hypertension were recently diagnosed and are being managed with insulin and α-methyldopa, with good control of both glycemia and blood pressure. Her obstetrician-gynecologist has been worried about possible secondary forms of hypertension and obtained a 24-hour urinary free cortisol measurement, which is elevated at 105 μg/24 h (<50 μg/24 h). She is referred to you for further evaluation of possible Cushing syndrome.

On physical examination, her blood pressure is 115/75 mm Hg and pulse rate is 72 beats/min. Her height is 66.5 in (169 cm), and weight is 209 lb (95 kg) (BMI = 33.2 kg/m²). She has some facial rounding and a small amount of retrocervical fat accumulation. On abdominal examination, she has a pregnant uterus with some pale stretch marks. There is minimal pedal edema.

Medications are insulins glargine and lispro; α-methyldopa, 250 mg twice daily; and prenatal vitamins. She has had minimal prenatal care and does not know if she had high blood pressure or diabetes before pregnancy. She has gained 19.8 lb (9 kg) so far during the pregnancy.

Which of the following is the best next step?
- A. Repeat 2 additional urinary free cortisol collections
- B. Perform a 1-mg dexamethasone suppression test
- C. Obtain 2 bedtime salivary cortisol levels
- D. Measure plasma ACTH
- E. Perform pituitary MRI without contrast

24 A 42-year-old woman seeks evaluation of hypophosphatemia. She reports longstanding fatigue, muscle weakness, and bone and joint pain requiring opioid medications for pain control. She also reports dental problems as a child. Despite treatment with phosphate and vitamin D supplementation, she continues to have mild to moderate symptoms. She is currently taking calcitriol, 1 mcg twice daily, and she has been adherent to her regimen of supplements. She has had 2 recent low-trauma tibial insufficiency fractures. She reports no nausea, vomiting, or diarrhea. She has 2 daughters who are also being evaluated for hypophosphatemia.

On physical examination, her height is 60 in (152.4 cm) and she has mild bowing of her lower extremities. Her examination findings are otherwise unremarkable.

Laboratory test results:
    Serum calcium = 10.2 mg/dL (8.2-10.2 mg/dL) (SI: 2.6 mmol/L [2.1-2.6 mmol/L])
    Serum phosphate = 1.4 mg/dL (2.3-4.7 mg/dL) (SI: 0.4 mmol/L [0.7-1.5 mmol/L])
    Serum creatinine = 1.0 mg/dL (0.6-1.1 mg/dL) (SI: 88.4 μmol/L [53.0-97.2 μmol/L])
    Serum intact PTH = 75 pg/mL (10-65 pg/mL) (SI: 75 ng/L [10-65 ng/L])
    Serum 25-hydroxyvitamin D = 43 ng/mL (30-80 ng/mL [optimal]) (SI: 107.3 nmol/L [74.9-199.7 nmol/L])
    Serum 1,25-dihydroxyvitamin D = 10 pg/mL (16-65 pg/mL) (SI: 26 pmol/L [41.6-169.0 pmol/L])
    Serum albumin = 3.9 g/dL (3.5-5.0 g/dL) (SI: 39 g/L [35-50 g/L])

Which of the following is the most appropriate next step in the management of this patient's hypophosphatemia?
- A. Increase her oral phosphate intake
- B. Increase the calcitriol dosage
- C. Start teriparatide therapy
- D. Switch to burosumab therapy
- E. Treat with intravenous phosphate

25 A 29-year-old transgender man is seeing you to establish care for management of gender-affirming hormone therapy. He socially transitioned as a transgender man at age 18 years and initiated testosterone injections at that time. He has not had any bleeding since starting injections, although he experiences some mild pelvic pain a few days before an injection. He and his wife notice a decline in mood right before each injection. He routinely donates blood because of elevated hemoglobin. His initial testosterone dosage was 200 mg every 2 weeks intramuscularly, but this was quickly reduced to 100 mg per dose. He finds injections painful, so he prefers to maintain the interval at every 2 weeks.

On review of family history, he mentions that his father has a platelet antibody condition and his paternal grandmother has a form of leukemia.

On physical examination, his height is 61.5 in (156.4 cm) and weight is 136.5 lb (62 kg) (BMI = 25.4 kg/m²). His blood pressure is 125/82 mm Hg. He is well-developed and masculinized with facial hair growth. There are well-healed chest surgery scars. No other pertinent findings are noted on examination.

You review his gender-affirming hormone therapy options and discuss lowering the dosage to 60 mg and switching to weekly subcutaneous injections to prevent erythrocytosis and symptoms before injections. You counsel the patient that subcutaneous injections should be less painful than intramuscular injections.

Laboratory test results:

Measurement	Timepoint and Testosterone Regimen		
	Baseline, 2 Days Before an Injection (Regimen: 100 mg every 2 weeks)	8 Weeks Later, 2 Days After Injection (Regimen: 60 mg weekly)	6 Weeks Later, Right Before Injection (Regimen: 50 mg weekly)
Total testosterone	423 ng/dL (SI: 14.7 nmol/L)	551 ng/dL (SI: 19.1 nmol/L)	243 ng/dL (SI: 8.4 nmol/L)
Hemoglobin	18.4 g/dL (SI: 184 g/L)	17.6 g/dL (SI: 176 g/L)	18.3 g/dL (SI: 183 g/L)
Bioavailable testosterone	...	139 ng/dL (SI: 12.2 nmol/L)	139 ng/dL (SI: 4.8 nmol/L)
Erythropoietin	...	...	6.8 mIU/mL

Reference ranges: total testosterone, 300-900 ng/dL (SI: 10.4-31.2 nmol/L); bioavailable testosterone, 83.0-257.0 ng/dL (SI: 2.88-8.92 nmol/L); hemoglobin, 13.8-17.2 g/dL (SI: 138-172 g/L); erythropoietin, 2.6-18.5 mIU/mL.

He undergoes a sleep study and has no apneic events or drops in oxygenation. Findings on echocardiography are normal. Findings on ultrasonography of the liver and spleen are normal.

Which of the following is the best next step in this patient's management?
A. Decrease the testosterone dosage to 40 mg every 2 weeks
B. Test for the *JAK2* V617F pathogenic variant
C. Switch to transdermal testosterone
D. Resume periodic phlebotomy/blood donation
E. Discontinue testosterone therapy

26 A 20-year-old woman is referred for management of inherited partial lipodystrophy and type 2 diabetes mellitus. She had normal body fat distribution as a young child. However, after puberty her pediatrician noted reduced adiposity in her extremities and trunk and increased adiposity in her neck and face. She was referred to pediatric endocrinology, and genetic testing revealed a pathogenic variant in the *LMNA* gene. Familial partial lipodystrophy type 2, or Dunnigan type lipodystrophy, was diagnosed. A year ago, she was admitted to the hospital with acute pancreatitis. Type 2 diabetes was diagnosed at that time. She is currently treated with metformin, 1000 mg twice daily, and fenofibrate, 145 mg daily.

Her mother has dyslipidemia, type 2 diabetes, and similar physical examination findings. Her father and younger brother are healthy.

On physical examination, she has a round face and fullness below the chin and in supraclavicular areas. Her extremities and trunk are muscular with reduced adiposity. There is no evidence of acanthosis nigricans or abdominal striae. The rest of her physical examination findings are normal.

Laboratory test results:
Hemoglobin A_{1c} = 7.6% (4.0%-5.6%) (60 mmol/mol [20-38 mmol/mol])
Total cholesterol = 260 mg/dL (<200 mg/dL [optimal]) (SI: 6.73 mmol/L [<5.18 mmol/L])
HDL cholesterol = 33 mg/dL (>60 mg/dL [optimal]) (SI: 0.85 mmol/L [>1.55 mmol/L])
LDL cholesterol, cannot be reported
Triglycerides = 1243 mg/dL (<150 mg/dL [optimal]) (SI: 14.0 mmol/L [<1.70 mmol/L])
Liver function tests, normal
Complete metabolic panel, normal
Fasting blood glucose = 188 mg/dL (70-99 mg/dL) (SI: 10.4 mmol/L [3.9-5.5 mmol/L])

In addition to counseling the patient on diet and exercise modification, which of the following is the best next step?
- A. Start insulin
- B. Start pioglitazone
- C. Start metreleptin
- D. Start adiponectin replacement
- E. Continue to monitor closely

27 A 49-year-old man is evaluated for poorly controlled hypertension despite treatment with maximum dosages of amlodipine, indapamide, and ramipril.

On physical examination, his blood pressure is 165/95 mm Hg. He has no other stigmata of endocrine dysfunction.

Laboratory tests confirm a diagnosis of primary aldosteronism, and further investigations are performed to determine whether he has unilateral or bilateral disease. Abdominal CT is shown (*see image*).

Adrenal venous sampling is performed (unstimulated [without cosyntropin], simultaneous sampling) (*see table*).

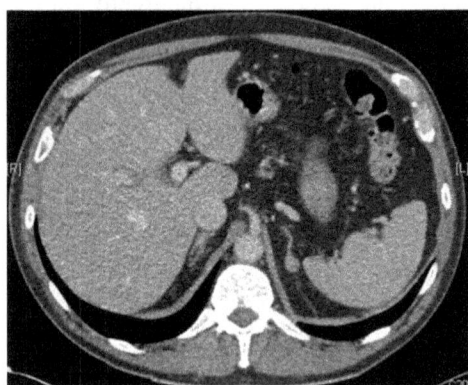

Location	Cortisol	Aldosterone	Aldosterone-to-Cortisol Ratio
Low inferior vena cava	8.5 µg/dL (SI: 234.4 nmol/L)	26.5 ng/dL (SI: 735.1 pmol/L)	3.1
Right adrenal vein	30.5 µg/dL (SI: 841.4 nmol/L)	51.3 ng/dL (SI: 1423.1 pmol/L)	1.7
Left adrenal vein	59.2 µg/dL (SI: 1633.2 nmol/L)	619.2 ng/dL (SI: 17,176.6 pmol/L)	10.5

Which of the following conclusions is best supported by these findings?
- A. The patient has bilateral primary aldosteronism with left-sided dominance
- B. The patient has unilateral primary aldosteronism due to a left aldosterone-producing adenoma
- C. The patient has unilateral primary aldosteronism due to a left aldosterone-producing adenoma with cortisol cosecretion
- D. The right adrenal vein has not been successfully cannulated
- E. Neither adrenal vein has been successfully cannulated and the procedure should be repeated with cosyntropin infusion

28 A 45-year-old woman seeks evaluation for hypercalcemia. She was well until 6 months ago when she noted the gradual onset of fatigue and increased thirst and polyuria. She has no notable clinical history except for hyperlipidemia treated with atorvastatin. She has no personal or family history of low-trauma fractures, calcium disorders, or nephrolithiasis. Until her calcium was noted to be elevated at 11 mg/dL (2.8 mmol/L) 4 weeks ago, she was also taking 1000 IU of vitamin D_3 daily.

Physical examination findings are normal, including no evidence of significant height loss since young adulthood, normal spinal curvature, and normal findings on respiratory and skin examinations.

Laboratory test results:
Serum calcium = 10.7 mg/dL (8.2-10.2 mg/dL (SI: 2.7 mmol/L [2.1-2.6 mmol/L])
Serum phosphate = 3.2 mg/dL (2.3-4.7 mg/dL) (SI: 1.0 mmol/L [0.7-1.5 mmol/L])
Serum magnesium = 1.9 mg/dL (1.5-2.3 mg/dL) (SI: 0.8 mmol/L [0.6-0.9 mmol/L])
Serum creatinine = 0.9 mg/dL (0.6-1.1 mg/dL) (SI: 79.6 µmol/L [53.0-97.2 µmol/L])
Serum albumin = 3.8 g/dL (3.5-5.0 g/dL) (SI: 38 g/L [35-50 g/L])

Serum intact PTH = 18 pg/mL (10-65 pg/mL) (SI: 18 ng/L [10-65 ng/L])
Plasma ionized calcium = 6.0 mg/dL (4.60-5.08 mg/dL) (SI: 1.5 mmol/L [1.2-1.3 mmol/L])
Serum 25-hydroxyvitamin D = 42 ng/dL (30-80 ng/mL [optimal]) (SI: 104.8 nmol/L [74.9-199.7 nmol/L])
Serum 1,25-dihydroxyvitamin D = 90 pg/mL (16-65 pg/mL) (SI: 234 pmol/L [41.6-169.0 pmol/L])
Urinary calcium = 450 mg/24 h (100-300 mg/24 h) (SI: 11.3 mmol/d [2.5-7.5 mmol/d])
Urinary creatinine = 1.2 g/24 h (1.0-2.0 g/24 h) (SI: 10.6 mmol/d [8.8-17.7 mmol/d])

Posteroanterior and lateral chest x-ray shows bilateral hilar prominence but no discrete lesions. Tuberculin skin test is negative.

Which of the following is the best next step in managing her calcium disorder?
  A. Alendronate
  B. Cinacalcet
  C. Zoledronic acid
  D. Prednisone
  E. Hydrochlorothiazide

29 A 43-year-old man with HIV infection, hypertension, obstructive sleep apnea, mixed hyperlipidemia, seizure disorder, and depression presents for management of medically complicated obesity.

The patient started gaining weight in his early 20s. Since then, his weight gain has been gradual. He is currently at his highest weight (304 lb [138 kg]). He has not participated in any commercial weight-loss programs, but he has tried adhering to different diets. When he took fenfluramine/phentermine in the past, he was able to lose 40 lb (18.2 kg). However, when he stopped the medication, he regained the weight.

The patient eats 3 meals daily: breakfast is usually oatmeal and coffee; lunch is meat with rice and potatoes; and dinner is either similar to lunch or a meal at a restaurant. Snacks include cakes, candy bars, and cookies. He eats large portions and sometimes returns for a second plate of food. He reports no episodes of binging or nocturnal eating. He drinks unsweetened tea, black coffee, water, and regular sodas. He has a gym membership and plans to start exercising on a regular basis. His medications include a single-tablet regimen for HIV (elvitegravir/cobicistat/emtricitabine/tenofovir alafenamide), lisinopril, levetiracetam, atorvastatin, and fluoxetine.

On physical examination, his blood pressure is 121/85 mm Hg and pulse rate is 79 beats/min. His height is 69.5 in (176.5 cm), and weight is 304 lb (138.2 kg) (BMI = 44.2 kg/m^2). He is in no acute distress. His heart sounds are normal, with a regular rate and rhythm, and he has no murmurs. His lungs are clear to auscultation bilaterally. His abdomen is soft and nontender. He has multiple weight-related stretch marks on his abdomen.

You recommend that he follow a low-calorie diet and track his food intake. You schedule an appointment with a dietitian for counseling.

In addition to lifestyle modifications, which of the following treatment options would you recommend next?
  A. Roux-en-Y gastric bypass
  B. Phentermine/topiramate
  C. Sleeve gastrectomy
  D. Naltrexone/bupropion
  E. Lorcaserin

30 Graves disease is diagnosed in a 24-year-old woman, and she elects to undergo therapy with radioactive iodine. In preparation for determination of her ^{131}I treatment dose, she has a radioactive iodine uptake and scan. The uptake is elevated at 70% at 24 hours. The scan shows homogeneous uptake but also a cold defect in the right lobe. Ultrasonography indicates that this corresponds to a suspicious nodule, which is determined by FNA biopsy to be papillary thyroid cancer. Following thyroidectomy and central neck dissection, the patient is found to have a 3-cm focus of cancer with gross extrathyroidal extension and involvement of 15 of 30 central compartment lymph nodes. All surgical margins are free of carcinoma. Her surgeon prescribes levothyroxine, and she comes to see you 4 weeks after the operation to discuss the next treatment steps.

Her physical examination findings are unremarkable, other than a healing cervical surgical scar. No abnormal cervical lymph nodes are palpable, and she appears clinically euthyroid.

Laboratory test results performed 2 weeks after surgery:
TSH = 0.34 mIU/L (0.5-5.0 mIU/L)
Free T_4 = 1.1 ng/dL (0.8-1.8 ng/dL) (SI: 14.2 pmol/L [10.30-23.17 pmol/L])
Thyroglobulin = 14.5 ng/mL (<1.0 ng/mL) (SI: 14.5 µg/L [<1.0 µg/L])
Thyroglobulin antibodies = 160 IU/mL (≤4.0 IU/mL) (SI: 160 kIU/L [≤4.0 kIU/L])
Thyroid-stimulating immunoglobulin = 400% (≤120% of basal activity)

You explain that after she has been treated with radioiodine, you intend to keep her serum TSH low to avoid stimulation of any residual thyroid cancer.

Which of the following could negatively affect this patient's prognosis with respect to her thyroid cancer?
A. Younger age
B. Surgery being performed for dual diagnoses of Graves disease and thyroid cancer
C. Presence of thyroglobulin antibodies
D. Elevated thyroid-stimulating immunoglobulin titer
E. Baseline thyroglobulin value of 14.5 ng/mL (14.5 µg/L)

31
A 53-year-old man is seen in the endocrinology clinic for evaluation and treatment of new-onset diabetes mellitus. He presented to the emergency department 8 days ago with abdominal pain, nausea, and emesis. Diabetic ketoacidosis was diagnosed. He was also treated for pancreatitis with intravenous fluids and analgesics and received intravenous insulin per protocol. Four days after admission, he was discharged on basal-bolus insulin therapy.

He has a history of stage IV malignant melanoma diagnosed 14 months ago. Treatment with ipilimumab and nivolumab was initiated 9 weeks ago, and he has been treated with this combination every 3 weeks (the most recent treatment was 2.5 weeks ago). He has never been diagnosed with pancreatitis in the past. He has hypertension treated with amlodipine and fosinopril and primary hypothyroidism treated with levothyroxine, 125 mcg daily. He does not smoke cigarettes. He occasionally drinks alcohol. Family history is not relevant except for a paternal first cousin with a history of diabetes mellitus (type unknown).

On physical examination, his height is 72 in (183 cm) and weight is 194 lb (88.2 kg) (BMI = 26.3 kg/m²). His blood pressure is 124/78 mm Hg, and pulse rate is 86 beats/min. Findings on examination of the heart, lungs, and abdomen are unremarkable. There are surgical scars on the posterior torso from resection of metastatic melanoma lesions.

Laboratory test results:
Hemoglobin A_{1c} = 9.2% (4.0%-5.6%) (77 mmol/mol [20-38 mmol/mol])
Plasma glucose = 182 mg/dL (70-99 mg/dL) (SI: 10.1 mmol/L [3.9-5.5 mmol/L])
C-peptide = 0.4 ng/mL (0.9-4.3 ng/mL) (SI: 0.13 nmol/L [0.30-1.42 nmol/L])
Creatinine = 1.0 mg/dL (0.7-1.3 mg/dL) (SI: 88.4 µmol/L [61.9-114.9 µmol/L])
Triglycerides = 145 mg/dL (<150 mg/dL) (SI: 1.64 mmol/L [<1.70 mmol/L])
TSH = 2.2 mIU/L (0.5-5.0 mIU/L)
Glutamic acid decarboxylase antibodies = <0.01 nmol/L (≤0.02 nmol/L)

Which of the following is the most likely diagnosis?
A. Secondary diabetes mellitus due to pancreatitis
B. Type 1 diabetes mellitus
C. Latent autoimmune diabetes in adults
D. Secondary diabetes mellitus associated with malignant melanoma
E. Type 2 diabetes mellitus

32 A 57-year-old woman presents for lipid management. She has no major medical problems. She has struggled with her weight over the years and has tried many diets. She recently started following a ketogenic diet (high-protein, high-fat, very low-carbohydrate), and she has lost about 15 lb (6.8 kg) over the past 3 months. However, a lipid panel obtained through her primary care provider's office revealed abnormal results. She has no history of abnormal lipid levels. There is no family history of cardiovascular disease. She does not smoke cigarettes, and she takes no medications or supplements.

On physical examination, her blood pressure is 134/88 mm Hg and pulse rate is 74 beats/min. Her height is 63 in (160 cm), and weight is 218 lb (99.1 kg) (BMI = 38.6 kg/m^2). The rest of her examination findings are normal except for abdominal adiposity.

Laboratory test results (sample drawn while fasting, on no treatment):

Measurement	2 Years Ago	Present
Total cholesterol	219 mg/dL (SI: 5.67 mmol/L)	345 mg/dL (SI: 8.94 mmol/L)
Triglycerides	158 mg/dL (SI: 1.79 mmol/L)	84 mg/dL (SI: 0.95 mmol/L)
HDL cholesterol	56 mg/dL (SI: 1.45 mmol/L)	64 mg/dL (SI: 1.66 mmol/L)
LDL cholesterol	131 mg/dL (SI: 3.39 mmol/L)	264 mg/dL (SI: 6.84 mmol/L)
Non-HDL cholesterol	163 mg/dL (SI: 4.22 mmol/L)	281 mg/dL (SI: 7.28 mmol/L)
Hemoglobin A$_{1c}$	6.2% (44 mmol/mol)	5.7% (39 mmol/mol)
Fasting plasma glucose	113 mg/dL (SI: 6.27 mmol/L)	95 mg/dL (SI: 5.27 mmol/L)
Creatinine	...	0.7 mg/dL (SI: 61.9 μmol/L)
TSH	...	2.8 mIU/L

Reference ranges: total cholesterol, <200 mg/dL (optimal) (SI: <5.18 mmol/L); triglycerides, <150 mg/dL (optimal) (SI: <1.70 mmol/L); HDL cholesterol, >60 mg/dL (optimal) (SI: >1.55 mmol/L); LDL cholesterol, <100 mg/dL (optimal) (SI: <2.59 mmol/L); non-HDL cholesterol, <130 mg/dL (optimal) (SI: <3.37 mmol/L); hemoglobin A$_{1c}$, 4.0%-5.6% (20-38 mmol/mol); plasma glucose, 70-99 mg/dL (SI: 3.9-5.5 mmol/L); creatinine, 0.6-1.1 mg/dL (SI: 53.0-97.2 μmol/L); TSH, 0.5-5.0 mIU/L.

Two years ago, her calculated 10-year risk of atherosclerotic cardiovascular disease was 2.8%. Her current risk could not be calculated due to significant hyperlipidemia.

Which of the following is the best next step in this patient's management?

A. Relax carbohydrate restriction and recheck lipids
B. Switch to a diet with healthy unsaturated fats and protein
C. Start statin therapy
D. Start PCSK9 inhibitor therapy
E. No intervention necessary now

33 A 70-year-old woman with chronic kidney disease presents for follow-up of osteoporosis. She has a history of an L2 vertebral compression fracture and has just completed a 2-year course of teriparatide therapy. A recent DXA scan revealed improving bone mineral density, with a T-score of –2.5 in the spine and –2.1 in the left femoral neck. She takes calcium and vitamin D supplementation. She is switched from teriparatide to denosumab therapy and receives her first injection at the time of her visit.

Laboratory test results at the time of the visit:
Serum calcium = 9.0 mg/dL (8.2-10.2 mg/dL) (SI: 2.3 mmol/L [2.1-2.6 mmol/L])
Serum phosphate = 5.0 mg/dL (2.3-4.7 mg/dL) (SI: 1.6 mmol/L [0.7-1.5 mmol/L])
Serum creatinine = 3.0 mg/dL (0.6-1.1 mg/dL) (SI: 265.2 μmol/L [53.0-97.2 μmol/L])
Glomerular filtration rate (estimated) = 17 mL/min per 1.73 m^2 (>60 mL/min per 1.73 m^2)
Serum intact PTH = 210 pg/mL (10-65 pg/mL) (SI: 210 ng/L [10-65 ng/L])

Serum 25-hydroxyvitamin D = 32 ng/mL (30-80 ng/mL [optimal]) (SI: 79.9 nmol/L [74.9-199.7 nmol/L])
Serum albumin = 3.6 g/dL (3.5-5.0 g/dL) (SI: 36 g/L [35-50 g/L])

Laboratory test results 2 weeks later:
    Serum calcium = 6.1 mg/dL (8.2-10.2 mg/dL) (SI: 1.5 mmol/L [2.1-2.6 mmol/L])
    Serum phosphate = 4.0 mg/dL (2.3-4.7 mg/dL) (SI: 1.3 mmol/L [0.7-1.5 mmol/L])
    Serum creatinine = 3.1 mg/dL (0.6-1.1 mg/dL) (SI: 274.0 μmol/L [53.0-97.2 μmol/L])
    Glomerular filtration rate (estimated) = 17 mL/min per 1.73 m^2 (>60 mL/min per 1.73 m^2)
    Serum intact PTH = 1348 pg/mL (10-65 pg/mL) (SI: 1348 ng/L [10-65 ng/L])
    Serum albumin = 3.6 g/dL (3.5-5.0 g/dL) (SI: 36 g/L [35-50 g/L])
    Serum magnesium, normal

Which of the following most likely explains these findings?
A. Primary hyperparathyroidism
B. Secondary hyperparathyroidism
C. Tertiary hyperparathyroidism
D. Parathyroid carcinoma
E. Hungry bone syndrome

34 A 26-year-old woman seeks evaluation for regular palpitations, heat intolerance, difficulty sleeping, and an 11-lb (5-kg) weight loss in the last 3 months.

On physical examination, her height is 65 in (165 cm) and weight is 135 lb (61.4 kg) (BMI = 22.5 kg/m^2). Her blood pressure is 135/85 mm Hg, and resting pulse rate is 110 beats/min and regular. She has a fine resting tremor and warm peripheral extremities. There is a small symmetric goiter but no signs of dysthyroid eye disease.

Laboratory test results:
    TSH = 2.4 mIU/L (0.5-5.0 mIU/L)
    Free T$_4$ = 3.2 ng/dL (0.8-1.8 ng/dL) (SI: 41.19 pmol/L [10.30-23.17 pmol/L])
    Free T$_3$ = 5.9 pg/mL (2.3-4.2 pg/mL) (SI: 9.06 pmol/L [3.53-6.45 pmol/L])

Which of the following is the most appropriate next step in this patient's management?
A. Contrast-enhanced pituitary MRI
B. Thyrotropin-releasing hormone test
C. Serum α-subunit measurement
D. *THRB* genetic testing
E. TSH dilution study

35 An 18-year-old woman with a 7-year history of type 1 diabetes mellitus is admitted to the hospital for diabetic ketoacidosis after presenting to the emergency department with dyspnea, tachycardia, nausea, and lethargy of acute onset. She had been in her usual state of health until the onset of symptoms, which worsened over several hours. Glucose levels at home were above the glucose meter detection limit.

Laboratory test results (sample drawn in the emergency department):
    pH = 7.09 (7.35-7.45)
    Pco$_2$ = 21 mm Hg (35-45 mm Hg) (SI: 2.8 kPa [4.7-6.0 kPa])
    Anion gap = 31 (<16)
    Serum urea nitrogen = 12 mg/dL (8-23 mg/dL) (SI: 4.3 mmol/L [2.9-8.2 mmol/L])
    Creatinine = 0.6 mg/dL (0.6-1.1 mg/dL) (SI: 53.0 μmol/L [53.0-97.2 μmol/L])
    Urinalysis, bland sediment with large ketones

On physical examination in the emergency department, her blood pressure is 112/72 mm Hg, pulse rate is 112 beats/min, and respiratory rate is 24 breaths/min. There are no other localizing signs. Mental status is normal. There is no evidence of hearing loss.

She reports being adherent to her basal insulin regimen, but admits to not taking bolus insulin. There is no history of microvascular complications or renal insufficiency. Her family history is notable for a paternal grandmother with type 2 diabetes. The patient's identical twin sister is healthy.

Treatment for diabetic ketoacidosis is initiated. Within 12 hours, urinary ketones decrease to "trace," the anion gap decreases to 16, and blood pH increases to 7.33. Over the next 12 hours, her anion gap ranges between 16 and 17 despite negative ketones on urinalysis. You are consulted because of the persistent anion gap acidosis.

Most recent laboratory test results:
Sodium = 143 mEq/L (136-142 mEq/L) (SI: 143 mmol/L [136-142 mmol/L])
Potassium = 3.8 mEq/L (3.5-5.0 mEq/L) (SI: 3.8 mmol/L [3.5-5.0 mmol/L])
Chloride = 108 mEq/L (96-106 mEq/L) (SI: 108 mmol/L [96-106 mmol/L])
Carbon dioxide = 19 mEq/L (22-28 mEq/L) (SI: 19 mmol/L [22-28 mmol/L])
Serum urea nitrogen = 2 mg/dL (8-23 mg/dL) (SI: 0.7 mmol/L [2.9-8.2 mmol/L])
Creatinine = 0.5 mg/dL (0.6-1.1 mg/dL) (SI: 44.2 μmol/L [53.0-97.2 μmol/L])
Glucose = 71 mg/dL (70-99 mg/dL) (SI: 3.9 mmol/L [3.9-5.5 mmol/L])
Serum osmolality = 285 mOsm/kg (275-295 mOsm/kg) (SI: 285 mmol/kg [275-295 mmol/kg])
Acetaminophen, undetectable
Salicylate, undetectable
Lactic acid = 32.4 mg/dL (5.4-20.7 mg/dL) (SI: 3.6 mmol/L [0.6-2.3 mmol/L])

Which of the following is the most likely additional contributor to metabolic acidosis in this patient?
A. Persistent β-hydroxybutyrate
B. Renal tubular acidosis type 4
C. Ethylene glycol poisoning
D. Diabetes due to mitochondrial defect
E. Elevated D-lactic acid

36 A 32-year-old woman who has had 3 miscarriages (G4P1) comes to see you because she is having a hard time getting pregnant. She has a healthy 4-year-old son and would like to have another child. Her obstetrician-gynecologist conducted an extensive workup for infertility and the findings were unremarkable. Her only surgical history is appendectomy at age 9 years. She takes occasional acetaminophen for abdominal pain during menstrual periods. She has not taken oral contraceptives for the past 1 year. Menarche was at age 10 years, and her periods have always been regular. Her family history is notable for lupus systemic erythematosus in her mother and hypothyroidism in her sister.

On physical examination, her blood pressure is 115/62 mm Hg and pulse rate is 70 beats/min. Her height is 64 in (162.6 cm), and weight is 126 lb (57.3 kg) (BMI = 21.6 kg/m²). Her thyroid gland is palpable. There is no cervical lymphadenopathy. She has patchy areas of hypopigmentation on her face, abdomen, hands, and legs. The rest of the examination findings are unremarkable.

Laboratory test results:
TSH = 3.0 mIU/L (0.5-5.0 mIU/L)
Free T$_4$ = 1.2 ng/dL (0.8-1.8 ng/dL) (SI: 15.4 pmol/L [10.30-23.17 pmol/L])
TPO antibodies = 85.0 IU/mL (<2.0 IU/mL) (SI: 85.0 kIU/L [<2.0 kIU/L])
Basic metabolic panel, normal

On the basis of current guidelines, which of the following is the best next step in this patient's management?
  A. Perform thyroid ultrasonography
  B. Initiate levothyroxine
  C. Initiate a gluten-free diet
  D. Perform a cosyntropin-stimulation test
  E. Assess Lupus anticoagulant and cardiolipin antibodies

37 A 65-year-old man is brought to the emergency department following a witnessed seizure. He has a history of metastatic gastrointestinal stromal tumor. He is unresponsive, and fingerstick glucose is noted to be less than 40 mg/dL (<2.2 mmol/L). The hypoglycemia is treated with D50, followed by a D10 infusion, and his blood glucose rises to the range of 100 to 150 mg/dL (5.6 to 8.3 mmol/L). His wife reports that he was lethargic over the past week. When the small-bowel gastrointestinal stromal tumor was diagnosed, he underwent surgery to resect 15 cm of the terminal ileum. Imatinib was initiated, and this was then switched to regorafenib because of disease progression. He did not receive glucocorticoids as part of his treatment. Hypoglycemia is not a well-established adverse effect of regorafenib.

On physical examination, his temperature is 98.4°F, blood pressure is 150/60 mm Hg, pulse rate is 81 beats/min, and respiratory rate is 14 breaths/min. His height is 69 in (175.3 cm), and weight is 136 lb (61.8 kg) (BMI = 20.1 kg/m^2). He is currently responding to questions. He has no hyperpigmentation of the lips, gums, or palms. A firm mass is palpable in the epigastric area. A colostomy is noted. The rest of the examination findings are normal.

Laboratory test results (after dextrose infusion started, 4 PM):
  Glucose = 87 mg/dL (SI: 4.8 mmol/L)
  Comprehensive metabolic panel, normal
  TSH = 4.1 mIU/L (0.5-5.0 mIU/L)
  ACTH = 14 pg/mL (10-60 pg/mL) (SI: 3.1 pmol/L [2.2-13.2 pmol/L])
  Cortisol = 5.7 μg/dL (2-14 μg/dL) (SI: 157.3 nmol/L [55.2-386.2 nmol/L])

The following laboratory test results are obtained when the dextrose drip is briefly discontinued:
  Insulin = <1 μIU/mL (3-19 μIU/mL) (SI: <6.9 pmol/L [9.7-97.2 pmol/L])
  C-peptide = <0.1 ng/mL (0.9-4.3 ng/mL) (SI: <0.03 nmol/L [0.30-1.42 nmol/L])
  Glucose = 42 mg/dL (SI: 2.3 mmol/L)

Abdominal CT shows a tumor encasing loops of bowel and carcinomatosis throughout the abdomen. The left adrenal gland is nodular (unchanged over past year), and the right adrenal gland appears normal. Mild left kidney hydronephrosis is noted.

A cosyntropin-stimulation test is performed and the results are normal. Serum glucose response to 1 mg of glucagon is greater than 25 mg/dL (>1.4 mmol/L).

Assessment of which of the following is most likely to determine the etiology of this patient's hypoglycemia?
  A. Insulin antibodies
  B. IGF-1 measurement
  C. IGF-2 measurement
  D. IGF-2-to-IGF-1 ratio
  E. Glucagon measurement

38 A 59-year-old woman presents with an 18-month history of gradually worsening hirsutism, mostly affecting her face and torso, and mild coarsening of her voice. There is no history of menstrual irregularity, subfertility, or hyperandrogenism during reproductive life. She underwent natural menopause at age 51 years and has never been on menopausal hormone therapy. Her medical history is notable for osteopenia and migraine headaches. She has no gastrointestinal symptoms or vaginal bleeding and her weight has been stable. She and her husband are both healthy and deny use of any illicit drugs. Her husband uses transdermal testosterone gel for "late-onset hypogonadism," but otherwise neither takes any medications.

On physical examination, her blood pressure is 134/82 mm Hg. Her height is 64 in (162.6 cm), and weight is 140 lb (63.6 kg) (BMI = 24 kg/m²). There is coarse terminal hair on her chin and abdomen and moderate frontal balding, but no clitoromegaly, skin atrophy, or striae. Muscle bulk is normal.

She has had repeatedly elevated total testosterone concentrations ranging from 100 to 230 ng/dL (SI: 3.5-8.0 nmol/L) (reference range, 8-60 ng/dL [SI: 0.3-2.1 nmol/L]).

Additional laboratory test results:
    LH = 7.5 mIU/mL (>30.0 mIU/mL) (SI: 7.5 IU/L [>30.0 IU/L])
    FSH = 22.2 mIU/mL (>30.0 mIU/mL) (SI: 22.2 IU/L [>30.0 IU/L])
    DHEA-S = 33.2 µg/dL (15-200 µg/dL) (SI: 0.9 µmol/L [0.41-5.42 µmol/L])
    17-hydroxyprogesterone after cosyntropin stimulation = 75.9 ng/dL (<217.8 ng/dL) (SI: 2.3 nmol/L [<6.6 nmol/L])

Transvaginal ultrasonography shows a 4-cm uterine fibroid, normal ovaries, and no evidence of ascites. CT of the abdomen and pelvis shows a 7-mm right adrenal adenoma with a radiodensity less than 10 Hounsfield units. There is no decrease in her serum testosterone concentration following GnRH-analogue suppression testing.

Which of the following is the most likely diagnosis?
    A. Polycystic ovary syndrome
    B. Late-onset congenital adrenal hyperplasia
    C. Androgen-secreting adrenal tumor
    D. Exposure to husband's testosterone gel
    E. Ovarian hyperthecosis

39 A 20-year-old woman is evaluated for oligomenorrhea and hirsutism. She describes a normal birth history and normal childhood development. Menarche occurred at age 11 years and her menses were regular until age 14 years when she developed oligomenorrhea. She had 6 to 9 menses per year from age 14 to 17, and 3 to 6 menses per year from age 17 to 20. In addition, she has noticed increased terminal hair growth on her chin, above her upper lip, and to a lesser degree on her upper chest. She is also bothered by increased facial acne and oily skin. She has no salt craving, hyperpigmentation, or orthostasis. She takes no medications. She is not interested in pregnancy at this time.

On physical examination, she is a well-appearing woman. Her blood pressure is 115/66 mm Hg, and pulse rate is 68 beats/min. Her height is 64 in (162.6 cm), and weight is 140 lb (63.6 kg) (BMI = 24 kg/m²). She has some facial hirsutism and acne without any overt signs or symptoms of Cushing syndrome.

Laboratory test results (sample drawn at 8 AM after overnight fast):
    Cortisol = 22 µg/dL (5-25 µg/dL) (SI: 606.9 nmol/L [137.9-689.7 nmol/L])
    17-Hydroxyprogesterone = 497 ng/dL (<80 ng/dL) (SI: 15.1 nmol/L [<2.42 nmol/L])
    DHEA-S = 545 µg/dL (44-332 µg/dL) (SI: 14.8 µmol/L [1.19-9.00 µmol/L])

A cosyntropin-stimulation test demonstrates an increase in the 17-hydroxyprogesterone concentration at the 60-minute mark (1545 ng/dL [46.8 nmol/L]). Nonclassic 21-hydroxylase deficiency is diagnosed.

Which of the following is the most appropriate first-line treatment?
    A. Nocturnal dexamethasone; monitor 17-hydroxyprogesterone levels
    B. Nocturnal prednisone; monitor 17-hydroxyprogesterone levels
    C. Prednisone and fludrocortisone in the morning
    D. Combined oral contraceptive pill
    E. Spironolactone

40 A 28-year-old man is referred for evaluation of hypercalcemia. He has had multiple episodes of kidney stones over the past 4 years. His dietary calcium intake is approximately 600 mg daily, and he does not take any calcium or vitamin D supplements. He has no history of fragility fractures or thyroid disease. He has an older brother who was diagnosed with peptic ulcer disease.

His physical examination findings are unremarkable.

Laboratory test results:
  Serum calcium = 13.2 mg/dL (8.2-10.2 mg/dL) (SI: 3.3 mmol/L [2.1-2.6 mmol/L])
  Serum phosphate = 2.1 mg/dL (2.3-4.7 mg/dL) (SI: 0.7 mmol/L [0.7-1.5 mmol/L])
  Serum creatinine = 1.1 mg/dL (0.7-1.3 mg/dL) (SI: 97.2 μmol/L [61.9-114.9 μmol/L])
  Serum intact PTH = 307 pg/mL (10-65 pg/mL) (SI: 307 ng/L [10-65 ng/L])
  Serum 25-hydroxyvitamin D = 26 ng/mL (30-80 ng/mL [optimal]) (SI: 64.9 nmol/L [74.9-199.7 nmol/L])
  Serum albumin = 4.2 g/dL (3.5-5.0 g/dL) (SI: 42 g/L [35-50 g/L])
  Urinary calcium = 310 mg/24 h (100-300 mg/24 h) (SI: 7.5 mmol/d [2.5-7.5 mmol/d])

A pathogenic variant in which of the following genes most likely explains his clinical presentation?
  A. *MEN1*
  B. *CASR*
  C. *RET*
  D. *CDC73*
  E. *VDR*

41 An 18-year-old man who is currently home from college is brought to the emergency department by his family because he has been experiencing palpitations and shortness of breath for several weeks. His symptoms worsened yesterday after he played basketball with his siblings. He also notes weight loss and hyperdefecation over the last several months.

On physical examination, he is anxious and confused. His temperature is 101°F and pulse rate is 160 beats/min. His respiratory rate is 25 breaths/min, and his breathing is shallow. He has obvious orbitopathy and a visible goiter. His thyroid gland is approximately 3 times normal size and a bruit is auscultated. His abdomen is tender to palpitation, and he vomits after being examined. Examination reveals moist skin, but no excoriations or bruising.

Review of his electronic medical record shows that he was prescribed methimazole therapy 7 months ago. He also had his wisdom teeth extracted 4 weeks ago. The family shares that the patient's mother has Graves disease, his younger brother has type 1 diabetes mellitus, and his sister has celiac disease. They cannot provide further details about the patient's medical situation.

Laboratory test results:
  TSH = <0.001 mIU/L (0.5-5.0 mIU/L)
  Free T$_4$ = 8.1 ng/dL (0.8-1.8 ng/dL) (SI: 104.2 pmol/L [10.30-23.17 pmol/L])
  Total T$_3$ = 900 ng/dL (70-200 ng/dL) (SI: 13.9 nmol/L [1.08-3.08 nmol/L])
  ALT = 80 U/L (10-40 U/L) (SI: 1.3 μkat/L [0.17-0.67 μkat/L])
  AST = 78 U/L (10-40 U/L) (SI: 1.3 μkat/L [0.33-0.80 μkat/L])
  Bicarbonate = 21 mEq/L (21-28 mEq/L) (SI: 17 mmol/L [21-28 mmol/L])
  Sodium = 137 mEq/L (136-142 mEq/L) (SI: 137 mmol/L [136-142 mmol/L])
  Potassium = 4.5 mEq/L (3.5-5.0 mEq/L) (SI: 4.5 mmol/L [3.5-5.0 mmol/L])

While in the emergency department, his mental status deteriorates further into delirium. He is admitted to the intensive care unit for treatment of thyroid storm.

Which of the following is the most likely precipitant of this patient's thyroid storm?
- A. Adrenal insufficiency
- B. Discontinuation of antithyroidal drugs
- C. Trauma
- D. Exercise
- E. Tooth extraction

42 A 22-year-old woman seeks help for management of obesity. The patient tells you that weight has been a problem since she was a child. She was born at term, with a normal birth weight (7.4 lb [3.4 kg]) after an uneventful pregnancy. Her motor and mental development was normal. However, around age 1 year she started gaining weight, and by age 3 she weighed 48 lb (22 kg) (>99th percentile for age). During elementary and middle school she was taller than her peers. She was screened for thyroid and adrenal disease in the past and all test results were normal. Her leptin level was elevated. The patient says she is hungry all the time and often feels hungry soon after eating a meal. She is currently in college.

On physical examination, her height is 66 in (168 cm) and weight is 387 lb (176 kg) (BMI = 62.3 kg/m²). She is in no distress and does not appear cushingoid. She has acanthosis nigricans with no hypopigmentation. She has brown hair. Her lungs are clear to auscultation bilaterally. On cardiac examination, heart sounds, rate, and rhythm are normal. She does not have polydactyly.

Given this patient's weight history, a genetic variant in which of the following genes or regions would best explain her clinical picture?
- A. Fat mass and obesity-associated gene (*FTO*)
- B. Proopiomelanocortin gene (*POMC*)
- C. Leptin gene (*LEP*)
- D. Melanocortin 4 receptor gene (*MC4R*)
- E. Prader-Willi critical region on chromosome 15

43 A 46-year-old woman is seen in the endocrinology clinic for evaluation and treatment of hypoglycemia. She was involved in a motor vehicle crash when the car she was driving sideswiped another vehicle. The airbag was not deployed, and there were no injuries to the patient or the other driver. Police and paramedics noted that she had slurred speech and was slow to respond to questions. The initial point-of-care glucose value at the scene of the accident was 42 mg/dL (2.3 mmol/L). She was treated with dextrose twice and transported to the emergency department. The episode occurred in the late morning on a day that she missed breakfast.

The initial glucose value in the emergency department was 138 mg/dL (7.7 mmol/L). The blood alcohol level was undetectable. During observation, a follow-up point-of-care glucose measurement was 57 mg/dL (3.2 mmol/L). Additional laboratory work was immediately ordered before she was treated for hypoglycemia (sample drawn at 12 PM).

Hemoglobin A_{1c} = 5.1% (4.0%-5.6%) (32 mmol/mol [20-38 mmol/mol])
Creatinine = 1.0 mg/dL (0.6-1.1 mg/dL) (SI: 88.4 μmol/L [53.0-97.2 μmol/L])
Estimated glomerular filtration rate = >60 mL/min per 1.73 m² (>60 mL/min per 1.73 m²)
TSH = 1.94 mIU/L (0.5-5.0 mIU/L)
Plasma glucose = 63 mg/dL (70-99 mg/dL) (SI: [3.5] mmol/L [3.9-5.5 mmol/L])
Insulin = 5.2 μIU/mL (1.4-14.0 μIU/mL) (SI: 36.1 pmol/L [9.7-97.2 pmol/L])
C-peptide = 3.6 ng/mL (0.9-4.3 ng/mL) (SI: 1.2 nmol/L [0.30-1.42 nmol/L])
Proinsulin = 154.6 pg/mL (26.5-176.4 pg/mL) (SI: 17.5 pmol/L [3.0-20.0 pmol/L])
Cortisol = 5.6 μg/dL (2.0-14.0 μg/dL) (SI: 154.6 nmol/L [55.2-386.2 nmol/L])

She consumed a sandwich and milk and was observed for 4 hours. There was no recurrence of hypoglycemia, and she was discharged home.

She has no history of diabetes mellitus or abdominal surgeries. Hypertension is treated with stable dosages of lisinopril and amlodipine. For the past 2 years, she has taken citalopram for depression. She does not smoke cigarettes. She has 1 glass of wine or beer 2 nights per week. She notes an unintentional weight loss of 24 lb (10.9 kg) over the last year.

On physical examination, she is alert and oriented. Her height is 65 in (165 cm) and weight is 184 lb (83.6 kg) (BMI = 30.6 kg/m^2). Her blood pressure is 132/83 mm Hg, and pulse rate is 78 beats/min. Findings on examination of the heart, lungs, and abdomen are unremarkable. Findings on neurologic examination are normal.

Which of the following is the best test to order now?
    A. Supervised fast in the hospital
    B. Mixed-meal test for hypoglycemia
    C. Abdominal CT
    D. Cosyntropin-stimulation test
    E. PET-CT of the chest, abdomen, and pelvis

44 A 22-year-old man with end-stage renal disease recently listed for renal transplant is referred to you for evaluation of a possible pituitary tumor. He has a history of reflux-mediated nephropathy. He developed bilateral breast enlargement with galactorrhea about 6 months ago that has progressively worsened. Laboratory testing 6 weeks ago showed markedly elevated prolactin (273.8 ng/mL [4-23 ng/mL] [SI: 11.9 nmol/L (0.17-1.00 nmol/L)]) and low serum testosterone (112 ng/dL [300-900 ng/dL] [SI: 3.9 nmol/L (10.4-31.2 nmol/L)]). At that time, he was prescribed cabergoline, 0.5 mg twice weekly, and he has had a marked decrease in galactorrhea and breast size. He has had no change in shoe or hand size. He has had acne for some time, treated by a dermatologist with tretinoin cream.

Current medications are calcium acetate, cinacalcet, metoprolol tartrate, and nifedipine.

On physical examination, his blood pressure is 132/64 mm Hg and pulse rate is 85 beats/min. His height is 64 in (162.6 cm), and weight is 148.5 lb (67.5 kg) (BMI = 25.5 kg/m^2). He has no facial features of acral enlargement and no sweaty palms. He has glandular breast tissue palpable bilaterally. There is no breast discharge. Testes are about 10 mL in volume bilaterally.

Current laboratory test results (on cabergoline):
    Prolactin = 5.5 ng/mL (4-23 ng/mL) (SI: 0.24 nmol/L [0.17-1.00 nmol/L])
    Testosterone = 660 ng/dL (300-900 ng/dL) (SI: 22.9 nmol/L [10.4-31.2 nmol/L])
    IGF-1= 375 ng/mL (116-341 ng/mL) (SI: 49.1 nmol/L [15.2-44.7 nmol/L])
    Thyroid function, normal

MRI without contrast documents a normal-sized pituitary gland.

You ask him to stop cabergoline for 1 month and then perform a GH suppression test (75 g of oral glucose). Results are shown (*see table*).

Measurement	Baseline	30 minutes	60 minutes	90 minutes	120 minutes
Glucose	93 mg/dL (SI: 5.2 mmol/L)	147 mg/dL (SI: 8.2 mmol/L)	118 mg/dL (SI: 6.5 mmol/L)	120 mg/dL (SI: 6.7 mmol/L)	91 mg/dL (SI: 5.1 mmol/L)
GH	16.6 ng/mL (SI: 16.6 µg/L)	7.8 ng/mL (SI: 7.8 µg/L)	3.9 ng/mL (SI: 3.9 µg/L)	2.2 ng/mL (SI: 2.2 µg/L)	1.2 ng/mL (SI: 1.2 µg/L)

Which of the following is the most appropriate next step in this patient's management?
    A. Perform an MRI with contrast and refer to neurosurgery
    B. Restart cabergoline
    C. Start pegvisomant
    D. Start a somatostatin receptor ligand
    E. No therapy now

45 A 21-year-old previously healthy man is referred after a recent hospitalization for acute pancreatitis. He developed sudden onset of upper abdominal pain after a large meal, and on presentation to the hospital he was found to have an elevated lipase level and a triglyceride concentration of 4100 mg/dL (46.33 mmol/L). Abdominal CT confirmed pancreatitis and also revealed hepatosplenomegaly. He reports a 12-lb (5.5-kg) weight gain over the past year as a junior in college. He does not smoke cigarettes or consume alcoholic beverages. His medical history is notable for markedly elevated triglycerides detected at age 8 years (up to 4250 mg/dL [48.03 mmol/L]) after frequent unexplained episodes of upper abdominal pain, and he saw a pediatric lipidologist who recommended a very low-fat diet at that time. His family history is unremarkable for cardiovascular disease or pancreatitis; both parents are alive and well. He has a 23-year-old sister who is healthy.

On physical examination, his blood pressure is 129/86 mm Hg and pulse rate is 65 beats/min. His height is 72 in (183 cm), and weight is 170 lb (77.3 kg) (BMI = 23.1 kg/m²). There are no xanthomas. Acanthosis nigricans is noted on the neck and in the axillae. The liver edge is palpable.

Laboratory test results (sample drawn while fasting, on no treatment):
  Total cholesterol = 494 mg/dL (<200 mg/dL [optimal]) (SI: 12.79 mmol/L [<5.18 mmol/L])
  Triglycerides = 3198 mg/dL (<150 mg/dL [optimal]) (SI: 36.14 mmol/L [<1.70 mmol/L])
  HDL cholesterol = 17 mg/dL (>60 mg/dL [optimal]) (SI: 0.44 mmol/L [>1.55 mmol/L])
  LDL cholesterol, unable to calculate
  Non-HDL cholesterol = 477 mg/dL (<130 mg/dL [optimal]) (SI: 12.35 mmol/L [<3.37 mmol/L])
  Apolipoprotein B = 63 mg/dL (50-110 mg/dL) (SI: 0.63 g/dL [0.5-1.1 g/dL])
  Lipoprotein (a) = 3 mg/dL (≤30 mg/dL) (SI: 0.11 μmol/L [≤1.07 μmol/L])
  Hemoglobin A$_{1c}$ = 4.4% (4.0%-5.6%) (25 mmol/mol [20-38 mmol/mol])
  Creatinine = 0.64 mg/dL (0.7-1.3 mg/dL) (SI: 56.6 μmol/L [61.9-114.9 μmol/L])
  TSH = 1.8 mIU/L (0.5-5.0 mIU/L)
  Fasting plasma glucose = 83 mg/dL (70-99 mg/dL) (SI: 4.6 mmol/L [3.9-5.5 mmol/L])

A pathogenic variant in the gene encoding which of the following proteins is most likely responsible for this clinical scenario?
  A. Apolipoprotein A-1
  B. Lipoprotein lipase
  C. LDL receptor
  D. Apolipoprotein B
  E. Apolipoprotein E

46 A 62-year-old man is evaluated for treatment-resistant hypertension. His blood pressure has escalated over the past 10 years and he requires 3 antihypertensive medications to control his blood pressure. A screening aldosterone value is 32 ng/dL (887.7 pmol/L) in the context of suppressed plasma renin activity of less than 0.6 ng/mL per h. An oral sodium suppression test reveals a 24-hour aldosterone excretion rate of 60 μg in the context of a 24-hour urinary sodium excretion of 250 mEq, thus confirming the diagnosis of primary aldosteronism.

Abdominal CT reveals nodularity of both adrenal glands, and adrenal venous sampling demonstrates evidence of bilateral autonomous aldosterone secretion. The patient is advised to start a mineralocorticoid receptor antagonist. His laboratory results and blood pressure parameters before and after starting spironolactone are shown (*see table*).

Parameters	Before Starting Spironolactone	3 Months After Starting Spironolactone
	Blood Pressure Medications: Amlodipine, 10 mg daily Lisinopril, 40 mg daily Labetalol, 200 mg twice daily	Blood Pressure Medications: Amlodipine, 10 mg daily Lisinopril, 40 mg daily Spironolactone, 50 mg daily
Blood pressure	154/96 mm Hg	138/82 mm Hg
Creatinine	1.12 mg/dL (SI: 99.0 µmol/L)	1.31 mg/dL (SI: 115.8 µmol/L)
Estimated glomerular filtration rate	74 mL/min per 1.73 m²	60 mL/min per 1.73 m²
Potassium	3.3 mEq/L (SI: 3.3 mmol/L)	3.8 mEq/L (SI: 3.8 mmol/L)
Plasma renin activity	<0.6 ng/mL h	<0.6 ng/mL per h
Aldosterone	32 ng/dL (SI: 887.7 pmol/L)	41 ng/dL (SI: 1137.3 pmol/L)

Which of the following treatment changes is indicated?

A. Increase the spironolactone dosage
B. Stop spironolactone
C. Stop spironolactone and initiate amiloride
D. Stop lisinopril
E. Stop lisinopril and initiate amiloride

47 A 40-year-old woman is referred for known medullary thyroid cancer. Two years ago, she had total thyroidectomy for a suspicious nodule, which revealed a 3.8-cm medullary thyroid carcinoma in the right lobe. No lymph nodes were removed.

After thyroidectomy, levothyroxine, 100 mcg daily, was started. Calcitonin and carcinoembryonic antigen (CEA) levels were measured periodically (*see table*). When her levels began to rise 6 months postoperatively, neck ultrasonography was performed and was unremarkable. One year postoperatively, she had repeated imaging that included neck ultrasonography, neck CT, chest CT, and abdominal CT. Several abnormal level VI lymph nodes were observed on neck CT, two 5-mm lung nodules were identified in the right upper lobe on chest CT, and no abnormal findings were observed on abdominal CT. She was not interested in another neck surgery.

You are now seeing her for the first time 2 years after thyroidectomy. Her calcitonin level is 320 pg/mL (93.4 pmol/L) and CEA level is 14 ng/mL (14 µg/L). You are concerned about the progression of medullary thyroid cancer. Repeated CT of the neck, chest, and abdomen show the same findings as last year. Her medical history is notable for a kidney stone at age 18 years. She takes levothyroxine, 112 mcg daily. She has occasional diarrhea.

On physical examination, her blood pressure is 110/70 mm Hg and pulse rate is 62 beats/min. Her height is 64 in (162.6 cm), and weight is 134 lb (60.9 kg) (BMI = 23 kg/m²). There is a well-healed scar at the base of her neck and no palpable cervical adenopathy. Physical examination findings are otherwise unremarkable.

Laboratory test results:
TSH = 2.2 mIU/L (0.5-5.0 mIU/L)
Free T$_4$ = 1.25 ng/dL (0.8-1.8 ng/dL) (SI: 16.1 pmol/L [10.30-23.17 pmol/L])

Calcitonin and CEA levels are summarized (*see table*).

	Time Point After Thyroidectomy				
Measurement	2 Months	6 Months	12 Months	18 Months	24 Months
Calcitonin	10 pg/mL (SI: 2.9 pmol/L)	80 pg/mL (SI: 23.4 pmol/L)	160 pg/mL (SI: 46.7 pmol/L)	250 pg/mL (SI: 73.0 pmol/L)	320 pg/mL (SI: 93.4 pmol/L)
CEA	...	6 ng/mL (SI: 6 µg/L)	10 ng/mL (SI: 10 µg/L)	12 ng/mL (SI: 12 µg/L)	14 ng/mL (SI: 14 µg/L)

Which of the following is the best next step in this patient's management?
 A. Start octreotide
 B. Start a tyrosine kinase inhibitor
 C. Perform ^{68}Ga DOTATATE PET-CT
 D. Perform contrast-enhanced liver MRI
 E. Increase the levothyroxine dosage to suppress TSH

48 A 48-year-old woman with a history of type 1 diabetes mellitus since age 14 years presents for follow-up. Her glycemic control has been fair, with hemoglobin A_{1c} levels in the range of 6% to 8% (42-64 mmol/mol) over the past 5 years. Her current hemoglobin A_{1c} value is 7.8% (62 mmol/mol). She has no known microvascular or macrovascular complications. She has a history of gastroesophageal reflux disease.

Her diabetes treatment consists of insulin glargine, 20 units every 12 hours; insulin aspart, 1 unit for every 12 g carbohydrate consumed and correction scale of 1 unit insulin aspart for every 25 mg/dL (1.4 mmol/L) glucose over 120 mg/dL (>6.7 mmol/L). Other medications are atorvastatin, 20 mg daily; multivitamin, 1 tablet daily; and omeprazole, 20 mg daily.

Her father has a history of coronary artery disease first diagnosed at age 60 years, and her mother has hypertension.

On physical examination, her blood pressure is 118/72 mm Hg and pulse rate is 79 beats/min. Her height is 62 in (157.5 cm), and weight is 199 lb (90.5 kg) (BMI = 36.4 kg/m^2). Except for obesity and mild abdominal lipohypertrophy, examination findings are normal.

Laboratory test results:
 Comprehensive metabolic panel, normal
 Total cholesterol = 139 mg/dL (<200 mg/dL [optimal]) (SI: 3.60 mmol/L [<5.18 mmol/L])
 HDL cholesterol = 51 mg/dL (>60 mg/dL [optimal]) (SI: 1.32 mmol/L [>1.55 mmol/L])
 LDL cholesterol = 53 mg/dL (<100 mg/dL [optimal]) (SI: 1.37 mmol/L [<2.59 mmol/L])
 Triglycerides = 75 mg/dL (<150 mg/dL [optimal]) (SI: 0.85 mmol/L [<1.70 mmol/L])
 Urine albumin-to-creatinine ratio = <16 mg/g creat (<30 mg/g creat)
 25-Hydroxyvitamin D = 28 ng/mL (30-80 ng/mL [optimal]) (SI: 69.9 nmol/L[74.9-199.7 nmol/L])

Before starting statin therapy 3 years ago, this patient's 10-year risk of cardiovascular disease based on a pooled risk cohort calculator was 1.1%.

Which of the following would you recommend in managing this patient's risk of cardiovascular disease?
 A. Recommend no changes
 B. Add aspirin
 C. Add aspirin and sucralfate
 D. Increase the atorvastatin dosage
 E. Add ezetimibe

49 A 39-year-old woman with acquired hypoparathyroidism is referred to you for recommendations regarding calcium management during pregnancy. She is presently 32 weeks' gestation with no maternal complications to date. Before this pregnancy, her hypoparathyroidism was well controlled on calcium citrate, 600 mg twice daily, and calcitriol, 0.50 mcg twice daily. She has continued this treatment regimen throughout her pregnancy.

Relevant laboratory values documented while on this regimen before pregnancy:
 Serum calcium = 9.2 mg/dL (8.2-10.2 mg/dL (SI: 2.3 mmol/L [2.1-2.6 mmol/L])
 Albumin = 4.0 g/dL (3.5-5.0 g/dL) (SI: 40 g/L [35-50 g/L])
 Urinary calcium = 235 mg/24 h (100-300 mg/24 h) (SI: 5.9 mmol/d [2.5-7.5 mmol/d])

Her medical history is notable for subtotal thyroidectomy for benign, multinodular goiter and postsurgical hypothyroidism and hypoparathyroidism. She takes levothyroxine, 100 mcg daily.

On physical examination, she appears well. Her abdomen is gravid. Chvostek testing is negative.

Updated laboratory test results:
    Serum calcium = 8.5 mg/dL (8.2-10.2 mg/dL (SI: 2.1 mmol/L [2.1-2.6 mmol/L])
    Serum phosphate = 4.0 mg/dL (2.3-4.7 mg/dL) (SI: 1.3 mmol/L [0.7-1.5 mmol/L])
    Serum magnesium = 2.0 mg/dL (1.5-2.3 mg/dL) (SI: 0.8 mmol/L [0.6-0.9 mmol/L])
    Serum creatinine = 0.9 mg/dL (0.6-1.1 mg/dL) (SI: 79.6 μmol/L [53.0-97.2 μmol/L])
    Serum albumin = 3.5 g/dL (3.5-5.0 g/dL) (SI: 35 g/L [35-50 g/L])
    Serum 25-hydroxyvitamin D = 35 ng/dL (30-80 ng/mL [optimal]) (SI: 87.4 nmol/L [74.9-199.7 nmol/L])
    Serum 1,25-dihydroxyvitamin D = 105 pg/mL (16-65 pg/mL) (SI: 273 pmol/L [41.6-169.0 pmol/L])
    Serum TSH = 1.5 mIU/L (0.5-5.0 mIU/L)
    Urinary calcium = 275 mg/24 h (100-300 mg/24 h) (SI: 6.9 mmol/d [2.5-7.5 mmol/d])
    Urinary creatinine = 1.5 g/24 h (1.0-2.0 g/24 h) (SI: 13.3 mmol/d [8.8-17.7 mmol/d])

Which of the following is the best next step in the management of this patient's hypoparathyroidism?
    A. Start cholecalciferol, 1000 IU daily
    B. Increase the calcium citrate dosage to 600 mg 3 times daily
    C. Decrease the calcitriol dosage to 0.5 mcg once daily
    D. Start hydrochlorothiazide, 12.5 mg daily
    E. Maintain current regimen

50 A 49-year-old woman is seeing you after years of being on cabergoline for a left-sided prolactin-secreting microadenoma diagnosed when she was having difficulty conceiving. She has been skipping periods every other month and experiencing hot flashes that interfere with sleep and work. She ran out of cabergoline 6 months ago and just recently saw her primary care physician for a routine physical. They are both wondering whether she needs to restart the cabergoline after more than 10 years of being on therapy or whether she is entering menopause. Her husband had a vasectomy 5 years ago. She would prefer to remain off cabergoline if it is no longer necessary.

Physical examination findings are normal.

Laboratory test results:
    TSH = 1.4 mIU/L (0.5-5.0 mIU/L)
    Prolactin = 46.7 ng/mL (4-30 ng/mL) (SI: 0.5 nmol/L [0.17-1.30 nmol/L])
    FSH = 44.5 mIU/mL (2.0-12.0 mIU/mL [follicular]) (SI: 44.5 IU/L [2.0-12.0 IU/L])
    Estradiol = 32 pg/mL (10-180 pg/mL [follicular]) (SI: 117.5 pmol/L [36.7-660.8 pmol/L])

Pituitary MRI is shown (*see image, coronal view*).

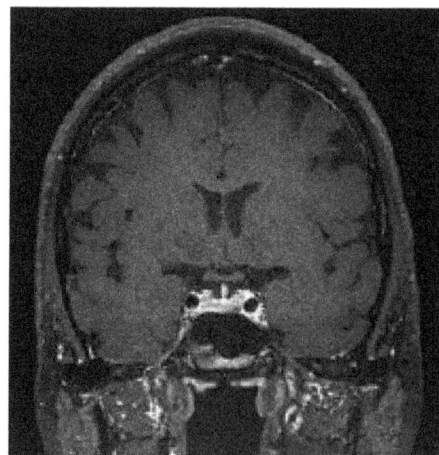

Which of the following is the best management plan?
    A. Restart cabergoline
    B. Restart cabergoline and estrogen replacement therapy
    C. Initiate estrogen replacement therapy
    D. Initiate vaginal estrogen therapy
    E. Monitor off therapy

51 A 46-year-old man is referred to you for management of panhypopituitarism 6 weeks after resection of a nonfunctioning pituitary tumor. He is currently taking replacement hydrocortisone, 15 mg in the morning and 5 mg in the afternoon; levothyroxine, 88 mcg daily; and desmopressin nasal spray twice daily. Testosterone and GH replacement have not been started.

The patient feels less energetic and has less stamina than before his surgery. He has no headaches or vision concerns. He has no symptoms suggestive of adrenal insufficiency.

On physical examination, his blood pressure is 134/78 mm Hg and pulse rate is 68 beats/min. His height is 69 in (175.3 cm), and weight is 150 lb (68.2 kg) (BMI = 22.1 kg/m^2). He has some mild gynecomastia, but examination findings are otherwise normal.

You reassess the patient's hormonal axes and confirm hypopituitarism. Postoperative MRI ordered by the patient's surgeon shows no evidence of residual tumor. You discuss testosterone and GH replacement with the patient. He elects to start testosterone therapy, but decides to defer GH therapy for now.

At a follow-up visit for reassessment of gonadal function, the patient states that he wishes to initiate GH therapy. GH therapy is started, and when you see him back in 2 months the patient is feeling well, although he has some new constipation and cold sensitivity. He has not had any additional changes in his treatment, and he maintains a consistent regimen for taking his medications.

Laboratory testing at each visit is shown (*see table*).

Analyte	Initial visit	1st Follow-Up Visit	2nd Follow-Up Visit
Comprehensive metabolic panel	Normal	Normal	...
Free T$_4$ (0.8-1.8 ng/dL [SI: 10.30-23.17 pmol/L])	1.5 ng/dL (19.3 pmol/L)	1.7 ng/dL (21.9 pmol/L)	0.7 ng/dL (9.0 pmol/L)
Testosterone (300-900 ng/dL [SI: 10.4-31.2 nmol/L])	150 ng/dL (5.2 nmol/L)	600 ng/dL (20.8 nmol/L)	560 ng/dL (19.4 nmol/L)
IGF-1 (91-246 ng/mL [SI: 11.9-32.2 nmol/L])	50 ng/mL (6.6 nmol/L)	40 ng/mL (5.2 nmol/L)	205 ng/mL (26.9 nmol/L)

Which of the following is the most likely cause of this patient's decreased free T$_4$ concentration following GH initiation?
A. Nonadherence to medical therapy
B. Impaired absorption of levothyroxine
C. Decreased thyroxine-binding globulin concentration
D. Increased conversion of T$_4$ to T$_3$
E. Increased body weight

52 A 60-year-old man with type 1 diabetes mellitus since age 30 years presents for a follow-up visit. His diabetes is complicated by retinopathy, neuropathy, coronary artery disease, and end-stage renal disease treated by peritoneal dialysis overnight, from approximately 8 PM to 8 AM. He brings the following data for the past 2 days:

Day	Time of Day						
	8 AM	12 PM	3 PM	6 PM	10 PM	3 AM	6 AM
Day 1	220 mg/dL (SI: 12.2 mmol/L)	112 mg/dL (SI: 6.2 mmol/L)	76 mg/dL (SI: 4.2 mmol/L)	97 mg/dL (SI: 5.4 mmol/L)	154 mg/dL (SI: 8.5 mmol/L)	210 mg/dL (SI: 11.7 mmol/L)	290 mg/dL (SI: 16.1 mmol/L)
Day 2	310 mg/dL (SI: 17.2 mmol/L)	156 mg/dL (SI: 8.7 mmol/L)	98 mg/dL (SI: 5.4 mmol/L)	102 mg/dL (SI: 5.7 mmol/L)	165 mg/dL (SI: 9.2 mmol/L)	250 mg/dL (SI: 13.9 mmol/L)	285 mg/dL (SI: 15.8 mmol/L)

The patient's continuous glucose monitor data show that the overnight glucose increase is gradual with no nocturnal hypoglycemia. He exercises by walking after lunch.

His treatment regimen consists of insulin glargine, 20 units at 8 AM and 10 PM, and insulin lispro for meals, 8 units plus medium-dose correction scale (adds 2 units of lispro per every glucose reading of 50 mg/dL above 150 mg/dL [>8.3 mmol/L]).

On physical examination, his blood pressure is 130/85 mm Hg and pulse rate is 80 beats/min. His height is 66.5 in (169 cm), and weight is 176 lb (80 kg) (dry weight) (BMI = 28 kg/m²). Examination findings are remarkable for a peritoneal catheter in the midabdomen and no evidence of infection.

Which of the following is the best next step in this patient's management?
   A. Increase his evening insulin glargine dose to 30 units
   B. Change his basal insulin to 40 units degludec, given at bedtime
   C. Change to insulin pump therapy
   D. Add an extra dose of insulin lispro at the start of peritoneal dialysis
   E. Change his evening basal insulin to 30 units of NPH

53 A 60-year-man presents to the emergency department because of fatigue, weakness, weight loss, and fever. He has a history of chronic lymphocytic leukemia and recently received chemotherapy with bendamustine and rituximab. The patient is admitted to the intensive care unit with a diagnosis of neutropenic fever.

On physical examination, his temperature is 102.5°F and pulse rate is 132 beats/min. He has left-sided neck swelling. He reports tenderness to palpation of both the left neck and the thyroid gland.

His white blood cell count is 66,900/μL (4500-11,000/μL) (SI: 66.9 × 10⁹/L [4.5-11.0 × 10⁹/L]) with 98% monocytes.

Initial CT imaging with intravenous contrast shows lymphomatous nodules throughout the lungs, spleen, liver, and kidney and a left-sided neck mass consistent with an abscess (*see image 1*). The thyroid gland is initially reported to be normal. Multiple treatments for the patient's lymphoma and infection are initiated. Thyroid function tests document severe thyrotoxicosis (*see table*). Radioiodine uptake cannot be done due to the patient's unstable condition.

Methimazole is initiated at a dosage of 30 mg every 8 hours, along with intravenous hydrocortisone and potassium iodide. Despite several days of methimazole therapy, the patient's free T₄ concentration continues to rise (*see table*). Repeated CT of the neck and abdomen show progression of widespread lymphomatous lesions. Diffuse lesions infiltrating the thyroid gland are also now noted (*see image 2*). Plasmapheresis or charcoal hemoperfusion are recommended to treat the patient's thyrotoxicosis, given the lack of response to methimazole. However, the patient dies of overwhelming sepsis before this therapy can be initiated.

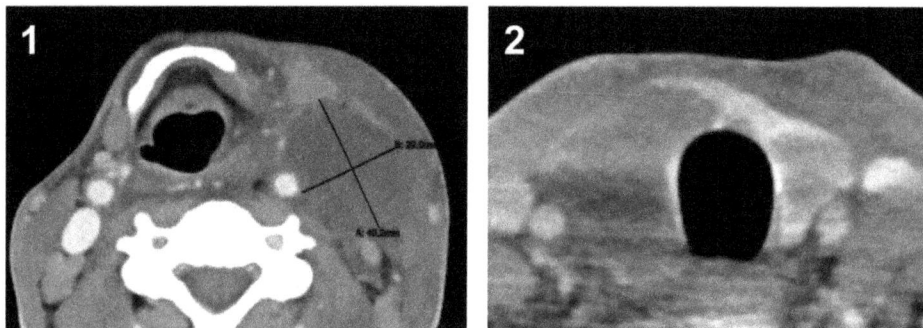

Image 1, CT of the neck showing a large left level 2 necrotic lymph node with extensive adjacent inflammatory changes, most likely representing an infected necrotic lymph node; the differential includes abscess. Image 2, Diffuse low-attenuation infiltrative lesions within the thyroid gland.

Time point	Admission	1 Day Later	2 Days Later	3 Days Later
TSH (0.5-5.0 mIU/L)	0.02 mIU/L	0.007 mIU/L	...	...
Free T₄ (0.8-1.8 ng/dL [SI: 10.30-23.17 pmol/L])	6.0 ng/dL (77.2 pmol/L)	6.7 ng/dL (86.2 pmol/L)	7.4 ng/dL (95.2 pmol/L)	>8 ng/dL (103.0 pmol/L)
Total T₃ (70-200 ng/dL [SI: 1.08-3.08 nmol/L])	...	244 ng/dL (3.8 nmol/L)	231 ng/dL (3.6 nmol/L)	229 ng/dL (3.5 nmol/L)

Which of the following laboratory tests would provide a potential explanation for the patient's lack of response to methimazole?
  A. Serum thyroglobulin measurement
  B. 24-Hour urinary iodine measurement
  C. Serum methimazole concentration
  D. Repeated white blood cell count
  E. Thyroid-stimulating immunoglobulin measurement

54 A 30-year-old woman is referred for evaluation of hypocalcemia. She reports that she has had a low serum calcium level since age 11 years and has been on longstanding calcium and vitamin D supplementation. She has no symptoms of hypocalcemia other than occasional perioral tingling. She has 2 first cousins (maternal uncle's children) who are very short and obese.

On physical examination, her height is 60 in (152.4 cm) and weight is 165 lb (75 kg) (BMI = 32.2 kg/m^2). She has foreshortened fourth metacarpal bones bilaterally. A subcutaneous hard nodule is palpated on her left forearm. Her examination findings are otherwise unremarkable.

Laboratory test results:
  Serum calcium = 8.0 mg/dL (8.2-10.2 mg/dL) (SI: 2.0 mmol/L [2.1-2.6 mmol/L])
  Serum phosphate = 4.5 mg/dL (2.3-4.7 mg/dL) (SI: 1.4 mmol/L [0.7-1.5 mmol/L])
  Serum creatinine = 0.8 mg/dL (0.7-1.3 mg/dL) (SI: 70.7 μmol/L [61.9-114.9 μmol/L])
  Serum intact PTH = 296 pg/mL (10-65 pg/mL) (SI: 296 ng/L [10-65 ng/L])
  Serum 25-hydroxyvitamin D = 42 ng/mL (30-80 ng/mL [optimal]) (SI: 104.8 nmol/L [74.9-199.7 nmol/L])
  Serum 1,25-dihydroxyvitamin D = 14 pg/mL (16-65 pg/mL) (SI: 36.4 pmol/L [41.6-169.0 pmol/L])
  Serum albumin = 3.9 g/dL (3.5-5.0 g/dL) (SI: 39 g/L [35-50 g/L])

Which of the following is the most likely diagnosis?
  A. Pseudohypoparathyroidism type 1a
  B. Pseudohypoparathyroidism type 1b
  C. Pseudohypoparathyroidism type 1c
  D. Pseudopseudohypoparathyroidism
  E. Hereditary resistance to vitamin D

55 A 35-year-old man presents with a 12-month history of increasing fatigue, low libido, and reduced shaving frequency. He reports low energy and an 8.8-lb (3.6-kg) weight gain, which he attributes to reduced physical activity. Eighteen months before presentation, he commenced carbamazepine for newly diagnosed grand mal seizures. His current maintenance dosage is 400 mg 3 times daily. Seizure activity has been well controlled. He reports undergoing normal puberty, and he has 2 children aged 10 and 7 years. His wife had no difficulty conceiving.

On physical examination, he has mildly reduced body hair, mild gynecomastia, and 16-mL testes bilaterally.

Laboratory test results (sample drawn at 8 AM while fasting):
  Serum total testosterone = 420 ng/dL (300-900 ng/dL) (SI: 14.6 nmol/L [10.4-31.2 nmol/L])
  Hemoglobin = 12.8 g/dL (13.8-17.2 g/dL) (SI: 128 g/L [138-172 g/L])
  Complete blood cell count, otherwise normal
  Serum electrolytes, normal
  Renal function, normal
  Liver enzymes, normal
  Thyroid function, normal

Which of the following is the best test to order now?
  A. Dihydrotestosterone measurement
  B. Estradiol measurement
  C. SHBG measurement
  D. Iron studies
  E. Prolactin measurement

56 A 70-year-old woman is seen in consultation for type 2 diabetes mellitus. Hypertension was diagnosed 2 years ago, and coronary artery disease with elective percutaneous transluminal coronary angioplasty of the left circumflex coronary artery was performed 1 year ago. She had a deep venous thrombosis 1 year ago. She also has gastroesophageal reflux disease and a compression fracture of the L5 vertebra.

Type 2 diabetes was diagnosed 2 years ago on the basis of routine testing. She was initially treated with metformin and required escalation of treatment with the addition of a sulfonylurea and insulin within 1 year. Her current hemoglobin A$_{1c}$ level is 8.1% (65 mmol/mol). She is adherent to dietary recommendations, but she has become more debilitated, which makes exercise difficult. This is frustrating to her, as her angina resolved after angioplasty and she thought she would exercise more. She also notes substantial weight gain of 18 lb (8.2 kg) in the last 3 years. Current medications include lisinopril, amlodipine, atorvastatin, detemir, glimepiride, rivaroxaban, and furosemide.

On physical examination, she is an elderly woman in a wheelchair. She is afebrile, blood pressure is 148/92 mm Hg, and pulse rate is 92 beats/min. Her height is 62 in (157.5 cm), and weight is 175 lb (79.5 kg) (BMI = 32 kg/m^2). Her oropharynx is clear, mucus membranes are moist, sclerae are anicteric, and conjunctivae are without pallor. There are no thyroid masses or cervical lymphadenopathy. Lungs are clear to auscultation bilaterally. On cardiovascular examination, she has a regular rate and rhythm. Point of maximal impulse is at the fifth intercostal space. There is bilateral trace nonpitting edema of the lower extremities up to the ankles. She has generalized weakness and is unable to get out of her wheelchair without assistance. Neurologic examination findings are otherwise nonfocal. Her mood is depressed. Skin is thin and there are ecchymoses on the exposed parts of lower and upper extremities.

Which of the following laboratory parameters(s) is most important to measure now?
  A. 24-Hour urinary free cortisol and midnight salivary cortisol
  B. Serum TSH and free T$_4$
  C. Glutamic acid decarboxylase, IA-2, and ZnT8 antibodies
  D. IGF-1
  E. Serum aldosterone and plasma renin activity

57 A 35-year-old man is admitted to the hospital under the care of the trauma team following a fall from a ladder. He has pain in the left flank and pink discoloration of urine. He has a history of epilepsy since childhood that is treated with carbamazepine. He takes no other regular medications.

On physical examination, his blood pressure is 165/105 mm Hg (confirmed on repeated measurements) and pulse rate is 80 beats/min and regular. Findings on cardiovascular and respiratory examination are otherwise normal. There is mild bruising of the left loin with tenderness to palpation. Fundoscopy documents grade 2 hypertensive changes.

Laboratory test results:
  Hemoglobin = 17.6 g/dL (13.8-17.2 g/dL) (SI: 176 g/L [138-172 g/L])
  Hematocrit = 54% (41%-51%) (SI: 0.54 [0.41-0.51])
  Platelet count = 232 × 10^3/μL (150-450 × 10^3/μL) (SI: 232 × 10^9/L [150-450 × 10^9/L])
  Serum sodium = 142 mEq/L (136-142 mEq/L) (SI: 142 mmol/L [136-142 mmol/L])
  Serum potassium = 3.8 mEq/L (3.5-5.0 mEq/L) (SI: 3.8 mmol/L [3.5-5.0 mmol/L])
  Serum creatinine = 1.0 mg/dL (0.7-1.3 mg/dL) (SI: 88.4 μmol/L [61.9-114.9 μmol/L])

Serum urea nitrogen = 26.5 mg/dL (8-23 mg/dL) (SI: 9.5 mmol/L
 [2.9-8.2 mmol/L])

Urinalysis = blood 1+, protein 2+

Abdominal CT is performed, and a left retroperitoneal mass is documented (*see image, arrow*).

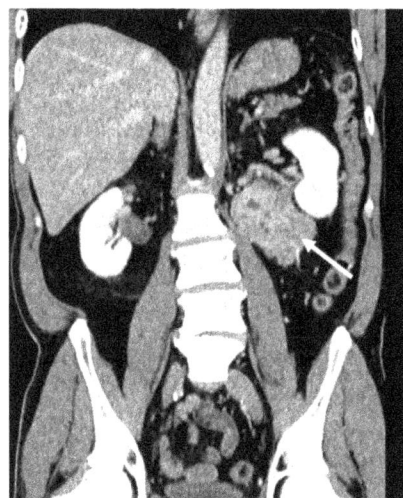

Which of the following is the most likely explanation for this patient's hypertension?

A. 11-Deoxycorticosterone–secreting adrenocortical carcinoma

B. Primary aldosteronism

C. Paraganglioma

D. Pheochromocytoma

E. Polycystic kidney disease

58 A 58-year-old man underwent total thyroidectomy at age 56 years, which revealed a 2.5-cm right papillary thyroid cancer, with extrathyroidal extension and vascular invasion. Seven of 8 lymph nodes had papillary thyroid cancer metastases with extranodal extension. He received 150 mCi of radioactive iodine and was prescribed levothyroxine, 150 mcg daily. At a follow-up visit 3 months later, he felt well. His TSH level was 1.0 mIU/L and thyroglobulin level was 3 ng/mL (3 μg/L) with no thyroglobulin antibodies. His levothyroxine dosage was increased to 175 mcg daily. Six months after thyroidectomy, his TSH level was 0.1 mIU/L and thyroglobulin level was 2.6 ng/mL (2.6 μg/L). A recombinant human TSH (rhTSH) radioactive iodine scan was negative. The stimulated thyroglobulin concentration was 10.0 ng/mL (10.0 μg/L). One year after thyroidectomy, his TSH level was 0.09 mIU/L and thyroglobulin level was 3.6 ng/mL (3.6 μg/L). Neck ultrasonography was unremarkable, and chest CT showed 2 small nodules in the right lung. Two years after thyroidectomy, his TSH level was 0.08 mIU/L and thyroglobulin level was 12.0 ng/mL (12.0 μg/L).

Which of the following is the best next step in this patient's management?

A. Administer hypothyroid radioiodine therapy with 150 mCi

B. Perform chest CT

C. Perform rhTSH ^{18}F-fluorodeoxyglucose PET/CT

D. Initiate tyrosine kinase inhibitor therapy

E. Increase the levothyroxine dosage to suppress TSH <0.01 mIU/L

59 A 70-year-old woman is referred for management of abnormal lipid levels. She has a 30-year history of elevated lipids. During the course of her medical care, statin therapy was recommended. She took atorvastatin, 20 mg daily, for several years with good response, but she developed bilateral muscle aches in her lower extremities about 5 years ago and discontinued the medication. Over the past year, simvastatin (40 mg daily) was attempted, but this resulted in similar adverse effects, with relief after stopping. She has no history of clinical atherosclerotic cardiovascular disease, and she has hypertension treated with hydrochlorothiazide. She has never smoked cigarettes and does not drink alcoholic beverages. Her family history is remarkable for several members with hyperlipidemia, including her mother (alive at age 91 years), sister (age 71 years), and brother (age 72 years and on lipid-lowering therapy). Her father had a stroke at age 73 years and is deceased. She has no children.

On physical examination, she appears anxious. Her blood pressure is 150/70 mm Hg, and pulse rate is 82 beats/min. Her height is 66 in (167.6 cm), and weight is 157 lb (71.4 kg) (BMI = 25.3 kg/m²). The rest of the examination findings are normal except for abdominal adiposity.

Laboratory test results (sample drawn while fasting, on no treatment):

Total cholesterol = 290 mg/dL (<200 mg/dL [optimal]) (SI: 7.51 mmol/L [<5.18 mmol/L])

Triglycerides = 263 mg/dL (<150 mg/dL [optimal]) (SI: 2.97 mmol/L [<1.70 mmol/L])

HDL cholesterol = 48 mg/dL (>60 mg/dL [optimal]) (SI: 1.24 mmol/L [>1.55 mmol/L])

LDL cholesterol = 189 mg/dL (<100 mg/dL [optimal]) (SI: 4.90 mmol/L [<2.59 mmol/L])

Non-HDL cholesterol = 242 mg/dL (<130 mg/dL [optimal]) (SI: 6.27 mmol/L [<3.37 mmol/L])

Apolipoprotein B = 145 mg/dL (50-110 mg/dL) (SI: 1.45 g/dL [0.5-1.1 g/dL])

Lipoprotein (a) = 3 mg/dL (≤30 mg/dL) (SI: 0.11 μmol/L [≤1.07 μmol/L])

Hemoglobin A$_{1c}$ = 4.4% (4.0%-5.6%) (25 mmol/mol [20-38 mmol/mol])

Creatinine = 0.69 mg/dL (0.6-1.1 mg/dL) (61.00 μmol/L [53.0-97.2 μmol/L])

TSH = 3.8 mIU/L (0.5-5.0 mIU/L)

Fasting plasma glucose = 103 mg/dL (70-99 mg/dL) (SI: 5.72 mmol/L [3.9-5.5 mmol/L])

Creatine kinase = 45 U/L (50-200 U/L) (SI: 0.75 μkat/L [0.84-3.34 μkat/L])

25-Hydroxyvitamin D = 24 ng/mL (30-80 ng/mL [optimal]) (SI: 59.9 nmol/L [74.9-199.7 nmol/L])

Her 10-year risk of atherosclerotic cardiovascular disease is 19%.

In addition to optimizing blood pressure management, which of the following medications should be started as the best next step in managing this patient's cardiovascular risk?

A. Rosuvastatin, 5 mg daily, and coenzyme Q10 supplementation

B. Rosuvastatin, 5 mg daily, and cholecalciferol, 2000 IU daily

C. Rosuvastatin, 5 mg daily

D. Marine omega-3 fatty acids, 4 g daily

E. Fenofibrate, 160 mg daily

60 A 67-year-old woman is seen in the endocrinology clinic for evaluation and treatment of type 1 diabetes mellitus. Diabetes was diagnosed at age 28 years after she presented with diabetic ketoacidosis. She has been treated with a basal-bolus insulin regimen for most of the past 15 years. Five years ago, she was treated with an insulin pump for 4 months. She developed diabetic ketoacidosis after a site change. Following appropriate treatment, she returned to a multidose subcutaneous insulin regimen. She has not been interested in restarting insulin pump therapy.

She has a history of hypoglycemia unawareness. Her glucose values drop to the range of 40 to 55 mg/dL (2.2-3.1 mmol/L) with few, if any, warning symptoms of hypoglycemia. In the last 7 months, she has had 3 episodes of severe hypoglycemia that required treatment by paramedics. Her husband has had to administer glucagon on numerous occasions—most recently 12 days ago.

She is currently administering 16 units of insulin degludec at 10 PM. She uses carbohydrate counting and administers 1 unit of insulin aspart per 15 g carbohydrates before meals. Her carbohydrate counting skills are excellent. She administers the insulin bolus about 10 minutes before meals. The glucose target is 100 to 140 mg/dL (5.6-7.8 mmol/L) and the correctional dose is 1 unit per 60 mg/dL (3.3 mmol/L) above the glucose target.

She takes simvastatin for hypercholesterolemia and levothyroxine, 88 mcg daily, for primary hypothyroidism. She does not smoke cigarettes. She has 3 glasses of wine per week. She has mild nonproliferative diabetic retinopathy as the only microvascular complication of diabetes.

On physical examination, her height is 68 in (173 cm) and weight is 144 lb (65.5 kg) (BMI = 21.9 kg/m^2). Her blood pressure is 118/72 mm Hg, and pulse rate is 64 beats/min. The thyroid gland is normal sized and no nodules are detected. Findings on examination of the heart, lungs, and abdomen are unremarkable. Findings on neurologic examination are normal.

Laboratory test results:

Hemoglobin A$_{1c}$ = 7.3% (4.0%-5.6%) (56 mmol/mol [20-38 mmol/mol])

Glucose = 122 mg/dL (70-99 mg/dL) (SI: 6.8 mmol/L [3.9-5.5 mmol/L])

Creatinine = 0.8 mg/dL (0.6-1.1 mg/dL) (SI: 70.7 μmol/L [53.0-97.2 μmol/L])

Estimated glomerular filtration rate = >60 mL/min per 1.73 m^2 (>60 mL/min per 1.73 m^2)

TSH = 2.1 mIU/L (0.5-5.0 mIU/L)

Cortisol (8 AM) = 12.8 μg/dL (5-25 μg/dL) (SI: 353.1 nmol/L [137.9-689.7 nmol/L])

ACTH = 42 pg/mL (10-60 pg/mL) (SI: 9.2 pmol/L [2.2-13.2 pmol/L])

Which of the following is the best treatment option for this patient who has hypoglycemia unawareness?
- A. Switch from insulin degludec to U300 insulin glargine
- B. Initiate intermittently viewed glucose monitoring
- C. Initiate real-time continuous glucose monitoring
- D. Change the glucose target to 140-190 mg/dL (7.8-10.5 mmol/L)
- E. Switch from the current insulin regimen to insulin pump therapy

61 An 18-year-old woman with a history of craniopharyngioma status post subtotal resection via craniotomy followed by radiation (total 5220 cGy) 5 years ago presents for transition to adult care from the pediatric endocrinology clinic.

The patient has a history of secondary hypogonadism, secondary hypothyroidism, and GH deficiency. Results from a recent cosyntropin-stimulation test were normal (peak post-cosyntropin serum cortisol = 24.7 μg/dL [681.4 nmol/L]). Her current medications include oral estrogen daily, progesterone 10 days a month, GH, and levothyroxine. Her current dosages of GH and levothyroxine are 1.2 mg daily and 125 mcg daily, respectively.

Laboratory test results;
   Free T_4 = 1.4 ng/dL (0.8-1.8 ng/dL) (SI: 18.0 pmol/L [10.30-23.17 pmol/L])
   IGF-1 = 483 ng/mL (162-541 ng/mL) (SI: 63.3 nmol/L [21.2-70.9 nmol/L])
   Prolactin = 34 ng/mL (4-30 ng/mL) (SI: 1.5 nmol/L [0.17-1.30 nmol/L])

On physical examination, her blood pressure is 124/69 mm Hg and pulse rate is 92 beats/min. Her height is 67.5 in (171.5 cm), and weight is 240 lb (109 kg) (BMI = 37 kg/m²). She has acanthosis nigricans in her axillary folds and silvery striae on her abdomen.

MRI shows no evidence of craniopharyngioma recurrence.

She is about to go to college, and she would prefer to use the transdermal estrogen patch. After discussing appropriate use of the patch, which of the following is the best next step?
- A. Change progesterone to daily dosing
- B. Increase the levothyroxine dosage by 20%
- C. Reduce the GH dosage by 50%
- D. Repeat the cosyntropin-stimulation test after 2 months
- E. Start cabergoline

62 A 50-year-old man is referred for evaluation and recommendations regarding nephrolithiasis. He was well until 6 months ago when he developed acute right-sided flank pain. Evaluation at a local emergency department revealed microscopic hematuria. His pain resolved with intravenous saline and analgesics over 4 hours, and a single renal stone was obtained on passage and was confirmed to be composed of calcium oxalate. Abdominal CT did not show evidence for residual nephrolithiasis. His medical history is unremarkable. He currently takes a multivitamin for seniors but no prescription medications. Family history is negative for nephrolithiasis or osteoporosis. He does not smoke cigarettes. He consumes 4 to 6 beers a week and does not drink soda. Review of systems is negative at this time for flank/abdominal pain, dysuria, or hematuria.

On physical examination, he appears well. He has no corneal calcifications. There is no elicitable costovertebral angle or abdominal tenderness. The rest of his examination findings are normal.

Laboratory test results:
   Serum calcium = 10.4 mg/dL (8.2-10.2 mg/dL (SI: 2.6 mmol/L [2.1-2.6 mmol/L])
   Serum phosphate = 3.8 mg/dL (2.3-4.7 mg/dL) (SI: 1.2 mmol/L [0.7-1.5 mmol/L])
   Serum magnesium = 2.1 mg/dL (1.5-2.3 mg/dL) (SI: 0.9 mmol/L [0.6-0.9 mmol/L])
   Serum albumin = 4.8 mg/dL (3.5-5.0 g/dL) (SI: 48 g/L [35-50 g/L])
   Serum creatinine = 1.0 mg/dL (0.7-1.3 mg/dL) (SI: 88.4 μmol/L [61.9-114.9 μmol/L])

Serum intact PTH = 55 pg/mL (10-65 pg/mL) (SI: 55 ng/L [10-65 ng/L])
Serum 25-hydroxyvitamin D = 48 ng/mL (30-80 ng/mL [optimal]) (SI: 119.8 nmol/L [74.9-199.7 nmol/L])
Urinary calcium = 200 mg/24 h (100-300 mg/24 h) (SI: 0.03 mmol/d [2.5-7.5 mmol/d])
Urinary creatinine = 1.2 g/24 h (1.0-2.0 g/24 h) (SI: 10.6 mmol/d [8.8-17.7 mmol/d])
Urinary sodium = 50 mEq/24 h (40-217 mEq/24 h) (SI: 50 mmol/d [40-217 mmol/d])
Urinary volume = 1.6 L/24 h

Which of the following is the most appropriate recommendation to manage this patient's nephrolithiasis?

A. Drink enough fluids to ensure at least 2 L of urine output daily
B. Start hydrochlorothiazide, 12.5 mg daily
C. Start a high-fiber diet (>25 g of fiber daily)
D. Refer to an endocrine surgeon for consideration of parathyroidectomy
E. Restrict dietary calcium intake to <200 mg daily

63 A 55-year-old woman with obstructive sleep apnea, severe gastroesophageal reflux disease, and depression returns for follow-up. For the past 4 months, she has been attending appointments in your clinic for help with weight loss. The first 4 weeks, she worked on changing her eating plan and starting an exercise program. Twelve weeks ago, when her weight was 193 lb (87.7 kg) and her BMI was 32 kg/m², you prescribed phentermine/topiramate. The main reason for prescribing this medication was to address her struggle with hunger. The first 2 weeks, she took phentermine/topiramate (3.75 mg/23 mg daily) and then she started the regular dosage of 7.5 mg/46 mg daily. She has been following up in your clinic every 4 weeks. During these visits, you have assessed for adverse effects of the weight-loss medication. She has reported dry mouth but no insomnia, tachycardia, or increased anxiety. Her other medications include famotidine, 20 mg daily, and bupropion extended release, 200 mg daily.

On physical examination today, her blood pressure is 132/78 mm Hg and pulse rate is 80 beats/min. Her weight is 189 lb (86 kg). The patient is in no distress, her lungs are clear to auscultation bilaterally, her heart sounds are regular in rate and rhythm (no murmurs detected), and she has no peripheral edema.

During the visit, you point out that since starting the weight-loss medication, she has lost 2% of her body weight.

Which of the following options would you recommend next?

A. Continue phentermine/topiramate at the current dosage
B. Continue phentermine/topiramate at the current dosage and add lorcaserin
C. Increase the current dosage of phentermine/topiramate to its maximum dosage
D. Stop phentermine/topiramate and start naltrexone/bupropion
E. Continue phentermine/topiramate at the current dosage and add liraglutide

64 A 22-year-old woman is brought to the emergency department because of vomiting. She was in the park with her friends when she began feeling tired and nauseated. Her friends brought her to the emergency department after she began having nonbilious, nonbloody emesis and appeared increasingly lethargic.

In the emergency department, her blood pressure is 190/100 mm Hg and pulse rate is 108 beats/min. Her height is 65 in (165 cm), and weight is 115 lb (52.3 kg) (BMI = 19.1 kg/m²). She appears diaphoretic, pale, and uncomfortable.

Her blood glucose concentration is 421 mg/dL (23.4 mmol/L).

She is admitted to the hospital where she receives hydration with saline, antiemetics, short-acting antihypertensive agents, and insulin. Her nausea and emesis resolve and her blood pressure and blood glucose normalize with these interventions.

The patient and her friends deny any illicit drug use, and she does not take any prescription medications or over-the-counter supplements.

Laboratory test results:

Plasma metanephrine = 1460 pg/mL (<99 pg/mL) (SI: 7.4 nmol/L [<0.50 nmol/L])

Plasma normetanephrine = 1227 pg/mL (<165 pg/mL) (SI: 6.7 nmol/L [<0.90 nmol/L])

24-Hour urine collection:

Volume = 1300 mL/24 h

Creatinine = 0.9 g/24 h (1.0-2.0 g/24 h) (SI: 8.0 nmol/d [11-138 nmol/d]]

Metanephrine = 9457 µg/24 h (<261 µg/24 h) (SI: 47,947 nmol/d [<1323 nmol/d])

Normetanephrine = 3749 µg/24 h (103-390 µg/24 h) (SI: 20,470 nmol/d [609-2306 nmol/d])

Epinephrine = 257 µg/24 h (<21 µg/24 h) (SI: 1402 nmol/d [<115 nmol/d])

Norepinephrine = 272 µg/24 h (<80 µg/24 h) (SI: 1609 nmol/d [<473 nmol/d])

Dopamine = 2086 µg/24 h (<400 µg/24 h) (SI: 13,609 nmol/d [<2610 nmol/d])

Which of the following is the most appropriate next step?

A. Toxicology screen for cocaine and tricyclic antidepressants

B. Fluorodeoxyglucose (FDG) PET scan

C. Meta-iodobenzylguanidine scan

D. Abdominal CT

E. ^{68}Ga DOTATATE PET scan

65 A 34-year-old man with a 10-year history of type 1 diabetes mellitus has been followed in your clinic for the past 2 years. He has fair glycemic control. He has no history of diabetic neuropathy. He reports that he had an eye examination at an external facility and was told he does not have retinopathy. He has taken lisinopril, 40 mg daily, for the 2 years you have been following him. The ACE inhibitor was prescribed for blood pressure control and renal protection since he had an elevated urine albumin-to-creatinine ratio. He has no history of cardiovascular disease. In addition to lisinopril, his current medications are insulin aspart via insulin pump and atorvastatin, 40 mg daily.

On physical examination, his blood pressure is 148/80 mm Hg and pulse rate is 82 beats/min. His height is 71 in (180 cm), and weight is 198 lb (90 kg) (BMI = 27.6 kg/m^2). The rest of the examination findings are normal.

Laboratory test results:

Hemoglobin A$_{1c}$ = 7.9% (4.0%-5.6%) (63 mmol/mol [20-38 mmol/mol])

Creatinine = 1.6 mg/dL (0.7-1.3 mg/dL) (SI: 114.9 µmol/L [61.9-114.9 µmol/L])

Urine albumin-to-creatinine ratio = >300 mg/g creat (<30 mg/g creat) (this ratio was 269 mg/g creat 1 year ago)

Urine protein = 2.4 g/24 h

Urine analysis:

Urine specific gravity = 1.015 (1.002-1.030)

pH = 6.0

Protein = 3+

Epithelial cells = 2

White blood cell count = 2 cells per high-power field

Red blood cell count = 8 cells per high-power field

Nitrates, negative

Leukocyte esterase, negative

Which of the following is the best next step in the management of this patient's proteinuria?

A. Intensify glucose control

B. Add an angiotensin-receptor blocker

C. Prescribe a low-protein diet

D. Perform renal biopsy

E. Doppler ultrasonography of renal arteries

66 A 23-year-old woman is diagnosed with thyroid cancer and elects to undergo minimally invasive thyroidectomy. After surgery, her surgeon prescribes levothyroxine therapy and orders a neck CT. She is then referred to an endocrinologist. When she presents for her first endocrinology visit, she informs you that she has just learned that she is pregnant based on a home pregnancy test. She has no other medical problems. She takes levothyroxine, 100 mcg daily.

On physical examination, she has a small healing thyroidectomy scar, a palpable midline mass, and palpable left-sided adenopathy. Her blood pressure is 124/75 mm Hg, and pulse rate is 75 beats/min. She appears clinically euthyroid.

Laboratory test results:

TSH = 0.3 mIU/L (0.5-5.0 mIU/L)

Free T$_4$ = 1.8 ng/dL (0.8-1.8 ng/dL) (SI: 23.2 pmol/L [10.30-23.17 pmol/L])

Total thyroglobulin = 31 ng/dL (<1.0 ng/mL)

β-hCG = 15,000 mIU/mL (>25 mIU/mL indicates positive pregnancy test) (SI: 15,000 IU/L [>25 IU/L])

You order neck ultrasonography. The images from both neck CT and ultrasonography are shown (*see images*).

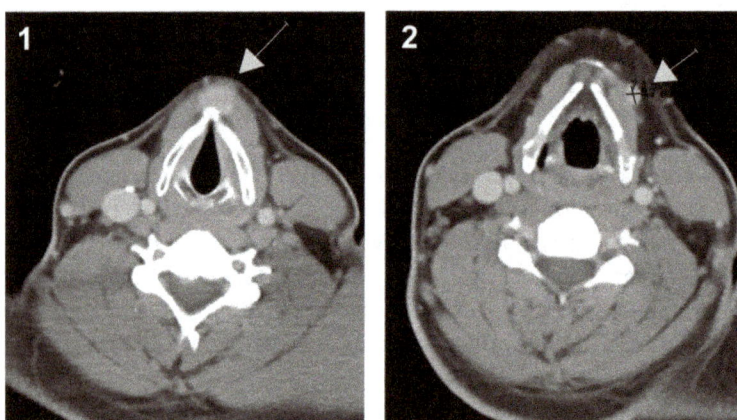

Image 1, Neck CT showing an irregularly shaped, heterogeneously enhancing mass lesion anterior to the mid-thyroid cartilage embedded within the strap muscles at the midline, which measures 13 × 15 mm (arrow). Image 2, Enhancing nodular foci associated with the left-sided strap muscles, the larger of which is seen in this image and measures 7 × 6 mm (arrow).

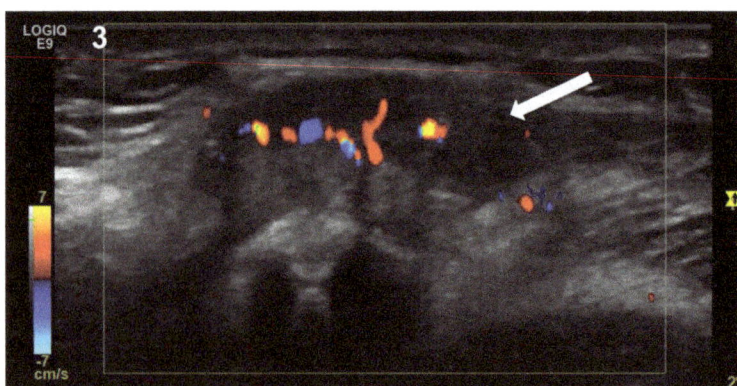

Image 3, Neck ultrasonography showing a sagittal view of heterogeneous, predominantly hypoechoic soft tissue within the anterior superior level 6 (central neck), just below the level of the mandible, measuring approximately 1.9 × 1.7 × 0.9 cm (arrow). There is internal vascularity. Additional suspicious left-sided lymph nodes were observed but are not shown on this image.

Which of the following would you recommend as the best next step in this patient's treatment?
  A. Referral for external beam radiation with uterine shielding
  B. Central and left neck dissection now
  C. Central and left neck dissection in the second trimester
  D. Central and left neck dissection in the third trimester
  E. Central and left neck dissection after delivery

67 A 29-year-old woman who is trying to conceive is referred for evaluation of secondary amenorrhea. Menarche was at age 12 years, and she initially had regular menses, occurring every 30 to 35 days. Since age 14 years, she has been on oral contraceptives because of painful periods. Within a few months of discontinuing birth control last year, she developed acne and irregular menses occurring every other month.

During an evaluation for irregular menses, nonclassic congenital adrenal hyperplasia and androgen excess were diagnosed. The following laboratory test results were documented:

TSH = 0.5 mIU/L (0.5-5.0 mIU/L)
Total testosterone = 30 ng/dL (8-60 ng/dL) (SI: 1.0 nmol/L [0.3-2.1 nmol/L])
Prolactin = 11 ng/mL (4-30 ng/mL) (SI: 0.48 nmol/L [0.17-1.30 nmol/L])
LH = 2.8 mIU/mL (0.5-18.0 mIU/mL [luteal]) (SI: 2.8 IU/L [05.18.0 IU/L])
DHEA-S = 418 µg/dL (44-332 µg/dL) (SI: 11.33 µmol/L [1.19-9.00 µmol/L])
Day 21 progesterone = 4.5 ng/mL (2.0-20.0 ng/mL [luteal]) (SI: 14.3 nmol/L [6.4-63.6 nmol/L])

Results of additional laboratory evaluation on day 3 of her menstrual cycle:
FSH = 4.5 mIU/mL (2.0-12.0 mIU/mL [follicular]) (SI: 4.5 IU/L [2.0-12.0 IU/L])
17-Hydroxyprogesterone = 2000 ng/dL (<80 ng/dL) (SI: 60.6 nmol/L [<2.42 nmol/L])
Estradiol = 29 pg/mL (10-180 pg/mL [follicular]) (SI: 106.5 pmol/L [36.7-660.8 pmol/L])
Day 3 progesterone = 4.1 ng/mL (≤1.0 ng/mL [follicular]) (SI: 13.0 nmol/L [≤3.2 nmol/L])

On physical examination, her height is 64 in (162.6 cm) and weight is 158 lb (71.8 kg) (BMI = 27.1 kg/m^2). Her blood pressure is 124/78 mm Hg. She has mild to moderate cystic acne along the jaw line. No violaceous striae or ecchymoses are observed. Terminal hair growth is present only on the upper lip and upper arms.

Which of the following should be initiated as the best next step in this patient's management?
  A. Spironolactone
  B. Metformin
  C. Dexamethasone
  D. Hydrocortisone
  E. Clomiphene

68 A 35-year-old Hispanic woman seeks evaluation and treatment of glucose intolerance. She had gestational diabetes mellitus with pregnancies at ages 27 and 32 years. She required insulin treatment during the first pregnancy. She was treated with insulin and metformin initially during the second pregnancy, but had gastrointestinal intolerance and had to stop metformin after 2 weeks of treatment. Eight weeks after her second pregnancy, she underwent a 75-g 2-hour oral glucose tolerance test. The fasting glucose value was 109 mg/dL (6.0 mmol/L), and the 2-hour postload glucose value was 176 mg/dL (9.8 mmol/L). She was instructed to follow a consistent carbohydrate diet. She requests a medication to prevent onset of diabetes.

She has not seen a dietician since the last pregnancy and does not follow the recommended diet. She does not engage in any regular exercise. She has hypothyroidism treated with levothyroxine, 75 mcg daily; anxiety treated with venlafaxine; and hypertension treated with lisinopril. She also has irritable bowel syndrome. An intrauterine device is in place for contraception. She does not smoke cigarettes and occasionally drinks alcohol.

Her mother, older brother, and maternal grandfather have diabetes. Her younger sister had gestational diabetes with a recent pregnancy.

On physical examination, her height is 64 in (163 cm) and weight is 231 lb (105 kg) (BMI = 39.6 kg/m^2). Her blood pressure is 136/78 mm Hg, and pulse rate is 86 beats/min. Examination findings are normal other than her thyroid gland, which is an estimated 25 g in size with no palpable nodules.

Laboratory test results:
 Hemoglobin A$_{1c}$ = 6.3% (4.0%-5.6%) (45 mmol/mol [20-38 mmol/mol])
 Fasting glucose = 115 mg/dL (70-99 mg/dL) (SI: 6.4 mmol/L [3.9-5.5 mmol/L])
 Creatinine = 1.1 mg/dL (0.6-1.1 mg/dL) (SI: 97.2 μmol/L [53.0-97.2 μmol/L])
 Estimated glomerular filtration rate = >90 mL/min per 1.73 m^2 (>60 mL/min per 1.73 m^2)
 TSH = 1.13 mIU/L (0.5-5.0 mIU/L)
 Urinary albumin = 12 μg/mg creat (30-300 μg/mg creat)

In addition to referring the patient to the nutritionist to review a diet plan and counseling her about intensive lifestyle modification, which of the following should be prescribed to prevent diabetes?
 A. Sitagliptin
 B. Acarbose
 C. Dulaglutide
 D. Pioglitazone
 E. Canagliflozin

69 A 58-year-old woman is referred to you for fatigue. She has a history of breast cancer, osteoporosis, and severe gastroesophageal reflux disease. Omeprazole, 20 mg daily, has been initiated. Esophagogastroduodenoscopy shows a 3-cm mass in the lower portion of her esophagus, and biopsy findings are consistent with esophageal cancer. She subsequently has a chest and abdominal CT, which identifies multiple liver metastases. She receives conventional chemotherapy with no regression of metastases. Intravenous pembrolizumab is initiated. You see her 2 weeks after her third cycle of pembrolizumab. Abdominal CT confirms reduction in the size of her esophageal tumor and liver metastases. She has been fatigued, but has no symptoms of gastroesophageal reflux disease, dysphagia, or chest pain.

On physical examination, her blood pressure is 110/60 mm Hg and pulse rate is 52 beats/min. Her height is 64 in (162.6 cm) and weight is 136 lb (61.8 kg) (BMI = 23.3 kg/m^2). She is in no acute distress. Her abdomen is soft and nontender. The rest of the examination findings are normal.

Laboratory test results:
 Basic metabolic panel, normal
 Complete blood cell count, normal
 25-Hydroxyvitamin D = 32 ng/mL (30-80 ng/mL [optimal]) (SI: 79.9 nmol/L [74.9-199.7 nmol/L])

Which of the following is the best next step in this patient's management?
 A. Measure ferritin
 B. Measure TSH and free T$_4$
 C. Measure TPO antibodies
 D. Start vitamin B$_{12}$ intramuscularly monthly
 E. Start prednisone

70 A 28-year-old man presents for evaluation of hypermagnesemia, which was first noted about a year ago. This persisted despite stopping an over-the-counter supplement containing magnesium. He feels well and does not currently take any medications or supplements. He has no history of fractures, kidney stones, or parathyroid disease. He has an older sister who underwent neck surgery last year.

His physical examination findings, including vital signs, are unremarkable.

Laboratory test results:

    Serum magnesium = 2.5 mg/dL (1.5-2.3 mg/dL) (SI: 1.0 mmol/L [0.6-0.9 mmol/L])

    Serum calcium = 10.2 mg/dL (8.2-10.2 mg/dL) (SI: 2.6 mmol/L [2.1-2.6 mmol/L])

    Serum phosphate = 3.1 mg/dL (2.3-4.7 mg/dL) (SI: 1.0 mmol/L [0.7-1.5 mmol/L])

    Serum creatinine = 1.0 mg/dL (0.6-1.1 mg/dL) (SI: 88.4 μmol/L [53.0-97.2 μmol/L])

    Serum intact PTH = 60 pg/mL (10-65 pg/mL) (SI: 60 ng/L [10-65 ng/L])

    Serum 25-hydroxyvitamin D = 30 ng/mL (30-80 ng/mL [optimal]) (SI: 74.9 nmol/L [74.9-199.7 nmol/L])

    Serum albumin = 3.7 g/dL (3.5-5.0 g/dL) (SI: 37 g/L [35-50 g/L])

Measuring which of the following is the best next step in the evaluation of this patient's hypermagnesemia?

    A. Morning serum cortisol

    B. Serum PTHrP

    C. Serum 1,25-dihydroxyvitamin D

    D. 24-Hour urinary magnesium

    E. 24-Hour urinary calcium

71 A 73-year-old woman seeks evaluation for a 6-week history of progressive tiredness, lethargy, and dizziness. For the last 24 hours, she has been nauseated and has vomited several times. She had breast carcinoma 20 years ago (treated with surgery and radiotherapy) and skeletal metastases 4 years ago (treated with chemotherapy and hormonal therapy). Her only current medication is an aromatase inhibitor. There is no other relevant medical history.

On physical examination, her height is 66 in (167.6 cm) and weight is 149 lb (67.7 kg) (BMI = 24 kg/m²). Her blood pressure is 90/60 mm Hg lying down and 70/40 mm Hg sitting, and pulse rate is 110 beats/min and regular. She appears pale and has dry mucous membranes and low venous pressure. There are no new findings on breast examination. The rest of the examination findings are normal.

Laboratory test results:

    Serum sodium = 140 mEq/L (136-142 mEq/L) (SI: 140 mmol/L [136-142 mmol/L])

    Serum potassium = 3.6 mEq/L (3.5-5.0 mEq/L) (SI: 3.6 mmol/L [3.5-5.0 mmol/L])

    Serum creatinine = 1.4 mg/dL (0.7-1.3 mg/dL) (SI: 123.8 μmol/L [61.9-114.9 μmol/L])

    Serum urea nitrogen = 28 mg/dL (8-23 mg/dL) (SI: 10.0 mmol/L [2.9-8.2 mmol/L])

    Blood glucose = 55 mg/dL (70-99 mg/dL) (SI: 3.1 mmol/L [3.9-5.5 mmol/L])

    Random serum cortisol = 1.0 μg/dL (SI: 27.6 nmol/L)

Initial management includes fluid resuscitation (intravenous 20% glucose and 0.9% sodium chloride) and intravenous hydrocortisone, 100 mg stat, followed by infusion of 8 mg/h. A urinary catheter is placed, and a brisk urine output is rapidly established.

Five hours later, her blood pressure cannot be detected, and a team is called for cardiac arrest. The capillary blood glucose concentration is 85 mg/dL (4.7 mmol/L).

Which of the following is the most likely explanation for the patient's collapse?

    A. Failure to commence fludrocortisone replacement

    B. Hypovolemia due to excessive urine output

    C. Inadequate hydrocortisone replacement

    D. Overly aggressive fluid resuscitation with cardiac decompensation

    E. Pulmonary embolism

72 A 66-year-old woman with a 20-year history of type 2 diabetes mellitus presents for follow-up. She has diabetic neuropathy but no other microvascular or macrovascular complications. At today's visit, her hemoglobin A_{1c} level is 7.3% (56 mmol/mol). Her medical history is notable for hypertension, dyslipidemia, elevated BMI, and seasonal allergies resulting in frequent cough. Her current medications are glimepiride, sitagliptin, metformin, exenatide, pravastatin, and pregabalin. She used to take ramipril; she does not remember why it was discontinued.

On physical examination, she is afebrile. Her blood pressure is 164/102 mm Hg, and pulse rate is 74 beats/min. Her height is 63.5 in (161.3 cm), and weight is 180 lb (81.7 kg) (BMI = 31.4 kg/m²). Examination findings are normal except for acanthosis nigricans on her neck and in the axillae bilaterally. She also has decreased protective sensation in her feet.

Laboratory test results:
   Sodium = 138 mEq/L (136-142 mEq/L) (SI: 138 mmol/L [136-142 mmol/L])
   Potassium = 4.0 mEq/L (3.5-5.0 mEq/L) (SI: 4.0 mmol/L [3.5-5.0 mmol/L])
   Serum urea nitrogen = 18 mg/dL (8-23 mg/dL) (SI: 6.4 mmol/L [2.9-8.2 mmol/L])
   Creatinine = 1.1 mg/dL (0.6-1.1 mg/dL) (SI: 97.2 μmol/L [53.0-97.2 μmol/L])
   Urine albumin-to-creatinine ratio = 24 mg/g creat (<30 mg/g creat)

Which of the following is the best next step in managing this patient's hypertension?
   A.   ACE inhibitor and angiotensin-receptor blocker
   B.   Angiotensin-receptor blocker and β-adrenergic blocker
   C.   Angiotensin-receptor blocker and calcium-channel blocker
   D.   Calcium-channel blocker and β-adrenergic blocker
   E.   ACE inhibitor and direct renin inhibitor

73 A 57-year-old man consults you for an increased hematocrit level documented while on testosterone replacement. He has been treated with testosterone using standard-dose topical testosterone gel for the past 12 months, following resection of a pituitary macroadenoma.

Laboratory test results before commencing testosterone (sample drawn at 8 AM while fasting):
   Serum testosterone = 50 ng/dL (300-900 ng/dL) (SI: 1.7 nmol/L [10.4-31.2 nmol/L]) and (repeated measurement 2 weeks
      later: 60 ng/dL [SI: 2.1 nmol/L])
   Serum LH = 0.2 mIU/mL (1.0-9.0 mIU/mL) (SI: 0.2 IU/L [1.0-9.0 IU/L])

He reports marked and sustained improvement of energy and libido since commencing testosterone replacement. While on treatment, he has experienced an increase in hematocrit from a baseline of 50% to 56% (0.50-0.56). Serum testosterone concentrations on treatment have ranged from 403 to 450 ng/dL (14.0-15.6 nmol/L). Other pituitary axes are treated appropriately. He is clinically well and has no headaches, dizziness, vision disturbances, or pruritus. He does not smoke tobacco.

On physical examination, his blood pressure is 120/74 mm Hg and pulse rate is 68 beats/min. His height is 70 in (177.8 cm) and weight is 202 lb (91.8 kg) (BMI = 29 kg/m²). There is no postural drop in blood pressure.

His primary care physician had previously ordered *JAK2* genetic testing, polysomnography, and high-resolution chest CT, all of which are unremarkable.

After withholding testosterone replacement for 3 months, his hematocrit decreases to 52% (0.52) and serum testosterone decreases to 30 ng/dL (1.0 nmol/L) with recurrence of hypogonadal symptoms. Two months after restarting testosterone gel at 50% of the standard replacement dose, serum testosterone rises to 190 ng/dL (6.6 nmol/L) and then to 230 ng/dL (8.0 nmol/L) 2 weeks later. Hematocrit is still 52% (0.52). He reports ongoing fatigue and low libido.

Which of the following is the best next step in this patient's management?
- A. Change his regimen to standard-dose intramuscular testosterone enanthate
- B. Change his regimen to hCG
- C. Increase topical testosterone and perform regular phlebotomy as needed
- D. Prescribe an aromatase inhibitor
- E. Stop testosterone treatment

74 A 55-year-old man comes to clinic for routine follow-up of osteogenesis imperfecta type 1, which was diagnosed when he presented with multiple lower-extremity fractures starting at age 3 years. He was treated with quarterly pamidronate therapy in childhood with a subsequent reduction in fracture frequency. His most recent therapy consisted of alendronate, 70 mg weekly, for 5 years, although he has been off alendronate for 2 years and has remained fracture free in the interim. His medical history is notable for hearing loss and multiple tooth loss with 4 dental implants. He currently takes a multivitamin; calcium citrate, 500 mg twice daily; and vitamin D_3, 400 IU twice daily. He takes no prescription medications. Family history is notable for osteogenesis imperfecta in his father and sister.

On physical examination, he appears well. His blood pressure is 120/50 mm Hg, and pulse rate is 82 beats/min. His height 69 in (175.3 cm) and is unchanged compared with measurements at previous visits. Examination reveals blue sclerae and multiple missing teeth. He has an audible diastolic murmur at the left sternal border. His chest is clear. Distal pulses are 2+ without bruits. There is no peripheral edema. The rest of the examination findings are normal, including normal spinal curvature without kyphosis.

Routine chemistries and 25-hydroxyvitamin D are normal. DXA scan documents the following results: lumbar spine T-score, –2.0; right femoral neck T-score, –2.2; and right total hip T-score, –1.7. Bone mineral density at the lumbar spine and total hip are unchanged compared with DXA results from 3 years ago on the same DXA machine.

Which of the following is the best next step in this patient's care?
- A. Refer to ophthalmology for slit-lamp examination
- B. Measure fasting serum C-telopeptide
- C. Administer zoledronic acid
- D. Restart alendronate
- E. Order 2-dimensional echocardiography

75 A 22-year-old woman is referred to you for evaluation of diabetes mellitus. Her medical history is notable for cystic fibrosis with pancreatic insufficiency, nasopharyngitis, *Pseudomonas aeruginosa* colonization, and *Aspergillus* infection. Her most recent pulmonary exacerbation requiring intravenous antibiotics was 7 months ago. Baseline FEV_1 is 60% predicted. Overall, she feels well and has no increased cough or hemoptysis. She reports adherence to her treatment regimen. During her most recent pulmonary exacerbation, she was treated with high-dosage glucocorticoids for 2 to 3 weeks, and her blood glucose values were elevated (175-250 mg/dL [9.7-13.9 mmol/L]). After hospital discharge, fingerstick blood glucose measurements at home ranged from 85 to 98 mg/dL (4.7-5.4 mmol/L) in the fasting state on 4 or 5 occasions.

On physical examination, her blood pressure is 112/68 mm Hg and pulse rate is 86 beats/min. Her height is 65 in (165 cm), and weight is 115 lb (52.3 kg) (BMI = 19.1 kg/m²).

Recent laboratory test results:
  Complete blood cell count, normal
  Basic metabolic panel, normal
  Fasting glucose = 90 mg/dL (70-99 mg/dL) (SI: 5.0 mmol/L [3.9-5.5 mmol/L])

To further assess her risk for diabetes mellitus, which of the following is the best next step?
  A.   No further testing needed
  B.   Glutamic acid decarboxylase antibody measurement
  C.   75-g oral glucose tolerance test, with fasting and 2-hour glucose values
  D.   Glycosylated hemoglobin measurement
  E.   Serum fructosamine measurement

76   A 21-year-old man is referred to the endocrine clinic with a 4-month history of progressive tiredness, lethargy, and weakness. He was previously fit and well. He takes no medications and has no history of substance use. There is no relevant family history.

On physical examination, his blood pressure is 105/75 mm Hg seated and 85/60 mm Hg standing. He has buccal and palmar pigmentation. There is increased tone in the lower limbs with slight weakness throughout. The rest of the physical examination findings are normal.

Laboratory test results:
  Serum sodium = 131 mEq/L (136-142 mEq/L) (SI: 131 mmol/L [136-142 mmol/L])
  Serum potassium = 5.4 mEq/L (3.5-5.0 mEq/L) (SI: 5.4 mmol/L [3.5-5.0 mmol/L])
  Serum creatinine = 0.9 mg/dL (0.7-1.3 mg/dL) (SI: 79.6 μmol/L [61.9-114.9 μmol/L])
  Serum urea nitrogen = 27.2 mg/dL (8-23 mg/dL) (SI: 9.7 mmol/L [2.9-8.2 mmol/L])
  Plasma ACTH = 1250 pg/mL (10-60 pg/mL) (SI: 275.0 pmol/L [2.2-13.2 pmol/L])
  Short cosyntropin-stimulation test (250 mcg):
      Baseline cortisol = 3.0 μg/dL (SI: 82.8 nmol/L)
      30-min cortisol = 4.8 μg/dL (SI: 132.4 nmol/L)

Which of the following tests is most likely to be helpful in identifying the underlying cause of his presentation?
  A.   21-Hydroxylase antibody assessment
  B.   Abdominal CT
  C.   HIV serology
  D.   Serum very long-chain fatty acids measurement
  E.   Sequencing of the *AIRE* gene

77   A 50-year-old woman with type 2 diabetes mellitus is admitted to the hospital with worsening lumbar back pain associated with lower-extremity weakness and urinary and fecal incontinence. She has a diagnosis of spinal stenosis. Home medications include insulin glargine, 60 units (200 units/cc) with a correction scale of insulin lispro before meals, which provides 1 unit per 50 mg/dL above 150 mg/dL (>8.3 mmol/L).

Her medical history is remarkable for lymphedema, bipolar disorder, asthma, and a motor vehicle crash 10 years ago that resulted in residual left-sided weakness. The patient is on long-term prednisone at a dosage between 10 and 50 mg daily due to asthma exacerbations, and she states that her blood glucose readings have been greater than 200 mg/dL (>11.1 mmol/L) for the last few weeks. She does not exercise because of back pain.

On physical examination, her height is 61.5 in (156.2 cm) and weight is 244 lb (111 kg) (BMI = 45.4 kg/m²). She has 0/5 muscle strength in her left lower extremity and tenderness throughout the entire length of her spine.

Laboratory test results:
  Hemoglobin A$_{1c}$ = 8.0% (4.0%-5.6%) (64 mmol/mol [20-38 mmol/mol])
  Serum urea nitrogen = 18 mg/dL (8-23 mg/dL) (SI: 6.4 mmol/L [2.9-8.2 mmol/L])
  Creatinine = 1.1 mg/dL (0.6-1.1 mg/dL) (SI: 97.2 μmol/L [53.0-97.2 μmol/L])

In the hospital, the patient is started on insulin glargine, 40 units at bedtime, and insulin lispro, 5 units with meals plus medium-dose correction scale (1 unit per 25 mg/dL above 150 mg/dL [>8.3 mmol/L]) before meals and at bedtime. She receives prednisone, 40 mg every morning at 10 AM. The graph shows her blood glucose pattern for the first 4 hospital days (*see image*).

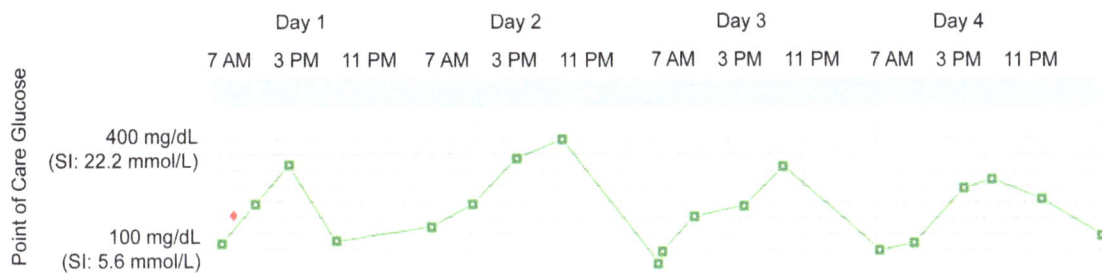

You are consulted to assist with her diabetes management in the hospital. Her prednisone dosage will remain 40 mg every morning. The patient is served a consistent carbohydrate diet.

Which of the following is the best next step to optimize this patient's glucose levels?

A. Begin an intravenous insulin infusion

B. Increase prandial insulin lispro to 8 units with meals

C. Increase correction scale to 2 units per 25 mg/dL above 150 mg/dL with meals

D. Change the timing of her basal insulin to the morning

E. Change her basal insulin dose to 40 units NPH in the morning

78 A 48-year-old woman is referred to you for a second opinion regarding Cushing syndrome. She initially presented with hypertension, osteoporosis associated with vertebral fractures, glucose intolerance, and an episode of deep venous thrombosis.

Laboratory test results during initial workup:

Urinary free cortisol = 152 μg/24 h (4-50 μg/24 h) (SI: 420 nmol/d [11-138 nmol/d])

Random plasma ACTH = 52 pg/mL (10-60 pg/mL) (SI: 11.4 pmol/L [2.2-23.2 pmol/L])

Cortisol following 1-mg dexamethasone suppression test = 5.4 μg/dL (SI: 149.0 nmol/L)

Bedtime salivary cortisol (2 collections) = 0.234 μg/dL and 0.147 μg/dL (<0.13 μg/dL) (SI: 6.46 nmol/L and 4.06 nmol/L [<3.6 nmol/L])

Pituitary MRI did not show an adenoma, and findings on chest and abdomen CT were normal. She underwent inferior petrosal sinus sampling, which failed to show a central-to-peripheral ACTH gradient before or after infusion of corticotropin-releasing hormone. A ^{68}Ga DOTATATE scan was negative for an ectopic source.

Current medications are calcium carbonate, ergocalciferol, losartan, metoprolol, alendronate, and tramadol, 50 mg as needed for pain.

On physical examination, she is a middle-aged woman with a cushingoid appearance. Her blood pressure is 172/90 mm Hg, and pulse rate is 92 beats/min. Her height is 64 in (162.5 cm), and weight is 189 lb (85.7 kg) (BMI = 32.4 kg/m²). She has some face rounding and a small amount of retrocervical fat accumulation, thin skin, and several bruises on her arms. There is no pedal edema.

Current laboratory test results:

Cortisol (4 PM) = 23 μg/dL (2-14 μg/dL) (SI: 634.5 nmol/L [55.2-386.2 nmol/L])

ACTH = 58 pg/mL (10-60 pg/mL) (SI: 12.8 pmol/L [2.2-13.2 pmol/L])

Potassium = 3.9 mEq/L (3.5-5.0 mEq/L) (SI: 3.9 mmol/L [3.5-5.0 mmol/L])

Which of the following is the best next step in this patient's management?
- A. ^{111}In octreotide scan
- B. Another inferior petrosal sinus sampling
- C. Another pituitary MRI with delayed images
- D. Adrenal-specific CT
- E. Abdominal and chest MRI

79 A 49-year-old woman is referred for very low lipid levels initially documented 11 years ago. She has an 8-year history of type 2 diabetes mellitus that is treated with metformin and no history of cardiovascular or neurologic disease. She takes no other medications. Her family history is remarkable for several members with type 2 diabetes on her mother's side. A maternal aunt with type 2 diabetes died of cryptogenic cirrhosis at age 52 years. The patient's 21-year-old son has low cholesterol and fatty liver disease. There is no family history of cardiovascular disease. She smokes 8 to 10 cigarettes daily and does not drink alcohol.

On physical examination, her blood pressure is 106/52 mm Hg and pulse rate is 70 beats/min. Her height is 69 in (175.3 cm), and weight is 240 lb (109 kg) (BMI = 35.4 kg/m^2). Central adiposity is present, there are no xanthomas, and the liver edge is palpable at the right costal margin. Neurologic examination reveals loss of ankle reflexes and monofilament sensation in both feet.

Laboratory test results (sample drawn while fasting, on no treatment):
    Total cholesterol = 84 mg/dL (<200 mg/dL [optimal]) (SI: 2.18 mmol/L [<5.18 mmol/L])
    Triglycerides = 64 mg/dL (<150 mg/dL [optimal]) (SI: 0.72 mmol/L [<1.70 mmol/L])
    HDL cholesterol = 48 mg/dL (>60 mg/dL [optimal]) (SI: 1.24 mmol/L [>1.55 mmol/L])
    LDL cholesterol = 21 mg/dL (<100 mg/dL [optimal]) (SI: 0.54 mmol/L [<2.59 mmol/L])
    Non-HDL cholesterol = 34 mg/dL (<130 mg/dL [optimal]) (SI: 0.88 mmol/L [<3.37 mmol/L])
    Apolipoprotein B = <40 mg/dL (50-110 mg/dL) (SI: 0.4 g/dL [0.5-1.1 g/dL])
    Hemoglobin A$_{1c}$ = 7.1% (4.0%-5.6%) (54 mmol/mol [20-38 mmol/mol])
    Creatinine = 0.84 mg/dL (0.6-1.1 mg/dL) (SI: 72.3 μmol/L [53.0-97.2 μmol/L])
    TSH = 1.8 mIU/L (0.5-5.0 mIU/L)
    Fasting plasma glucose = 132 mg/dL (70-99 mg/dL) (SI: 7.3 mmol/L [3.9-5.5 mmol/L])
    ALT = 52 U/L (10-40 U/L) (SI: 0.86 μkat/L [0.17-0.67 μkat/L])
    AST = 41 U/L (20-48 U/L) (SI: 0.68 μkat/L [0.33-0.80 μkat/L])

Which of the following is the best next step in this patient's management?
- A. Measure levels of vitamins A, D, and E
- B. Perform liver ultrasonography
- C. Obtain complete blood cell count with peripheral smear
- D. Perform serum protein electrophoresis
- E. Perform genetic testing for pathogenic variants in the *PCSK9* gene

80 A 71-year-old man is evaluated for treatment-resistant hypertension. He has elevated blood pressure despite the use of 3 antihypertensive medications. He is otherwise asymptomatic. He has no palpitations, sweating, anxiety, or headaches. He specifically has had no episodic symptoms or spells.

Laboratory test results:
    ACTH (8 AM) = 17 pg/mL (10-60 pg/mL) (SI: 3.7 pmol/L [2.2-13.2 pmol/L])
    Cortisol (8 AM) = 19.7 μg/dL (5-25 μg/dL) (SI: 543.5 nmol/L [137.9-689.7 nmol/L])
    Aldosterone = 9 ng/dL (4-21 ng/dL) (SI: 249.7 pmol/L [111.0-582.5 pmol/L]
    Plasma renin activity = 1.4 ng/mL per h (0.6-4.3 ng/mL per h)
    Plasma normetanephrine = 2747 pg/mL (<165 pg/mL) (SI: 15.00 nmol/L [<0.90 nmol/L])
    Plasma metanephrine = 39 pg/mL (<99 pg/mL) (SI: 0.20 nmol/L [<0.50 nmol/L])

Urinary free cortisol = 29 μg/24 h (<4-50 μg/24 h) (SI: 80 nmol/d [11-138 nmol/d])
DHEA-S = 20.7 μg/dL (25-131 μg/dL) (SI: 0.56 μmol/L [0.68-3.55 μmol/L])

Abdominal CT reveals bilateral adrenal masses (*see image, arrows*). There is a 6.8 × 5.3 × 6.7-cm left adrenal mass. This mass is described as having an unenhanced attenuation of 33.5 Hounsfield units. Following contrast administration and a 15-minute washout period, there is 45% absolute washout and 24% relative washout. In addition, a 2.3 × 1.8 × 1.4-cm right adrenal mass is identified (*see image, arrows*). This mass is described as having an unenhanced attenuation of –15 Hounsfield units. Following contrast administration and a 15-minute washout period, there is 63% absolute washout and 75% relative washout.

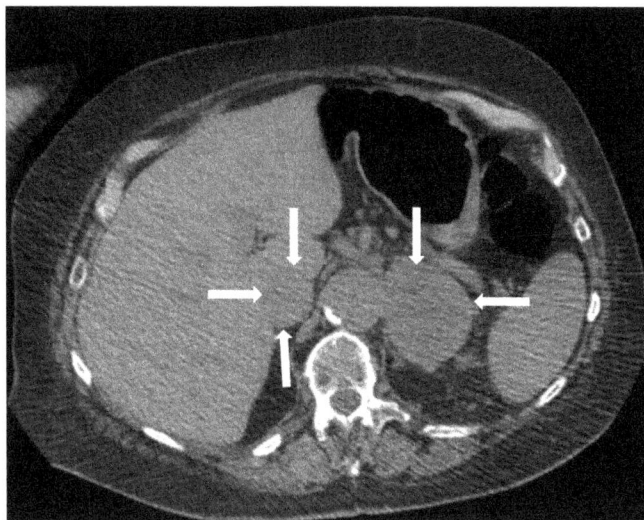

Which of the following is the most appropriate recommendation?
A. Right adrenalectomy
B. Left adrenalectomy
C. Bilateral adrenalectomy
D. Repeated imaging in 3 months
E. Biopsy of the right adrenal mass

81 A 35-year-old woman with a history of hypothyroidism, vitamin D deficiency, and asthma is referred to you for management of hypothyroidism. Her current regimen is levothyroxine, 125 mcg daily, which she takes on an empty stomach. Six months ago, she was on levothyroxine dosage of 100 mcg daily, and her primary care physician increased the dosage due to elevated TSH. She also uses an albuterol inhaler for asthma and takes vitamin D, 50,000 IU weekly.

On physical examination, her weight is 125 lb (56.8 kg) and height is 61 in (155 cm) (BMI = 23.6 kg/m^2). She has mild thyromegaly. The rest of her examination findings are unremarkable.

Laboratory test results:
TSH = 9.0 mIU/L (0.5-5.0 mIU/L)
Free T$_4$ = 1.0 ng/dL (0.8-1.8 ng/dL) (SI: 12.9 pmol/L [10.30-23.17 pmol/L])
Free T$_3$ = 2.3 pg/mL (2.3-4.2 pg/mL) (SI: 3.53 pmol/L [3.53-6.45 pmol/L]
TPO antibodies = 100.0 IU/mL (<2.0 IU/mL) (SI: 100.0 kIU/L [<2.0 kIU/L])
25-Hydroxyvitamin D = 20 ng/mL (30-80 ng/mL [optimal]) (SI: 49.9 nmol/L [74.9-199.7 nmol/L])
Basic metabolic panel, normal

Which of the following is the best next step in this patient's management?
A. Increase the levothyroxine dosage to 150 mcg daily
B. Start liothyronine, 12.5 mcg daily
C. Increase the vitamin D dosage to 50,000 IU twice weekly
D. Levothyroxine absorption test
E. Measure tissue transglutaminases IgA and IgG

82 A 28-year-old man with type 2 diabetes mellitus is seen in the emergency department for asthma exacerbation. Antibiotics and inhaled glucocorticoids were started 2 days ago for an upper respiratory tract infection, and he now seeks help because of persistent symptoms. The endocrine service is called to address hyperglycemia because he is going to be started on oral steroids. Over the past 2 years, his hemoglobin A_{1c} level has been in the range of 7.6% (60 mmol/mol).

In the emergency department, his blood glucose concentration is 350 mg/dL (19.4 mmol/L). Following intravenous glucocorticoids and nebulizer therapy, he feels better. The plan is to discharge him on antibiotic therapy (for 1 week) and oral prednisone, 40 mg in the morning (for 2 weeks). Inhaled steroids will most likely be restarted after this 2-week treatment period.

His current diabetes regimen consists of metformin, 1000 mg twice daily.

On physical examination, his temperature is 100.6°F (38.1°C), blood pressure is 117/78 mm Hg, and pulse rate is 108 beats/min. His height is 66 in (167.6 cm), and weight is 184 lb (83.6 kg) (BMI = 39.7 kg/m²). He has tachypnea and mild tachycardia, but he is speaking in full sentences. He appears comfortable and is not using accessory muscles to breathe. Expiratory wheezes are heard bilaterally on lung examination. The rest of his examination findings are normal.

You instruct him to check his blood glucose before meals and at bedtime.

Which of the following medications should be added to his regimen to ensure adequate blood glucose control while on glucocorticoid therapy?

- A. Insulin aspart on a supplemental scale at mealtimes
- B. Liraglutide
- C. Insulin glargine
- D. SGLT-2 inhibitor
- E. Insulin 70/30 twice daily

83 A 32-year-old woman wishes to undergo thyroidectomy for definitive treatment of her Graves disease. Graves disease was diagnosed 5 months ago, and she was initially treated with β-adrenergic blockers and methimazole and now requires 15 mg of methimazole daily to maintain her free T_4 and total T_3 levels slightly above the normal range. She describes difficulty adhering to her methimazole regimen, but believes she will be adherent to daily thyroid hormone therapy.

On physical examination during her surgical consultation, her blood pressure is 124/78 mm Hg and pulse rate is 90 beats/min. She has evidence of orbitopathy and a visible goiter. On palpation, her thyroid gland is twice normal size with a spongy texture. There is a soft bruit. Examination findings are otherwise unremarkable with normal deep tendon reflexes.

Laboratory evaluations now and at the time of diagnosis are shown (*see table*).

Thyroid Function Tests	5 Months Ago	At Surgical Consultation
TSH (0.5-5.0 mIU/L)	<0.001 mIU/L	0.15 mIU/L
Free T_4 (0.8-1.8 ng/dL [SI: 10.30-23.17 pmol/L])	7.0 ng/dL (SI: 90.1 pmol/L)	2.0 ng/dL (SI: 25.7 pmol/L)
Total T_3 (70-200 ng/dL [SI: 1.08-3.08 nmol/L])	500 ng/dL (SI: 7.7 nmol/L)	280 ng/dL (SI: 4.3 nmol/L)
Thyroid-stimulating immunoglobulin (≤120%)	300%	...

Because of religious reasons, the patient states that she will not consider administration of blood products during the perioperative period, even if it were medically indicated.

Which of the following is the best therapy to minimize the risk of blood loss during this patient's thyroidectomy?
- A. Initiate high-dosage steroids
- B. Increase the methimazole dosage
- C. Initiate rituximab
- D. Initiate lithium
- E. Initiate potassium iodide

84 A 20-year-old woman with Turner syndrome is referred by her pediatric endocrinologist for transition to adult care. Coarctation of the aorta was diagnosed at age 5 years and was repaired at age 8 years. In annual follow-up, her cardiologist noted that her height was falling on the growth chart and puberty was delayed. This led to an endocrinology referral at which time karyotype analysis was performed and Turner syndrome was diagnosed. She brings a copy of her chromosomal analysis describing 45,X/46,XX. She was treated with GH and achieved a height of 63 in (160 cm) before initiation of oral estrogen therapy at age 14 years. She has menses with micronized progesterone given every month for 12 days. Primary hypothyroidism was diagnosed at age 12 years. Her regimen of oral estrogen was transitioned to the transdermal estrogen patch in recent years, and she does not have any symptoms of vaginal dryness or hot flashes. She is a college freshman. Although she is currently not sexually active, she has been in the past and has always used condoms. She has been told that pregnancy is not possible.

On physical examination, she is a well-developed, well-nourished woman. Her height is 63 in (160 cm) and weight is 159 lb (72.3 kg) (BMI = 28.2 kg/m²). Her blood pressure is 119/71 mm Hg. She has no physical features of Turner syndrome.

Recent laboratory test results:
    TSH = 4.8 mIU/L (0.5-5.0 mIU/L)
    FSH = 43.0 mIU/mL (2.0-12.0 mIU/mL [follicular]) (SI: 43.0 IU/L [2.0-12.0 IU/L])
    25-Hydroxyvitamin D = 37 ng/mL (30-80 ng/mL [optimal]) (SI: 95.4 nmol/L [74.9-199.7 nmol/L])

Which of the following should be part of her annual evaluation?
- A. Fasting glucose and/or hemoglobin A_{1c} measurements
- B. Morning ACTH and cortisol measurements
- C. Tissue transglutaminase IgA antibody assessment
- D. PTH and calcium measurements
- E. IGF-1 measurement

85 A 34-year-old woman is being seen in clinic for treatment of type 1 diabetes mellitus. She has had diabetes since age 20 years. Diabetes-related complications include a history of background retinopathy and mild peripheral neuropathy. She has hypoglycemia unawareness and was started on insulin pump therapy and a continuous glucose monitor 2 years ago. Her hemoglobin A_{1c} level has ranged between 7.3% and 8.2% (56-66 mmol/mol) over the past 18 months.

She does not smoke cigarettes or drink alcohol.

On physical examination, her height is 64 in (163 cm) and weight is 154 lb (70 kg) (BMI = 26.4 kg/m²). Her blood pressure is 102/72 mm Hg, and pulse rate is 72 beats/min. Examination findings are normal except for mildly reduced sensation to monofilament touch and vibrational sense in each foot.

Laboratory test results:
    Hemoglobin A_{1c} = 8.4% (4.0%-5.6%) (68 mmol/mol [20-38 mmol/mol])
    Creatinine = 0.8 mg/dL (0.6-1.1 mg/dL) (SI: 70.7 µmol/L [53.0-97.2 µmol/L])
    TSH = 1.4 mIU/L (0.5-5.0 mIU/L)
    Urinary albumin = 12 µg/mg creat (30-300 µg/mg creat)
    2-week mean fingerstick glucose = 184 mg/dL (SI: 10.2 mmol/L)
    2-week mean glucose (sensor data) = 172 mg/dL (SI: 9.5 mmol/L)

She uses an insulin-to-carbohydrate ratio of 1 unit per 10 g carbohydrate before meals and boluses insulin 10 to 15 minutes before she eats a meal. Her meals are usually consumed at 8 AM, 12 PM, and 5:30 PM. The glucose goal is 90 to 130 mg/dL (5.0-7.2 mmol/L). The correction is 1 unit per 80 mg/dL (4.4 mmol/L) above the glucose target. The total insulin amount per day is 22.6 units. The average bolus and correctional insulin together is 12 units/day.

Basal insulin rates are as follows:

12:00 AM-4:00 AM	0.350 units/h
4:00 AM-7:30 AM	0.700 units/h
7:30 AM-12:00 PM	0.400 units/h
12:00 PM-4:00 PM	0.375 units/h
4:00 PM-8:00 PM	0.650 units/h
8:00 PM-12:00 AM	0.250 units/h

Data from her continuous glucose monitor are shown (*see image*). Mealtimes are indicated with blue arrows.

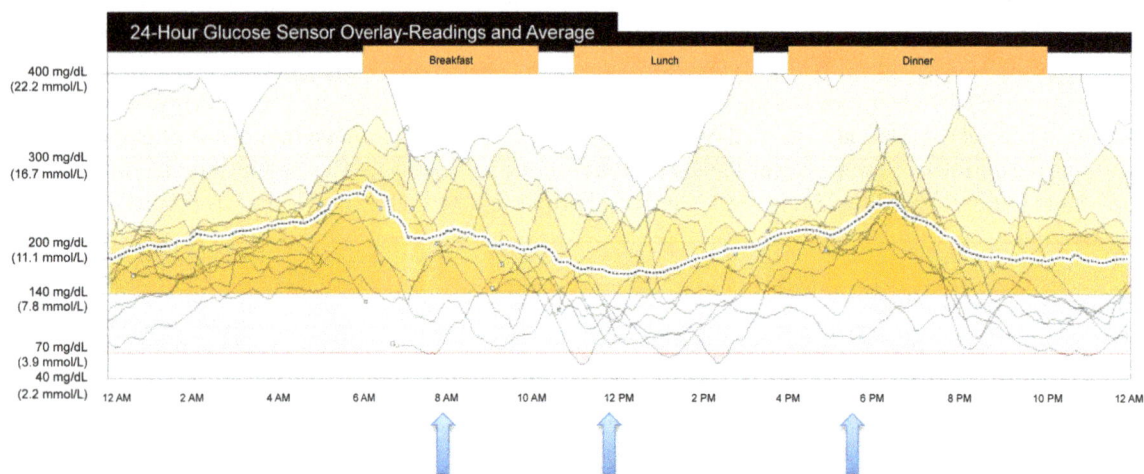

In addition to referring the patient for review of carbohydrate counting, which of the following is the best approach to manage her diabetes?
- A. Change the insulin-to-carbohydrate ratio to 1 unit per 8 g carbohydrates before each meal
- B. Change the insulin-to-carbohydrate ratio to 1 unit per 8 g carbohydrates at 7:30 AM and 5 PM
- C. Increase the basal insulin rate at midnight, 4 AM, and 4 PM
- D. Increase the basal insulin rate at midnight, 4 AM, and 7:30 AM
- E. Increase the basal insulin rate at midnight and change the insulin-to-carbohydrate ratio to 1 unit per 8 g carbohydrates at 7:30 AM and 5 PM

86 A 56-year-old woman with hypertension, hypercholesterolemia, chronic kidney disease, and obstructive sleep apnea seeks your assistance with weight loss. About 14 years ago, she started gaining weight. At that time, she was involved in a motor vehicle crash and she was unable to ambulate for 6 months. The patient has not followed any commercial weight-loss programs, but has tried diets on her own. She is able to adhere to a meal plan for a few weeks, but then she becomes bored of eating the same foods, due to the restriction in macronutrient composition in the meal plans she has tried. She would like to follow a long-term program. She has not taken any weight-loss medications. On a typical day, breakfast is an English muffin with bacon and egg, lunch is either fried chicken and a salad with ranch dressing or a cheeseburger with French fries, and dinner is meat with 2 sides (eg, macaroni and cheese and green beans). She eats out 3 nights a week. She reports eating large portions. She drinks sugar-free beverages only.

On physical examination, her blood pressure is 105/66 mm Hg and pulse rate is 64 beats/min. Her height is 63.5 in (161.3 cm), and weight is 256 lb (116.5 kg) (BMI = 44.6 kg/m^2). She is in no distress and she does not look cushingoid. Her lungs are clear to auscultation bilaterally, her heart sounds are normal, and her heart has a regular rate and rhythm. Her abdomen is soft and nontender. She has no peripheral edema.

Laboratory test results:
    Creatinine = 1.6 mg/dL (0.6-1.1 mg/dL) (SI: 141.4 mmol/L [53.0-97.2 mmol/L])
    Estimated glomerular filtration rate = 36 mL/min per 1.73 m² (>60 mL/min per 1.73 m²)
    TSH = 1.5 mIU/L (0.5-5.0 mIU/L)
    Total cholesterol = 215 mg/dL (<200 mg/dL [optimal]) (SI: 5.57 mmol/L [<5.18 mmol/L])
    Triglycerides = 146 mg/dL (<150 mg/dL [optimal]) (SI: 1.65 mmol/L [<1.70 mmol/L])
    HDL-cholesterol = 41 mg/dL (>60 mg/dL [optimal]) (SI: 1.06 mmol/L [>1.55 mmol/L])
    LDL-cholesterol =145 mg/dL (<100 mg/dL [optimal]) (SI: 3.76 mmol/L [<2.59 mmol/L])

Which of the following dietary plans would you recommend for this patient?
    A. Very low-calorie diet (<800 calories per day)
    B. Low-calorie diet (1200 calories per day)
    C. Ketogenic diet
    D. Low-fat diet (<30% of daily calories)
    E. High-protein diet (1 g/kg)

87 A 45-year-old woman is referred to you for evaluation of hypercalcemia on serial laboratory testing, dating back at least 10 years. She has marked fatigue and diffuse bony pain, but has no polydipsia, polyuria, or confusion. She has a history of hypertension but is otherwise healthy. She has no history of renal stones, fractures, or craniocervical irradiation. She takes only a multivitamin and baby aspirin daily. She is an only child and has no children of her own, and her parents are deceased. Her family history is negative for known parathyroid disease, endocrine tumors (pituitary, pancreatic, or adrenal), nephrolithiasis, or osteoporosis.

On physical examination, she appears healthy. She has lost 1 in (2.5 cm) in height since her adult maximum height was recorded. Neck examination is negative for masses or nodules. She has no kyphosis or vertebral tenderness. There is no bony or soft-tissue tenderness to palpation. The rest of the examination findings are unremarkable.

Laboratory test results:
    Serum calcium = 11.2 mg/dL (8.2-10.2 mg/dL (SI: 2.8 mmol/L [2.1-2.6 mmol/L])
    Serum phosphate = 3.5 mg/dL (2.3-4.7 mg/dL) (SI: 1.1 mmol/L [0.7-1.5 mmol/L])
    Serum magnesium = 2.7 mg/dL (1.5-2.3 mg/dL) (SI: 1.1 mmol/L [0.6-0.9 mmol/L])
    Serum albumin = 4.2 mg/dL (3.5-5.0 g/dL) (SI: 42 g/L [35-50 g/L])
    Serum creatinine = 0.8 mg/dL (0.6-1.1 mg/dL) (SI: 70.7 µmol/L [53.0-97.2 µmol/L])
    Serum intact PTH = 85 pg/mL (10-65 pg/mL) (SI: 85 ng/L [10-65 ng/L])
    Serum 25-hydroxyvitamin D = 30 ng/mL (30-80 ng/mL [optimal]) (SI: 74.9 nmol/L [74.9-199.7 nmol/L])
    Urinary calcium = 75 mg/24 h (100-300 mg/24 h) (SI: 74.9 mmol/d [2.5-7.5 mmol/d])
    Urinary creatinine = 1.2 mg/24 h (1.0-2.0 g/24 h) (SI: 10.6 mmol/d [8.8-17.7 mmol/d])
    Urinary volume = 1600 mL/24 h

Before referral to your clinic, she underwent a ⁹⁹Tc sestamibi parathyroid scan (*see image*).

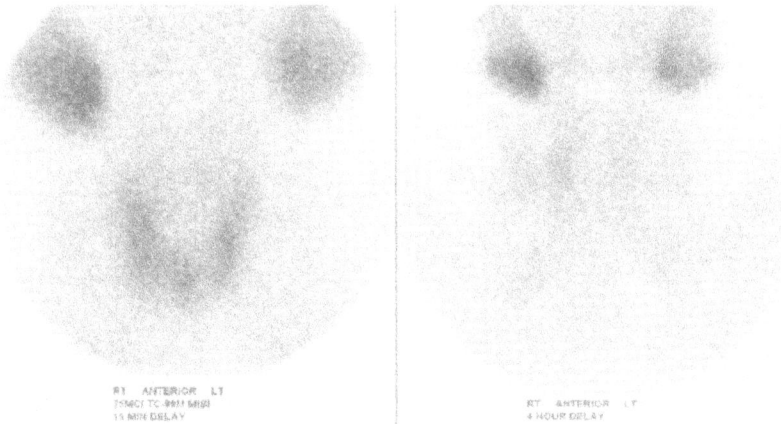

On the basis of this patient's clinical presentation, which of the following is the best next step in her management?
- A. Start cinacalcet
- B. Start pregabalin
- C. Administer pamidronate
- D. Refer to an endocrine surgeon for consideration of neck exploration
- E. Reassure the patient that no additional investigation or treatment is indicated

88 A 58-year-old man is referred for progressive metastatic papillary thyroid carcinoma. His initial radioiodine scan while hypothyroid (TSH = 65 mIU/L) showed radioiodine-refractory disease despite an elevated thyroglobulin value of 10 ng/mL (10 µg/L). He was then found to have lung nodules on chest CT. During follow-up visits, he underwent recombinant human TSH (rhTSH) PET/CT imaging, which revealed multiple fluorodeoxyglucose-avid nodules in both lungs. His thyroglobulin value after rhTSH injections was 150 ng/mL (150 µg/L), and it later increased to 600 ng/mL (600 µg/L) (*see table*). He has now become short of breath.

After a long discussion, he agrees to start lenvatinib. Ten weeks after starting this medication, he starts feeling tired, but he otherwise tolerates it well. He has normal libido. He has no polyuria, polydipsia, or sweating.

His medications include levothyroxine, 150 mcg daily; multivitamin, 1 tablet daily; and losartan, 100 mg daily. He confirms that he takes levothyroxine every day on an empty stomach and waits 1 hour before eating.

Measurement	Timing		
	6 Weeks After Surgery	6 Months After Surgery	12 Months After Surgery
TSH	65 mIU/L	0.1 mIU/L	0.09 mIU/L
Thyroglobulin	10 ng/mL (SI: 10 µg/L)	45 ng/mL (SI: 45 µg/L) (150 ng/mL [SI: 150 µg/L] after rhTSH injections)	600 ng/mL (SI: 600 µg/L)
Thyroglobulin antibodies	Negative	Negative	Negative

On physical examination, his blood pressure is 125/68 mm Hg and pulse rate is 70 beats/min. There is no palpable mass in his neck, and lung examination reveals scattered rales bilaterally. He has no lower-extremity edema.

Laboratory test results:

White blood cell count = 5000/µL (4500-11,000/µL) (SI: 5.0 × 10^9/L [4.5-11.0 × 10^9/L])
Hemoglobin = 11.0 g/dL (13.8-17.2 g/dL) (SI: 110 g/dL [138-172 g/L])
Platelet count = 160 × 10^3/µL (150-450 × 10^3/µL) (SI: 160 × 10^9/L [150-450 × 10^9/L])
Sodium = 138 mEq/L (136-142 mEq/L) (SI: 138 mmol/L [136-142 mmol/L])
Potassium = 3.9 mEq/L (3.5-5.0 mEq/L) (SI: 3.9 mmol/L [3.5-5.0 mmol/L])
Glucose = 87 mg/dL (70-99 mg/dL) (SI: 4.8 mmol/L [3.9-5.5 mmol/L])
Creatinine = 1.0 mg/dL (0.7-1.3 mg/dL) (SI: 88.4 µmol/L [61.9-114.9 µmol/L])
Calcium = 8.9 mg/dL (8.2-10.2 mg/dL) (SI: 2.2 mmol/L [2.1-2.6 mmol/L])

Which of the following should be measured in this patient?
- A. TSH
- B. 8-AM cortisol
- C. Vitamin D
- D. 8-AM testosterone
- E. Hemoglobin A$_{1c}$

89 A 72-year-old man seeks your advice regarding testosterone treatment. He reports low libido and fatigue. He has well-controlled hypertension treated with an ACE inhibitor and no history of cardiovascular disease or diabetes mellitus. He reports stable nocturia (twice nightly) and an occasionally weak urinary stream.

On physical examination, his height is 69 in (175.3 cm) and weight is 210 lb (95.5 kg) (BMI = 31 kg/m²). His blood pressure is 132/84 mm Hg. He has normal body hair, and testes are 20 mL bilaterally.

Laboratory test result (sample drawn at 8 AM while fasting):
  Total testosterone = 250 ng/dL (300-900 ng/dL) (SI: 8.7 nmol/L [10.4-31.2 nmol/L]) (repeated measurement 1 week later = 234 ng/dL [SI: 8.1 nmol/L])

DXA documents T-scores of 1.2 at the lumbar spine, 0.6 at the total hip, and –0.3 at the femoral neck.

As you counsel this patient, which of the following is the most likely effect(s) of starting testosterone in his case?
  A. Reduced risk of falls
  B. Reduced nocturia and improved urinary flow
  C. Reduced coronary artery plaque volume
  D. Improved bone density
  E. Improved memory

90 A 38-year-old man is referred for evaluation of hypoglycemia. He underwent Roux-en-Y gastric bypass surgery 12 months ago for treatment of obesity. Before this procedure, he had no known glucose problems—no diabetes or hypoglycemia. The patient now describes shakiness and sweating approximately 1 hour after any meal that contains more than 1 serving of carbohydrates. The symptoms are generally self-limited and resolve after 2 hours. He treats the condition by avoiding carbohydrates. He reports being in a motor vehicle crash where he lost control of his car. He does not recall the circumstances of the event, except waking up after hitting a guardrail. The event occurred 90 minutes after drinking a milk shake.

The patient's primary care physician performs a mixed-meal glucose challenge (60% carbohydrates, 25% protein, 15% fat) that includes 90 g of carbohydrates in the form of bread and potatoes. The results of the test are shown (*see figure*).

The patient takes no regular medications.

On physical examination, his blood pressure is 140/85 mm Hg and pulse rate is 75 beats/min. His height is 68 in, and weight is 242 lb (110 kg) (BMI = 36.8 kg/m²) (weight is reduced from 286 lb [130 kg] 1 year ago). Examination findings are otherwise normal.

Which of the following is the most likely cause of this patient's symptoms and hypoglycemia?
  A. A diet that is too high in carbohydrates
  B. Malabsorption of carbohydrates
  C. Malabsorption of fat
  D. Insulinoma
  E. Overactive secretion of GLP-1

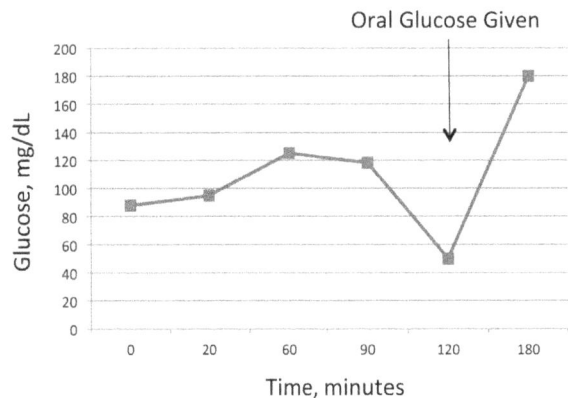

91 A 26-year-old man with no notable medical history reports that over the past 2 years he has been experiencing headaches. Brain MRI shows a sellar mass with some suprasellar extension abutting the optic chiasm with possible right cavernous sinus invasion (*see images*).

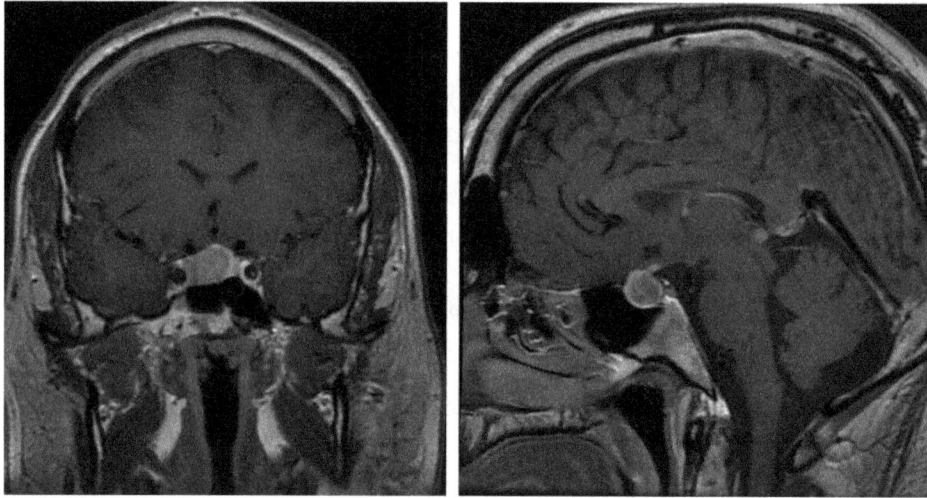

Over the last 12 months, he has had a 40-lb (18.2-kg) weight gain, absent sex drive, and erectile dysfunction. He and his partner would like to conceive in the next year.

On physical examination, his blood pressure is 119/69 mm Hg and pulse rate is 80 beats/min. His height is 70 in (177.8 cm), and weight is 222 lb (100.9 kg) (BMI = 31.9 kg/m²). Visual fields by confrontation are normal. There is no obvious gynecomastia. Patellar reflexes are absent bilaterally. Testes are 8 mL bilaterally.

Laboratory test results:
Prolactin = 1125 ng/mL (4-23 ng/mL) (SI: 48.9 nmol/L [0.17-1.00 nmol/L])
Cortisol (8 AM) = 15.8 µg/dL (5-25 µg/dL) (SI: 435.9 nmol/L [137.9-689.7 nmol/L])
TSH = 2.46 mIU/L (0.5-5.0 mIU/L)
Free T$_4$ = 0.76 ng/dL (0.8-1.8 ng/dL) (SI: 9.8 pmol/L [10.30-23.17 pmol/L])
Testosterone = 174 ng/dL (300-900 ng/dL) (SI: 6.0 nmol/L [10.4-31.2 nmol/L])
IGF-1 = 216 ng/mL (117-321 ng/mL) (SI: 28.3 nmol/L [15.3-42.1 nmol/L])
LH = 3.8 mIU/mL (1.0-9.0 mIU/mL) (SI: 3.8 IU/L [1.0-9.0 IU/L])
FSH = 5.6 mIU/mL (1.0-13.0 mIU/mL) (SI: 5.6 IU/L [1.0-13.0 IU/L])

He is started on cabergoline, 0.5 mg orally twice weekly. Three months later, his prolactin and free T$_4$ levels have normalized at 4.6 ng/mL (0.2 nmol/L) and 1.1 ng/dL (14.2 pmol/L), respectively. MRI shows mass shrinkage by approximately 30%. Testosterone remains low at 158 ng/dL (5.5 nmol/L). He still has reduced libido.

Which of the following is the best next step in this patient's management?
  A. Maintain current regimen
  B. Start hCG therapy
  C. Start testosterone replacement
  D. Start clomiphene
  E. Start an aromatase inhibitor

92 A dermatologist refers a 59-year-old woman after diagnosing androgenetic alopecia. The patient has a history of breast cancer diagnosed 7 years ago. She had her last period at that time. Hair thinning started at the temples and progressed to the top of her scalp. She notes new terminal hair growth on the chin and inner thighs. Before menopause, she had normal menses and no difficulties conceiving. She has no history of glucose intolerance and never had terminal hair growth before menopause.

Medications include levothyroxine for primary hypothyroidism diagnosed 10 years ago.

On physical examination, her height is 64 in (162.5 cm) and weight is 147 lb (66.8 kg) (BMI = 25.2 kg/m^2). Her blood pressure is 124/76 mm Hg. She has terminal hair growth on the upper lip. There is hair loss on the crown of her head, as well as a receding hairline. Her thyroid gland is palpable with swallowing without nodules or enlargement. On cardiac examination, there is a regular rate and rhythm. There is an audible S$_1$ and S$_2$ without murmurs, rubs, or gallops. Lungs are clear to auscultation. Her abdomen is nondistended, soft, and nontender with positive bowel sounds. There is no hepatosplenomegaly or masses. She has no cyanosis, clubbing, or edema of the extremities. Reflexes are 2+ without delay.

Laboratory test results:
    TSH = 1.5 mIU/L (0.5-5.0 mIU/L)
    Free T$_4$ = 1.3 ng/dL (0.8-1.8 ng/dL) (SI: 16.73 pmol/L [10.30-23.17 pmol/L])
    Prolactin = 18.7 ng/mL (4-30 ng/mL) (SI: 0.81 nmol/L [0.17-1.30 nmol/L])
    Total testosterone = 68 ng/dL (8-60 ng/dL) (SI: 2.4 nmol/L [0.3-2.1 nmol/L])
    DHEA-S = 257 µg/dL (15-200 µg/dL) (SI: 6.96 µmol/L [0.41-5.42 µmol/L])
    Androstenedione = 137 ng/dL (30-200 ng/dL) (SI: 4.78 nmol/L [1.05-6.98 nmol/L])
    FSH = 94.0 mIU/mL (>30.0 mIU/mL [postmenopausal]) (SI: 94.0 IU/L >30.0 IU/L)

A 48-hour low-dose dexamethasone suppression test is performed with the following results:
    Cortisol = <1.0 µg/dL (SI: 26.6 nmol/L)
    DHEA-S = 63.2 µg/dL (SI: 1.71 µmol/L)
    Androstenedione = 47 ng/dL (SI: 1.64 nmol/L)
    Total testosterone = 63.2 ng/dL (SI: 2.2 nmol/L)

Abdominal CT demonstrates a 1.9 × 1.0-cm nodule with features consistent with a benign adenoma.

Which of the following is the best next step in this patient's management?
A. Start a GnRH analogue
B. Start spironolactone
C. Perform pelvic ultrasonography
D. Perform ovarian/adrenal venous sampling
E. Perform MRI of the abdomen/pelvis

93 A 56-year-old man returns for routine follow-up of type 2 diabetes mellitus. Diabetes was diagnosed at age 43 years. His glycemic control was poor for the first 10 years after diagnosis, but over the last 3 years, he has substantially improved his adherence to lifestyle and medication recommendations and his hemoglobin A$_{1c}$ level has ranged from 6.7% to 7.0% (50-53 mmol/mol). Medications include liraglutide, 1.2 mg daily; metformin, 2000 mg daily; insulin glargine, 25 units daily; lisinopril, 30 mg daily; and atorvastatin, 20 mg daily. Glucose meter download shows that he checks glucose 3 times daily with a mean glucose value of 138 mg/dL (7.7 mmol/L).

On physical examination, his blood pressure is 138/78 mm Hg and pulse rate is 92 beats/min. His height is 68 in (172.7 cm), and weight is 205 lb (93.2 kg) (BMI = 31.2 kg/m^2). Pertinent findings include mild acanthosis nigricans at the base of the neck, absence of Achilles tendon reflexes, and normal monofilament and vibratory sensation.

Laboratory test results:
    Urinary albumin-to-creatinine ratio = 85 mg/g creat (<30 mg/g creat)
    Renal function, normal
    Total cholesterol = 190 mg/dL (<200 mg/dL [optimal]) (SI: 4.92 mmol/L [<5.18 mmol/L])
    LDL cholesterol = 102 mg/dL (<100 mg/dL [optimal]) (SI: 2.64 mmol/L [<2.59 mmol/L])
    HDL cholesterol = 34 mg/dL (>60 mg/dL [optimal]) (SI: 0.88 mmol/L [>1.55 mmol/L])
    Triglycerides = 280 mg/dL (<150 mg/dL [optimal]) (SI: 3.16 mmol/L [<1.70 mmol/L])

Ophthalmologic examination reveals moderate nonproliferative diabetic retinopathy.

Which of the following interventions will have the greatest effect on reducing progression of diabetic retinopathy in this patient?
- A. Increase the atorvastatin dosage
- B. Add fenofibrate
- C. Add verapamil
- D. Add rapid-acting insulin analogue with meals
- E. Add aspirin

94 You detect a right-sided thyroid nodule in a 34-year-old woman during a follow-up appointment for management of polycystic ovary syndrome. Ultrasonography shows a solitary thyroid nodule with a TI-RADS (Thyroid Imaging Reporting and Data System) score of 5. Results of FNA biopsy document a follicular lesion of undetermined significance. Testing for gene mutations to determine the risk of cancer returns favoring malignancy. Tests of the patient's thyroid function 3 months ago show a TSH value of 2.1 mIU/L.

Your surgical colleague suggests to the patient that either total thyroidectomy or a right lobectomy would be a reasonable treatment option. The patient schedules a follow-up appointment to discuss her surgical options with you. She has no additional medical problems. Her family history is notable for her mother and sister having Hashimoto thyroiditis.

On physical examination, you confirm the presence of the 2-cm, right-sided thyroid nodule. No other nodules or abnormal lymph nodes are palpable. Her blood pressure is 120/68 mm Hg, and pulse rate is 60 beats/min. She appears clinically euthyroid.

The patient states that she has friends who have required thyroid hormone replacement after thyroid surgery. Many of them have not felt well while taking thyroid hormone. She is willing to undergo right lobectomy, but her primary goal is to avoid needing thyroid hormone after surgery.

What additional evaluation would be useful to help predict whether this patient will require thyroid hormone replacement following right lobectomy?
- A. TPO antibody titer
- B. Free T_4 measurement
- C. Total T_3 measurement
- D. Repeated serum TSH measurement
- E. Serum thyroglobulin measurement

95 A 56-year-old woman with epilepsy is referred for evaluation of osteoporosis, which was diagnosed based on a screening bone density test done 2 months ago (lowest T-score of –2.6 at the lumbar spine ([Z-score –2.4]). She recently sustained a Colles fracture of her right wrist after falling. She reports diffuse bony pain and muscle weakness. She has limited dietary calcium intake and does not take any calcium or vitamin D supplements. She had surgical menopause at age 45 years. She has no family history of osteoporosis.

On physical examination, her height is 63 in (160 cm) and weight is 124 lb (56.4 kg) (BMI = 22 kg/m²). She is unable to rise from a chair without using her arms. She uses a cane to assist with ambulation.

Laboratory test results:
    Serum calcium = 8.0 mg/dL (8.2-10.2 mg/dL) (SI: 2.0 mmol/L [2.1-2.6 mmol/L])
    Serum phosphate = 2.2 mg/dL (2.3-4.7 mg/dL) (SI: 0.7 mmol/L [0.7-1.5 mmol/L])
    Serum creatinine = 0.7 mg/dL (0.6-1.1 mg/dL) (SI: 61.9 μmol/L [53.0-97.2 μmol/L])
    Serum intact PTH = 80 pg/mL (10-65 pg/mL) (SI: 80 ng/L [10-65 ng/L])
    Serum 25-hydroxyvitamin D = 6 ng/mL (30-80 ng/mL [optimal]) (SI: 15.0 nmol/L [74.9-199.7 nmol/L])
    Serum 1,25-dihydroxyvitamin D = 35 pg/mL (16-65 pg/mL) (SI: 91 pmol/L [41.6-169.0 pmol/L])
    Serum albumin = 3.4 g/dL (3.5-5.0 g/dL) (SI: 34 g/L [35-50 g/L])
    Serum alkaline phosphatase = 150 U/L (50-120 U/L) (SI: 2.51 μkat/L [0.84-2.00 μkat/L])
    Urinary calcium = 30 mg/24 h (100-300 mg/24 h) (SI: 0.8 mmol/d [2.5-7.5 mmol/d])

In addition to dietary counseling and calcium supplementation, which of the following should be recommended?
- A. Vitamin D
- B. Vitamin D for 3 months, then start alendronate
- C. Vitamin D for 3 months, then start zoledronic acid
- D. Vitamin D for 3 months, then start denosumab
- E. Vitamin D for 3 months, then start teriparatide

96 A 44-year-old woman with prediabetes, hypothyroidism, and depression seeks assistance with weight loss. Her medications include metformin, levothyroxine, and paroxetine. During your initial visit, you recommend that she change her meal plan, start tracking her food intake, and initiate an exercise routine. Four weeks later, she returns to clinic and has lost 6 lb (2.7 kg), but at subsequent follow-up visits she has not lost additional weight. The patient reports the main barrier to adhering to her meal plan is hunger. She thinks about food all the time.

You discuss her options and she agrees to start a weight-loss medication. One day after initiating the medication, she experiences tremors, diaphoresis, and diarrhea. She stops all her medications and the symptoms resolve. Currently, she is taking only levothyroxine.

On physical examination, her blood pressure is 113/71 mm Hg, pulse rate is 64 beats/min, and temperature is 97°F. Her height is 63.5 in (161.3 cm), and weight is 189 lb (88.6 kg) (BMI = 33 kg/m²). She is well developed and well nourished. Her lungs are clear to auscultation bilaterally. Heart sounds are regular, and she has no murmurs. Her neurologic examination is grossly intact. Deep tendon reflex are 2+.

The addition of which of the following medications most likely contributed to this patient's symptoms?
- A. Lorcaserin
- B. Liraglutide
- C. Phentermine
- D. Orlistat
- E. Topiramate

97 A 48-year-old man is being seen in the endocrinology clinic for follow-up of diabetes mellitus. Diabetes and hemochromatosis were both diagnosed 7 years ago. His most recent hemoglobin A_{1c} measurement was 6.8% (51 mmol/mol) obtained 2 weeks ago. He is currently taking metformin, 2000 mg daily, and he administers insulin glargine once daily (36 units at bedtime). Mild peripheral neuropathy is his only microvascular diabetes complication. He has hemolytic anemia, compensated cirrhosis of the liver, and hypertension. He is being treated with losartan/hydrochlorothiazide (100/25 mg daily). He has a history of recurrent urinary tract infections, but he is not currently taking an antibiotic. He is being treated with topical testosterone for hypogonadism. He does not smoke cigarettes or drink alcohol.

His father has hemochromatosis and diabetes mellitus.

On physical examination, his height is 70 in (178 cm) and weight is 204 lb (92.7 kg) (BMI = 29.3 kg/m²). His blood pressure is 138/87 mm Hg, and pulse rate is 82 beats/min. Findings on heart, lung, and vascular examinations are normal. The liver edge is palpable at the right costal margin and is nontender. There is mildly reduced sensation to vibrational sense in each foot. Ankle reflexes are reduced.

Laboratory test results:
   Creatinine = 1.4 mg/dL (0.7-1.3 mg/dL) (SI: 123.8 μmol/L [61.9-114.9 μmol/L])
   TSH = 1.8 mIU/L (0.5-5.0 mIU/L)
   Free T_4 = 1.2 ng/dL (0.8-1.8 ng/dL) (SI: 15.4 pmol/L [10.30-23.17 pmol/L])
   Albumin = 3.7 g/dL (3.5-5.0 g/dL) (SI: 37 g/L [35-50 g/L])
   ALT = 32 U/L (10-40 U/L) (SI: 0.53 μkat/L [0.17-0.67 μkat/L])
   AST = 42 U/L (20-48 U/L) (SI: 0.70 μkat/L [0.33-0.80 μkat/L])
   Urinary albumin = 6.0 μg/mg creat (30-300 μg/mg creat)

Fingerstick glucose readings (point of care) are shown (*see table*).

Day	Breakfast	Lunch	Dinner	Bedtime
Monday	97 mg/dL (SI: 5.4 mmol/L)	187 mg/dL (SI: 10.4 mmol/L)	189 mg/dL (SI: 10.5 mmol/L)	197 mg/dL (SI: 10.9 mmol/L)
Tuesday	113 mg/dL (SI: 6.3 mmol/L)	194 mg/dL (SI: 10.8 mmol/L)	208 mg/dL (SI: 11.5 mmol/L)	212 mg/dL (SI: 11.8 mmol/L)
Wednesday	106 mg/dL (SI: 5.9 mmol/L)	198 mg/dL (SI: 11.0 mmol/L)	206 mg/dL (SI: 11.4 mmol/L)	217 mg/dL (SI: 12.0 mmol/L)
Thursday	102 mg/dL (SI: 5.7 mmol/L)	192 mg/dL (SI: 10.7 mmol/L)	201 mg/dL (SI: 11.1 mmol/L)	196 mg/dL (SI: 10.9 mmol/L)
Friday	109 mg/dL (SI: 6.0 mmol/L)	175 mg/dL (SI: 9.7 mmol/L)	188 mg/dL (SI: 10.4 mmol/L)	203 mg/dL (SI: 11.3 mmol/L)

In addition to referring the patient to the nutritionist to review a diabetic meal plan, which of the following is the best approach to manage his diabetes?

A. Start empagliflozin
B. Start dulaglutide
C. Increase the insulin glargine dosage
D. Stop insulin glargine and start mixed insulin (70/30) twice daily
E. No treatment changes needed as hemoglobin A_{1c} is at goal

98 A 53-year-old man with a history of nonfunctioning pituitary macroadenoma is seen for follow-up 6 months after transsphenoidal surgery. Secondary hypogonadism was diagnosed 2 years ago, and he has since been on testosterone replacement (at the time, his primary care physician had documented normal prolactin, LH, and FSH). Only more recently, when he developed headaches, did his primary care physician order brain MRI, which showed a sellar mass (*see left image [preoperative]*). With the exception of central hypogonadism, his primary care physician reports that preoperatively he had documented normal pituitary function, including normal results from a cosyntropin-stimulation test, although these laboratory results are not available to you. The mass was successfully removed (*see right image [postoperative]*).

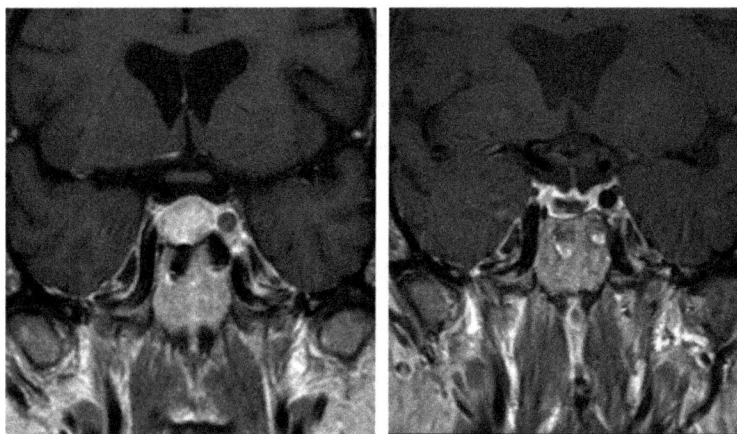

Pathology confirmed a pituitary adenoma, with negative staining for GH, ACTH, and prolactin.

At his clinic appointment today, the patient reports that he is not feeling well. He has been having a hard time performing his duties at work and feels fatigued. His only medication is testosterone gel (1.62%, 4 pump presses daily).

On physical examination, his blood pressure is 127/86 mm Hg and pulse rate is 79 beats/min. His height is 75 in (190.5 cm), and weight is 347 lb (157.7 kg) (BMI = 43.4 kg/m²). His examination findings are normal except for obesity and small testes (8 mL bilaterally).

Laboratory test results:

Cortisol (8 AM) = 15.8 μg/dL (5-25 μg/dL) (SI: 435.9 nmol/L [137.9-689.7 nmol/L])

Prolactin = 8.7 ng/mL (4-23 ng/mL) (SI: 0.38 nmol/L [0.17-1.00 nmol/L])

IGF-1 = 187 ng/mL (84-233 ng/mL) (SI: 24.5 nmol/L [11.0-30.5 nmol/L])

TSH = 1.2 mIU/L (0.5-5.0 mIU/L)

Free T$_4$ = 0.9 ng/dL (0.8-1.8 ng/dL) (SI: 11.6 pmol/L [10.30-23.17 pmol/L])

Testosterone = 475 ng/dL (300-900 ng/dL) (SI: 16.5 nmol/L [10.4-31.2 nmol/L])

Comprehensive metabolic panel, normal

Which of the following is the best next step in this patient's management?
A. Perform another cosyntropin-stimulation test
B. Perform a GH-stimulation test
C. Increase the testosterone dosage
D. Switch to injectable testosterone
E. Start levothyroxine

99 A 60-year-old woman presents with concerns of weight gain, muscle weakness, and worsening hypertension. She describes a 66-lb (30-kg) weight gain over the course of a year, with the development of abdominal obesity, a buffalo hump, and facial fullness.

On physical examination, her blood pressure is 120/68 mm Hg and pulse rate is 68 beats/min. Her height is 60.6 in (154 cm), and weight is 179.7 lb (81.7 kg) (BMI = 34.4 kg/m^2). She has a cushingoid appearance, moon facies, a dorsocervical fat pad, violaceous striae on the abdomen, and multiple ecchymoses.

Laboratory test results:

Urinary free cortisol = 191 μg/24 h (<45 μg/24 h) (SI: 527.2 nmol/d [11-138 nmol/d])

8 AM cortisol after overnight 1-mg dexamethasone = 21.5 μg/dL (SI: 593.1 nmol/L)

Late-night salivary cortisol, markedly elevated on 4 consecutive nights

Random morning ACTH = <5 pg/mL (10-60 pg/mL) (SI: <1.1 pmol/L [2.2-13.2 pmol/L])

Abdominal CT reveals a 1.7 × 2.4-cm right adrenal adenoma (*see image, arrow*). The left adrenal gland appears normal. Adrenal Cushing syndrome is diagnosed, and she is advised to undergo laparoscopic right adrenalectomy.

Which of the following describes the most likely postoperative steroid strategy that this patient will require?
A. No further glucocorticoids postoperatively
B. Short-duration taper (days-to-weeks) of supplemental glucocorticoid therapy
C. Short-duration taper (days-to-weeks) of supplemental glucocorticoid and mineralocorticoid therapy
D. Long-duration taper (weeks-to-months) of supplemental glucocorticoid therapy
E. Long-duration taper (weeks-to-months) of supplemental glucocorticoid and mineralocorticoid therapy

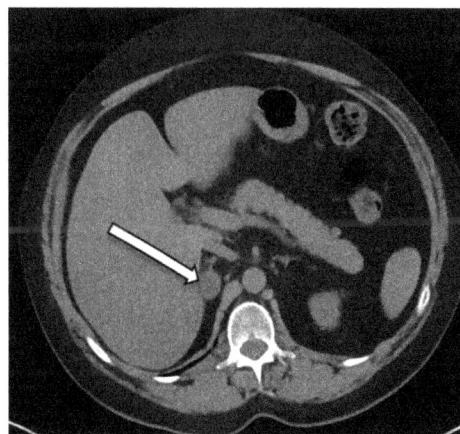

100 A 72-year-old man with hypertension, mitral valve insufficiency, coronary artery disease (status post coronary artery bypass grafting x3), and hyperlipidemia undergoes mitral valve replacement and the maze procedure. Postoperatively, he develops atrial fibrillation with a heart rate of 170 beats/min and is started on intravenous amiodarone. Two days later, his treatment is switched to amiodarone, 200 mg orally twice daily. At his follow-up visit with his cardiologist 3 months later, his pulse rate is 116 beats/min and irregularly irregular. He has shortness of breath at rest. He has also noticed loose stools and has lost 10 lb (4.5 kg) despite good appetite. His cardiologist orders thyroid function testing and refers him to you. His TSH level was 0.5 mIU/L 1 year ago.

TSH = <0.01 mIU/L (0.5-5.0 mIU/L)
Free T$_4$ = 5.0 ng/dL (0.8-1.8 ng/dL) (SI: 64.4 pmol/L [10.30-23.17 pmol/L])
Free T$_3$ = 7.0 pg/mL (2.3-4.2 pg/mL) (SI: 10.8 pmol/L [3.53-6.45 pmol/L])
Thyroid radioiodine uptake = 1% at 24 hours

His current medications are amiodarone, 200 mg twice daily; lisinopril, 20 mg daily; metoprolol XL, 50 mg daily; rivaroxaban, 5 mg twice daily; and atorvastatin, 40 mg daily.

On physical examination, he has a slightly enlarged thyroid gland that is firm, irregular, and nontender. He has an irregularly irregular heart rate at 126 beats/min and no lower-extremity edema. There is mild tremor in his hands.

In addition to increasing his β-adrenergic blocker dosage, which of the following is the most appropriate treatment?
A. Methimazole
B. Methimazole and prednisone
C. Prednisone
D. Total thyroidectomy
E. Radioiodine treatment

101 A 22-year-old woman with a 4-year history of type 1 diabetes mellitus calls the office requesting advice. She has been on insulin pump therapy for 4 years and her hemoglobin A$_{1c}$ values have been in the range of 7.2% to 8.4% (55-68 mmol/mol) for the past 2 years. She has no known diabetes-related complications and has not had any episodes of diabetic ketoacidosis since her initial presentation. She now reports that her blood glucose values have been running high since early this morning, with measurements increasing from 190 mg/dL (10.5 mmol/L) upon awakening at 6:30 AM to 382 mg/dL (21.2 mmol/L) when she checked at 3 PM before calling you. She reports that she has entered her carbohydrate consumption and glucose readings as usual. Her urine is positive for moderate ketones. She has had no nausea, vomiting, or fever. She changed her infusion set yesterday at 11 AM, and there is no tenderness or redness at the insertion site and no pump errors or messages.

Her pump settings are as follows:
Midnight to 6 AM: 0.8 units/h
6 AM to 6 PM: 1.1 units/h
6 PM to midnight: 1.0 units/h
Insulin-to-carbohydrate ratio: 1 unit to 8 g carbohydrate
Correction: 1 unit per 30 mg/dL above 150 mg/dL (>8.3 mmol/L)

Which of the following should you advise as the best next step?
A. Go to the closest emergency department for intravenous fluids
B. Increase her basal rate by 30%
C. Immediately change insulin, reservoir, infusion set, and infusion site, then administer correction bolus using fresh supplies
D. Administer a correction bolus via insulin syringe
E. Remove the pump and administer insulin glargine

102 A 54-year-old man is referred by his primary care physician for management of cardiovascular risk. He has a history of heterozygous familial hypercholesterolemia. At age 26 years, he developed chest pain and underwent 2-vessel coronary bypass. He has been treated with lipid-lowering medications since that time. His current regimen includes rosuvastatin, 40 mg daily; ezetimibe, 10 mg daily; and niacin, 1500 mg daily. He has had no other events and does not have angina, shortness of breath, or other cardiac symptoms. He has treated hypertension and prediabetes. He does not smoke cigarettes, and he occasionally drinks alcohol.

On physical examination, his blood pressure is 118/72 mm Hg and pulse rate is 62 beats/min. His height is 68.5 in (174 cm), and weight is 282 lb (128.2 kg) (BMI = 42.2 kg/m^2). He has marked abdominal adiposity.

Laboratory test results (sample drawn while fasting, on therapy):
Total cholesterol = 181 mg/dL (<200 mg/dL [optimal]) (SI: 4.69 mmol/L [<5.18 mmol/L])
Triglycerides = 104 mg/dL (<150 mg/dL [optimal]) (SI: 2.69 mmol/L [<1.70 mmol/L])
HDL cholesterol = 33 mg/dL (>60 mg/dL [optimal]) (SI: 0.85 mmol/L [>1.55 mmol/L])
LDL cholesterol = 127 mg/dL (<100 mg/dL [optimal]) (SI: 3.29 mmol/L [<2.59 mmol/L])
Non-HDL cholesterol = 148 mg/dL (<130 mg/dL [optimal]) (SI: 3.83 mmol/L [<3.37 mmol/L])
Lipoprotein (a) = 3 mg/dL (≤30 mg/dL) (SI: 0.11 µmol/L [≤1.07 µmol/L])
Hemoglobin A$_{1c}$ = 6.3% (4.0%-5.6%) (45 mmol/mol [20-38 mmol/mol])
Creatinine = 0.7 mg/dL (0.7-1.3 mg/dL) (SI: 61.9 µmol/L [61.9-114.9 µmol/L])
TSH = 2.8 mIU/L (0.5-5.0 mIU/L)
Fasting plasma glucose = 118 mg/dL (70-99 mg/dL) (SI: 6.5 mmol/L [3.9-5.5 mmol/L])

In addition to stopping niacin, which of the following is the best next step in this patient's cardiovascular risk management?
A. No changes needed now
B. Add marine omega-3 fatty acids
C. Add metformin
D. Add semaglutide
E. Add evolocumab

103 A 25-year-old man is referred to you for evaluation of left thigh pain. His medical history is unremarkable except for late childhood onset of lower-extremity bowing and bilateral genu varus. Approximately 6 months ago, he developed left medial lateral thigh pain without antecedent trauma. The pain is worse with ambulation and has intensified over 3 to 4 months. A plain radiograph is shown (*see image*).

His family history is negative for bone disease but is notable for nephrolithiasis in his father and paternal uncle. Review of systems is negative for other bone pain, dyspnea, cough, rashes, or relevant dental history.

On physical examination, he appears well. Findings on examination of the head, eyes, ears, nose, and throat are normal, as are those from chest, cardiac, and abdominal examination. He does have moderate tenderness to palpation over the lateral proximal mid left thigh, as well as mild tenderness to firm palpation of both anterior mid tibias.

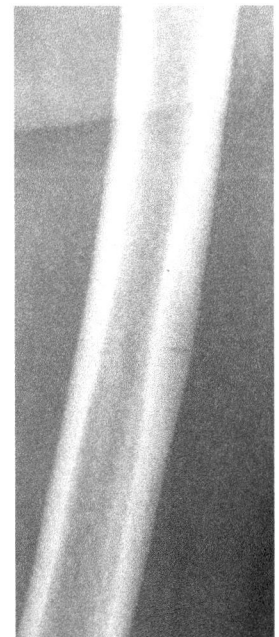

Laboratory test results:
Serum calcium = 9.5 mg/dL (8.2-10.2 mg/dL (SI: 2.4 mmol/L [2.1-2.6 mmol/L])
Serum phosphate = 1.9 mg/dL (2.3-4.7 mg/dL) (SI: 0.6 mmol/L [0.7-1.5 mmol/L])
Serum magnesium = 2.1 mg/dL (1.5-2.3 mg/dL) (SI: 0.7 mmol/L [0.6-0.9 mmol/L])
Serum albumin = 4.4 mg/dL (3.5-5.0 g/dL) (SI: 44 g/L [35-50 g/L])
Serum creatinine = 1.0 mg/dL (0.7-1.3 mg/dL) (SI: 88.4 µmol/L [61.9-114.9 µmol/L])
Serum alkaline phosphatase = 165 U/L (50-120 U/L) (SI: 2.76 µkat/L [0.84-2.00 µkat/L])
Serum intact PTH = 15 pg/mL (10-65 pg/mL) (SI: 15 ng/L [10-65 ng/L])
Serum 25-hydroxyvitamin D = 35 ng/mL (30-80 ng/mL [optimal]) (SI: 87.4 nmol/L [74.9-199.7 nmol/L])

Serum 1,25-dihydroxyvitamin D = 140 pg/mL (16-65 pg/mL) (SI: 364 pmol/L [41.6-169.0 pmol/L])
Urinary calcium = 450 mg/24 h (100-300 mg/24 h) (SI: 11.3 mmol/d [2.5-7.5 mmol/d])
Urinary creatinine = 1.0 mg/24 h (1.0-2.0 g/24 h) (SI: 8.8 mmol/d [8.8-17.7 mmol/d])
Urinary volume = 1500 mL/24 h

On the basis of his clinical presentation, which of the following is the most appropriate therapy for his skeletal disorder?
A. Elemental phosphorus
B. Elemental phosphorus and calcitriol
C. Asfotase alfa
D. Hydrochlorothiazide
E. Teriparatide

104 A 78-year-old woman has had diabetes mellitus for 22 years. Three months ago, she underwent urologic surgery for a renal stone and her serum creatinine level increased to 1.8 mg/dL (159.1 μmol/L) and has remained at this level, as documented by 2 subsequent measurements. Her estimated glomerular filtration rate is 29 mL/min per 1.73 m². She has no known diabetes complications. Her current diabetes medications are metformin, 1000 mg twice daily, and glipizide, 2.5 mg daily. Other medications include lisinopril, 10 mg daily, and atorvastatin, 10 mg daily.

Laboratory test results:
Hemoglobin A$_{1c}$ = 8.3% (4.0%-5.6%) (67 mmol/mol [20-38 mmol/mol])
Serum urea nitrogen = 25 mg/dL (8-23 mg/dL) (SI: 8.9 mmol/L [2.9-8.2 mmol/L])
Creatinine = 1.8 mg/dL (0.6-1.1 mg/dL) (SI: 159.1 μmol/L [53.0-97.2 μmol/L])
Glucose = 185 mg/dL (70-99 mg/dL) (SI: 10.3 mmol/L [3.9-5.5 mmol/L])

On physical examination, her height is 65 in (165 cm) and weight is 110 lb (50 kg) (BMI = 18.3 kg/m²). Her blood pressure is 153/70 mm Hg, and pulse rate is 90 beats/min.

Which of the following is the best next step?
A. Discontinue metformin and glipizide and start low-dosage basal insulin
B. Discontinue metformin and start a GLP-1 receptor agonist
C. Reduce the metformin dosage to 500 mg twice daily
D. Discontinue metformin and continue glipizide
E. Discontinue metformin and start an SGLT-2 inhibitor

105 A 60-year-old man presents to the emergency department with new left lower-quadrant pain. Abdominal CT with intravenous contrast is performed to evaluate for diverticulitis. An incidental 2.2-cm left adrenal mass is identified and is described as round and with an attenuation value of 41 Hounsfield units.

Two months later, his primary care physician orders another abdominal CT with a contrast washout protocol. The 2.6 × 2.6 × 2.2-cm left adrenal mass is again noted (*right image, arrow*) and is described as oval and solid without calcifications or hemorrhage. The unenhanced attenuation value is 24 Hounsfield units; the attenuation value 1 minute after intravenous contrast is 61 Hounsfield units; and the attenuation value 15 minutes after contrast is 29 Hounsfield units. The absolute washout is calculated as 87% and the relative washout is calculated as 53%. The right adrenal gland is normal in appearance (*left image, arrow*).

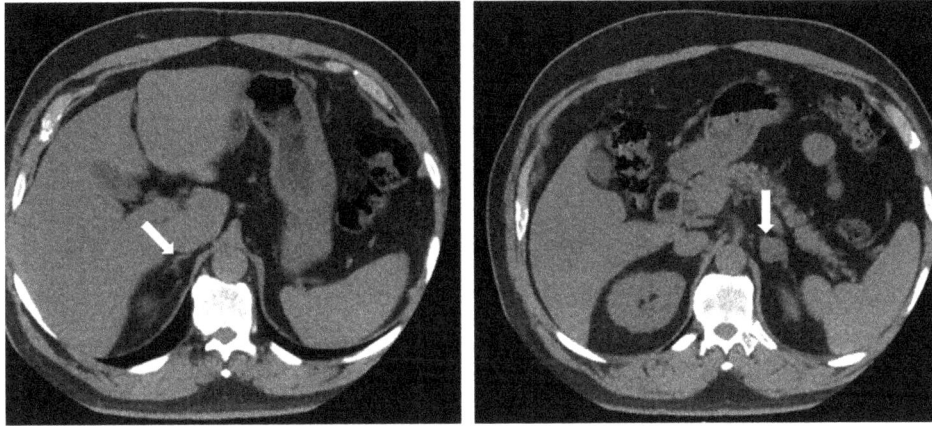

The left adrenal mass is most likely to be which of the following?
A. Adrenocortical adenoma
B. Adrenocortical carcinoma
C. Metastasis from extraadrenal malignancy
D. Myelolipoma
E. Pheochromocytoma

106 You are asked to consult on a 71-year-old man for a nonsuppressible serum testosterone level. High-risk localized prostate cancer was diagnosed 12 months before consultation. Following diagnosis, he was treated with external beam radiation therapy and adjuvant androgen deprivation therapy using the GnRH analogue goserelin. Four months later, despite adherence to goserelin therapy, his serum testosterone was not adequately suppressed (144 ng/dL [300-900 ng/dL; castration range <29 ng/dL] [SI: 5.0 nmol/L (10.4-31.2 nmol/L; castration range <1.0 nmol/L)]). He was subsequently switched to an alternative GnRH analogue, leuprolide, without adequate reduction in his serum testosterone 3 months later (155 ng/dL [5.4 nmol/L]). Consequently, bilateral orchidectomy was performed. Two months later, his serum testosterone remained detectable (150 ng/dL [5.2 nmol/L]). On review of symptoms, he describes mild fatigue but no hot flashes.

On physical examination, he has a tanned appearance. His height is 64 in (162.5 cm), and weight is 164 lb (74.5 kg) (BMI = 28.1 kg/m²).

Current laboratory test results:
Serum testosterone = 167 ng/dL (SI: 5.8 nmol/L)
LH = 0.5 mIU/mL (1.0-9.0 mIU/mL) (SI: 0.5 IU/L [1.0-9.0 IU/L])
DHEA-S = 340 µg/dL (25-131 µg/dL) (SI: 9.2 µmol/L [0.68-3.55 µmol/L])
PSA = 0.8 ng/mL (therapeutic target, <0.03 ng/mL) (SI: SI: 0.8 µg/L [<0.03 µg/L])

Which of the following serum measurements should you assess next?
A. hCG
B. SHBG
C. 17α-hydroxyprogesterone
D. Estradiol
E. Dihydrotestosterone

107 A 21-year-old woman with polycystic ovary syndrome is referred to endocrinology for management of irregular menses. After menarche at age 12 years, the patient had regular menses until she started college. She skipped months at a time, alternating between unpredictable periods and more frequent bleeding, which prompted her to visit the university health service for evaluation and treatment. After polycystic ovary syndrome was diagnosed, she initiated oral contraceptives (1 year ago). Six months ago, she had a pulmonary embolism, following which oral contraceptives were discontinued. Anticoagulation was limited to 3 months for a provoked episode. Her periods are irregular again, and she would like to learn about her treatment options. She is not sexually active.

She has a family history of venous thromboembolic disease. Her mother and sister have a history of lower-extremity deep venous thrombosis in the context of surgery. There is no family history of diabetes.

On physical examination, her height is 64 in (162.5 cm) and weight is 125 lb (56.8 kg) (BMI = 21.5 kg/m²). She has no signs of hirsutism.

Health records she brought from the university health service reveal mildly elevated total testosterone and normal prolactin, thyroid function, 17-hydroxyprosterone, and fasting glucose.

Which of the following is the best treatment for this patient to restore more regular menstrual cycles?
- A. Metformin
- B. Spironolactone
- C. Combined oral contraceptives with anticoagulation
- D. Micronized progesterone daily
- E. Medroxyprogesterone

108 A 26-year-old woman is referred to you for abnormal results of thyroid function tests, with a question as to whether she should be treated with thyroid hormone. She was an athlete in college and she became concerned about her weight at that time. She no longer exercises, but she is very fearful about weight gain. She follows a low-fat, nondairy, vegetarian diet including large quantities of carrots and celery. She has had amenorrhea for 2 years, but has no other medical conditions. She takes no medications.

On physical examination, the patient appears extremely thin. Her height is 65 in (165 cm), and weight is 102 lb (46.4 kg) (BMI = 17 kg/m²). Her blood pressure is 104/65 mm Hg, and pulse rate is 70 beats/min. She has generalized yellow discoloration of the skin, lanugo is present on her face, and calluses are present across her knuckles. Her thyroid gland is at the lower end of the normal size range and is firm without discrete nodules. Her ankle reflexes are slightly sluggish.

Serial laboratory evaluations obtained by her previous physician are shown (*see table*).

Thyroid Function Tests	2 Years Ago (weight 88 lb [40 kg])	1 Year Ago (weight 92.4 lb [42 kg])	Currently (weight 101.2 lb [46.4 kg])
TSH (0.5-5.0 mIU/L)	0.2 mIU/L	0.25 mIU/L	0.3 mIU/L
Free T₄ (0.8-1.8 ng/dL [SI: 10.30-23.17 pmol/L])	0.7 ng/dL (SI: 9.0 pmol/L)	0.8 ng/dL (SI: 12.3 pmol/L)	0.7 ng/dL (SI: 9.0 pmol/L)
Total T₃ (70-200 ng/dL [SI: 1.08-3.08 nmol/L])	50 ng/dL (SI: 0.77 nmol/L)	60 ng/dL (SI: 0.92 nmol/L)	60 ng/dL (SI: 0.92 nmol/L)
Reverse T₃ (10-24 ng/dL [SI: 0.15-0.37 nmol/L])	30 ng/dL (SI: 0.46 nmol/L)	35 ng/dL (SI: 0.54 nmol/L)	32 ng/dL (SI: 0.49 nmol/L)
TPO antibodies (<2.0 IU/mL [SI: <2.0 kIU/L])	1.0 IU/mL (SI: 1.0 kIU/L)	...	...

Which of the following is most likely contributing to the patient's abnormal thyroid function?
- A. Altered kisspeptin signaling
- B. Decreased hepatic type 1 deiodinase activity
- C. Decreased hepatic type 3 deiodinase activity
- D. Increased TSH pulsatility
- E. Increased hypothalamic thyrotropin-releasing hormone expression

109 A 35-year-old man was diagnosed with type 2 diabetes mellitus 1 year ago. His hemoglobin A_{1c} level was 7.2% (55 mmol/mol) at diagnosis. He has managed his blood glucose with dietary modification and exercise, and he has lost 15 lb (6.8 kg). His hemoglobin A_{1c} level at today's visit is 6.7% (50 mmol/mol).

He wants to discuss his family history of prostate cancer, which was diagnosed in his father at age 68 years. The patient has recently read about an increased risk of cancer in patients with type 2 diabetes. He wants to know whether there are possible treatments that would reduce his risk of prostate cancer.

How would you counsel the patient to reduce his risk of prostate cancer?
A. No specific therapy
B. Start metformin
C. Start glipizide
D. Start pioglitazone
E. Start insulin

110 A 47-year-old physician accompanies his wife to her visit for management of a thyroid nodule. You note that his hands are large and his jaw is protruding; before they leave, you mention to him in private the possibility that he has acromegaly. He sees his primary care physician, who measures serum his IGF-1 level on 2 occasions—both values return mildly elevated (1.1 and 1.25 times the upper normal limit). He returns to your office to be formally evaluated. He has always had large hands. For many years, he has been told that he snores loudly. He does not sweat excessively. He has had hypertension for about 5 years, and it is well controlled on lisinopril, 40 mg daily, and metoprolol, 50 mg daily.

On physical examination, his blood pressure is 112/74 mm Hg and pulse rate is 66 beats/min. His height is 73 in (185.4 cm), and weight is 288 lb (131 kg) (BMI = 38 kg/m²). He has no increased teeth spacing, no thyroid enlargement, and no skin tags on his neck.

You order a 2-hour GH-suppression test with 75 g of glucose.

Measurement	Baseline	30 Minutes	60 Minutes	90 Minutes	120 Minutes
Glucose	88 mg/dL (SI: 4.9 mmol/L)	160 mg/dL (SI: 8.9 mmol/L)	122 mg/dL (SI: 6.8 mmol/L)	118 mg/dL (SI: 6.5 mmol/L)	101 mg/dL (SI: 5.6 mmol/L)
GH	1.1 ng/mL (SI: 1.1 µg/L)	1.1 ng/mL (SI: 1.1 µg/L)	1.0 ng/mL (SI: 1.0 µg/L)	1.1 ng/mL (SI: 1.1 µg/L)	1.2 ng/mL (SI: 1.2 µg/L)

Before you have an opportunity to discuss the results with him, he has his office partner order a pituitary MRI with and without gadolinium. This shows a normal pituitary gland.

Which of the following is the best next step in this patient's management?
A. Repeat the GH-suppression test after stopping metoprolol
B. Measure IGFBP-3
C. Measure free IGF-1
D. Measure plasma GHRH
E. No further evaluation

111 A 68-year-old man with a history of esophageal stricture presents for evaluation and management of an elevated alkaline phosphatase level documented on routine blood testing. He does not have any bony pain and has not had any fractures. He has no history of thyroid disease. He takes a daily supplement containing 800 mg of calcium and 1000 IU of cholecalciferol.

On physical examination, there are no palpable bony abnormalities and there is no tenderness to palpation of his spine and hips.

Laboratory test results:

Serum calcium = 9.0 mg/dL (8.2-10.2 mg/dL) (SI: 2.3 mmol/L [2.1-2.6 mmol/L])

Serum phosphate = 2.6 mg/dL (2.3-4.7 mg/dL) (SI: 0.8 mmol/L [0.7-1.5 mmol/L])

Serum creatinine = 0.84 mg/dL (0.7-1.3 mg/dL) (SI: 74.3 μmol/L [61.9-114.9 μmol/L])

Serum 25-hydroxyvitamin D = 39 ng/mL (30-80 ng/mL [optimal]) (SI: 97.3 nmol/L [74.9-199.7 nmol/L])

Serum albumin = 4.1 g/dL (3.5-5.0 g/dL) (SI: 41 g/L [35-50 g/L])

Serum total alkaline phosphatase = 393 U/L (50-120 U/L) (SI: 6.56 μkat/L [0.84-2.00 μkat/L])

Serum bone-specific alkaline phosphatase = 130.3 μg/L (≤24.4 μg/L)

His imaging results are shown (*see images*).

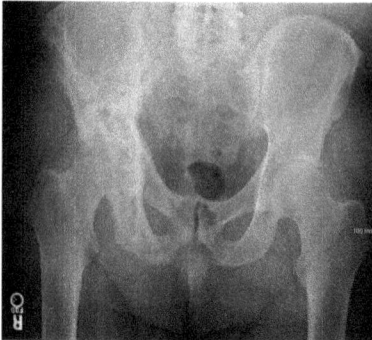

Plain x-ray of the pelvis (anteroposterior view).

Which of the following is the best treatment choice for this patient?

A. Risedronate

B. Zoledronic acid

C. Denosumab

D. Calcitonin

E. No treatment is necessary because he is asymptomatic

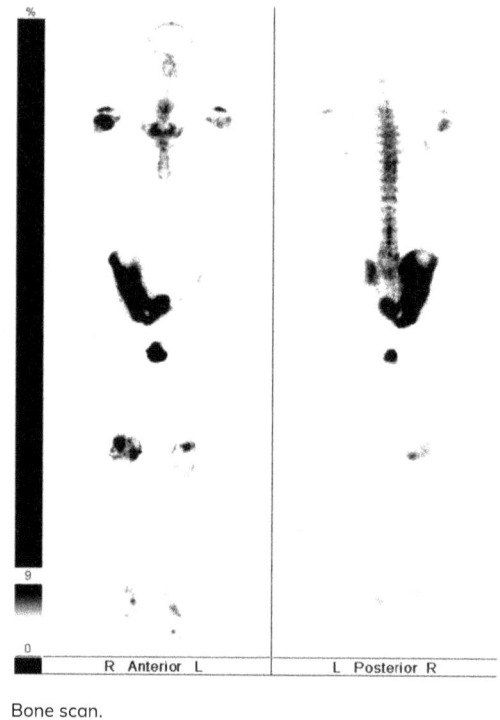

Bone scan.

112 A 38-year-old man with obstructive sleep apnea who underwent Roux-en-Y gastric bypass 7 years ago is referred by his primary care physician. At the time of his surgery, his weight was 275 lb (125 kg) (BMI = 43 kg/m²). Due to frequent travel, he has not been seen for follow-up on a consistent basis. He reports adherence to his regimen of minerals and vitamins. He currently takes a multivitamin and calcium citrate. Three years ago, he became a vegetarian.

On review of systems, he reports hair loss and intermittent diarrhea. On physical examination, his blood pressure is 113/75 mm Hg and pulse rate is 70 beats/min. His height is 67.5 in (171.5 cm), and weight is 195 lb (88.6 kg) (BMI = 30.1 kg/m²). He is in no distress. Lungs are clear to auscultation. On cardiac examination, his heart sounds are normal and rate and rhythm are regular. His abdomen is soft and nontender and bowel sounds are present. He has multiple white stretch marks.

Laboratory test results:

Complete blood cell count, normal

Kidney function, normal

Liver function, normal

Micronutrient measurements:

Cobalamin (vitamin B₁₂) = 650 pg/mL (180-914 pg/mL) (SI: 480 pmol/L [133-674 pmol/L])

Copper = 0.85 μg/mL (0.75-1.45 μg/mL) (SI: 13.4 μmol/L [11.8-22.8 μmol/L])

Iron = 75 μg/dL (50-150 μg/dL) (SI: 13.4 μmol/L [9.0-26.8 μmol/L])

Ferritin = 120 ng/mL (15-200 ng/mL) (SI: 443.8 pmol/L [33.7-449.4 pmol/L])

Folate = 7.0 ng/mL (≥4.0 ng/mL) (SI: 7.0 µg/L [≥4.0 µg/L])

Thiamine (vitamin B$_1$) = 4.5 µg/dL (2.5-7.5 µg/dL) (SI: 133 nmol/L [74-222 nmol/L])

Zinc = 0.46 µg/mL (0.66-1.10 µg/mL) (SI: 7.0 µmol/L [10.1-16.8 µmol/L])

In addition to starting this patient on zinc, 60 mg twice daily, which of the following would you recommend?

A. Cobalamin

B. Iron

C. Folic acid

D. Thiamine

E. Copper

113 A 58-year-old man is admitted to the medical intensive care unit with hypoxic ventilatory failure secondary to pneumonia. He is sedated and intubated for ventilatory support. He is initially on vasopressors for circulatory support, but then transitions to maintenance intravenous fluids. On the second hospital day, he is extubated. On the third hospital day, he is transferred to a progressive care unit.

His medical history is notable for diabetes mellitus and hypertension. His medications before admission included glipizide, metformin, and nifedipine. His hemoglobin A$_{1c}$ level measured at admission was 8.4% (68 mmol/mol). A carbohydrate-controlled diet is initiated, and he is reportedly eating well. However, his blood glucose values range from 200 to 250 mg/dL (11.1-13.9 mmol/L), and you are consulted for diabetes management. There was prerenal azotemia on admission, but his kidney function is now improving (*see table*).

Measurement	On Admission	Current
Serum urea nitrogen	48 mg/dL (SI: 17.1 mmol/L)	32 mg/dL (SI: 11.4 mmol/L)
Creatinine	2.2 mg/dL (SI: 194.5 µmol/L)	1.2 mg/dL (SI: 106.1 µmol/L)

Reference ranges: serum urea nitrogen, 8-23 mg/dL (SI: 2.9-8.2 mmol/L); creatinine, 0.7-1.3 mg/dL (SI: 61.9-114.9 µmol/L).

Which of the following treatment regimens would be most appropriate?

A. Resume metformin and glipizide

B. Administer subcutaneous insulin aspart every 4 to 6 hours as needed on a correctional scale

C. Administer insulin glargine + correctional aspart every 4 to 6 hours only

D. Administer insulin glargine + fixed-dose insulin aspart with meals and on a correctional scale

E. Administer insulin glargine only

114 An 18-year-old woman seeks evaluation for a 12-month history of secondary amenorrhea and reduced vision in her left eye for the last 3 months.

On physical examination, her height is 65 in (165 cm) and weight is 111 lb (50.5 kg) (BMI = 18.5 kg/m^2). Her blood pressure is 95/60 mm Hg. Visual acuity is 20/30 (6/9) in the right eye and 20/120 (6/36) in the left eye. Visual fields demonstrate bilateral inferior quadrantanopia. She has normal secondary sexual characteristics.

Laboratory test results:

Prolactin = 67 ng/mL (4-30 ng/mL) (SI: 2.91 nmol/L [0.17-1.30 nmol/L])

TSH = 0.8 mIU/L (0.5-5.0 mIU/L)

Free T$_4$ = 0.7 ng/dL (0.8-1.8 ng/dL) (SI: 9.01 pmol/L [10.30-23.17 pmol/L])

Serum cortisol (9 AM) = 4.0 µg/dL (5-25 µg/dL) (SI: 110.4 nmol/L [137.9-689.7 nmol/L])

IGF-1 = 125 ng/mL (162-541 ng/mL) (SI: 16.4 nmol/L [21.2-70.9 nmol/L])

FSH = 1.9 mIU/mL (2.0-12.0 mIU/mL [follicular]) (SI: 1.9 IU/L [2.0-12.0 IU/L])

LH = 2.3 mIU/mL (1.0-18.0 mIU/mL [follicular]) (SI: 2.3 IU/L [1.0-18.0 IU/L])

Estradiol = 25 pg/mL (10-180 pg/mL [follicular]) (SI: 91.8 pmol/L [36.7-660.8 pmol/L])

MRI of the sella (T1 postcontrast) is shown (*see image*).

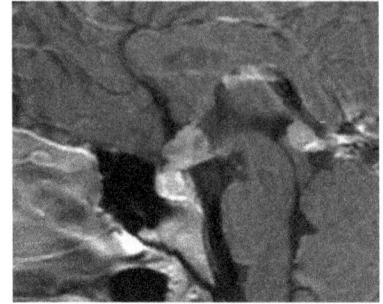

Which of the following is the most likely diagnosis?
A. Craniopharyngioma
B. Germinoma
C. Nonfunctioning pituitary adenoma
D. Rathke cleft cyst
E. Suprasellar meningioma

115 A 42-year-old man presents with epigastric and right flank pain. Abdominal CT reveals a 10-cm left adrenal mass. There are no signs of masses or metastases in the liver or lungs. There is no indication of thrombus in the vena cava or renal vein. He undergoes a radical left adrenalectomy with nephrectomy, and the pathology reveals adrenocortical carcinoma. The pathology report indicates that the tumor is 10 cm in largest diameter, and the Ki67 index is 25%. There is focal vascular invasion, and the tumor abuts the peripheral margin of the surgical specimen. Two of 10 lymph nodes from the periadrenal retroperitoneum are positive for malignant cells. There is no tumor in the kidney sample. CT imaging 7 days after the surgery shows no evidence of the residual tumor. The patient recovers fully within 14 days.

Which of the following recommendations is the most appropriate treatment now?
A. No further therapy; surveillance imaging in 3 months
B. Etoposide, doxorubicin, cisplatin
C. Streptozotocin
D. Adjuvant mitotane monotherapy
E. Mitotane in addition to etoposide, doxorubicin, cisplatin

116 A 24-year-old woman was initially evaluated 3 years ago for a macroprolactinoma. At the time of diagnosis, her prolactin level was 1796 ng/mL (4-30 ng/mL) (SI: 78.1 nmol/L [0.17-1.30 nmol/L]), and MRI showed a 1.5-cm mass abutting the optic chiasm, but with no compression or displacement and no obvious cavernous sinus invasion. She responded very well to cabergoline, and her prolactin rapidly normalized. Six months later, a follow-up MRI showed significant tumor shrinkage. She is currently taking cabergoline, 0.25 mg twice weekly, which she is tolerating well. Current pituitary MRI shows no obvious evidence of residual pituitary adenoma. Her prolactin level is now 5.1 ng/mL (0.22 nmol/L). Her periods are normal while on oral contraceptives.

On physical examination, she is a well-nourished young woman in no distress. Her blood pressure is 114/63 mm Hg, and pulse rate is 77 beats/min. Her height is 60 in (152.4 cm), and weight is 118.5 lb (53.9 kg) (BMI = 23.1 kg/m^2).

At today's visit, she states that she and her partner would like to conceive fairly soon, if possible.

Which of the following is the best next step?
A. Discontinue oral contraceptives, continue cabergoline
B. Discontinue both oral contraceptives and cabergoline
C. Discontinue oral contraceptives and change from cabergoline to bromocriptine
D. Advise delaying pregnancy at least 2 years to allow for a 5-year cabergoline course
E. Continue current regimen and recommend referral for donor egg in vitro fertilization

117 A 33-year-old man with Klinefelter syndrome desires fertility. He is otherwise healthy, and apart from long-term testosterone replacement with intramuscular testosterone undecanoate, he takes no regular medications. He reports good libido and sexual function.

On physical examination, his blood pressure is 110/70 mm Hg. His height is 72 in (183 cm), and weight is 185 lb (kg) (BMI = 25.1 kg/m²). He appears well androgenized, with normal muscle bulk and body hair. There is no palpable gynecomastia. Testes are 2 mL bilaterally and firm to palpation. His serum trough testosterone concentrations consistently range from 375 to 403 ng/dL (SI: 13.0-14.0 nmol/L) (therapeutic range for trough testosterone 288-432 ng/dL [SI: 10.0-15.0 nmol/L]).

Laboratory test results:
 Complete blood cell count, normal
 Renal function, normal
 Liver function, normal
 Semen analysis, azoospermia

Which of the following is the best next step regarding this patient's goal of fertility?
 A. Recommend use of donor semen
 B. Stop testosterone treatment and start a selective estrogen-receptor modulator
 C. Stop testosterone treatment and start hCG
 D. Switch to transdermal testosterone treatment at 50% of the standard replacement dosage
 E. Recommend testicular sperm extraction and intracytoplasmic sperm injection

118 A 37-year-old man is seen in the emergency department for nausea and vomiting. He has type 1 diabetes mellitus complicated by gastroparesis. He has been intermittently seen by a gastroenterologist who had prescribed metoclopramide, 10 mg 3 times daily before meals. The patient reports that his nausea and bloating were well controlled until 5 days ago when the nausea worsened, accompanied by daily vomiting. His current insulin regimen consists of insulin degludec, 20 units daily, and insulin lispro as needed for meals using a sliding scale. His primary care physician recommended that he seek care at the emergency department. You are consulted to evaluate his gastroparesis.

On physical examination, he is afebrile. His blood pressure is 110/70 mm Hg, pulse rate is 96 beats/min, and respiratory rate is 18 breaths/min and unlabored. His height is 66 in (167.5 cm), and weight is 136.5 lb (62 kg) (BMI = 22 kg/m²). He has decreased sensation in his feet bilaterally. He has a dry mouth and tongue.

Laboratory test results (sample drawn while in the emergency department):
 Serum glucose = 285 mg/dL (70-99 mg/dL) (SI: 15.8 mmol/L [3.9-5.5 mmol/L])
 Sodium = 139 mEq/L (136-142 mEq/L) (SI: 139 mmol/L [136-142 mmol/L])
 Potassium = 3.8 mEq/L (3.5-5.0 mEq/L) (SI: 3.8 mmol/L [3.5-5.0 mmol/L])
 Chloride = 96 mEq/L (96-106 mEq/L) (SI: 96 mmol/L [96-106 mmol/L])
 Bicarbonate = 24 mEq/L (21-28 mEq/L) (SI: 24 mmol/L [21-28 mmol/L])
 Hemoglobin A_{1c} = 10.5% (4.0%-5.6%) (91 mmol/mol [20-38 mmol/mol])
 TSH = 2.12 mIU/L (0.5-5.0 mIU/L)

In addition to giving intravenous fluids and replacing electrolytes, which of the following is the best next step in this patient's management?
 A. Admit to the hospital and treat his nausea with parenteral ondansetron
 B. Perform a cosyntropin-stimulation test
 C. Discharge home and change his diet to small frequent meals
 D. Discharge home and change metoclopramide to oral erythromycin
 E. Perform a urinalysis

119 A 50-year-old woman is referred to you for assistance in the management of hypercalcemia. She presented to her primary care physician with 3 months of abnormal vaginal bleeding and lower abdominal fullness, as well as gradually worsening fatigue and mental confusion. CT at that time revealed a 9 × 11-cm heterogeneously enhancing mass involving the uterine fundus, with evidence of likely metastatic disease involving the retroperitoneal lymph nodes and the lungs. Whole-body bone scanning was negative for evidence of skeletal metastases. Uterine biopsy documented poorly differentiated endometrial carcinoma.

Laboratory test results:
    Serum calcium = 13.0 mg/dL (8.2-10.2 mg/dL (SI: 3.3 mmol/L [2.1-2.6 mmol/L])
    Serum phosphate = 2.5 mg/dL (2.3-4.7 mg/dL) (SI: 0.8 mmol/L [0.7-1.5 mmol/L])
    Serum albumin = 3.0 mg/dL (3.5-5.0 g/dL) (SI: 30 g/L [35-50 g/L])
    Serum urea nitrogen = 42 mg/dL (8-23 mg/dL) (SI: 15.0 mmol/L [2.9-8.2 mmol/L])
    Serum creatinine = 1.4 mg/dL (0.6-1.1 mg/dL) (SI: 123.8 µmol/L [53.0-97.2 µmol/L])
    Serum intact PTH = 12 pg/mL (10-65 pg/mL) (SI: 12 ng/L [10-65 ng/L])
    Plasma PTHrP = 7.5 pmol/L (<2.0 pmol/L)
    Serum 25-hydroxyvitamin D = 28 ng/mL (30-80 ng/mL [optimal]) (SI: 69.9 nmol/L [74.9-199.7 nmol/L])
    Serum 1,25-dihydroxyvitamin D = 30 pg/mL (16-65 pg/mL) (SI: 78.0 pmol/L [41.6-169.0 pmol/L])

She is initially treated with hydration, which resolves her azotemia. She then receives zoledronic acid, 4 mg intravenously, and starts pembrolizumab, with a subsequent fall in her corrected serum calcium to 10.5 mg/dL (2.6 mmol/L) after 4 days. She is seen in the oncology clinic 2 weeks after hospital discharge, at which time her serum calcium level is 12.8 mg/dL (3.2 mmol/L) with a serum creatinine level of 1.0 mg/dL (88.4 µmol/L). She is given a second dose of zoledronic acid, 4 mg intravenously. Upon follow-up 10 days later, she is found to have a serum calcium level of 13.2 mg/dL (3.3 mmol/L), along with worsening confusion, polyuria, and polydipsia.

In addition to intravenous hydration, which of the following is the best choice to manage this patient's hypercalcemia?
    A. Furosemide
    B. Pamidronate
    C. Denosumab
    D. Calcitonin
    E. Prednisone

120 A 63-year-old woman with type 2 diabetes mellitus, mixed hyperlipidemia, major depression, and obstructive sleep apnea is referred by her sleep medicine physician for assistance with weight loss. In the past, the patient tried a commercial weight-loss program. However, after participating actively for 6 months, she did not lose weight, but actually gained 5 lb (2.3 kg). She also took an over-the-counter supplement (garcinia cambogia) to help decrease her appetite, but she did not lose weight. Most days, she skips breakfast and has 2 large meals. For the past 12 months, about once a week, she has an episode when her meals last about 2 hours, during which she eats large portions. She usually eats alone because she is embarrassed about the amount she is eating. At the end of a meal, she feels uncomfortably full. She knows that her weight is a problem and she is ashamed by how much she eats. She is currently not participating in an exercise program. Her medications are metformin, 1000 mg twice daily; bupropion, 200 mg daily; and atorvastatin, 40 mg daily.

On physical examination, her blood pressure is 140/78 mm Hg and pulse rate is 60 beats/min. Her height is 63 in (160 cm), and weight is 210 lb (95.5 kg) (BMI = 37.2 kg/m²). The patient is in no distress. Her lungs are clear to auscultation bilaterally. On cardiac examination, her heart sounds are normal and rate and rhythm are regular. Her abdomen is soft and nontender. She has no rashes.

Laboratory test result:
    Hemoglobin A$_{1c}$ = 6.0% (4.0%-5.6%) (42 mmol/mol [20-38 mmol/mol])

If you were to recommend a medication for this patient, which of the following would you choose?

    A. Empagliflozin

    B. Phentermine

    C. Lorcaserin

    D. Fluoxetine

    E. Liraglutide

ENDOCRINE SELF-ASSESSMENT PROGRAM 2020

Part II

ANSWER: D) Teriparatide

This postmenopausal woman has severe osteoporosis (very low T-scores and a right hip fragility fracture) in the setting of end-stage liver disease. She is a liver transplant candidate and is already at high risk of future fracture before transplant; furthermore, she is expected to have significant decline in her bone mineral density within the first 6 months after she receives a liver transplant. The high-turnover state documented after liver transplant is thought to be due to a combination of factors, including resolution of the liver disease, use of glucocorticoid therapy, and the development of secondary hyperparathyroidism due to possible renal effects of the immunosuppressant therapy. This is in contrast to the decreased bone formation and low turnover typically seen before liver transplant. Pretransplant laboratory evaluation of patients with end-stage liver disease has shown decreased serum concentrations of 25-hydroxyvitamin D (since vitamin D is hydroxylated in the liver by hepatic 25-hydroxylase), PTH, and osteocalcin when compared with concentrations of healthy controls. However, there are no pretransplant variables that reliably predict posttransplant bone loss and fracture in individual patients. Subsequent recovery of bone mineral density at the spine has been documented following liver transplant in patients receiving no treatment for bone disease, reaching pretransplant values at about 2 years after transplant and staying stable thereafter. However, vertebral fracture risk remains high after liver transplant regardless of changes in bone mineral density.

As with any other patient with osteoporosis, she should be counseled on fall prevention, as well as receive pharmacologic therapy for osteoporosis, with the most appropriate drug chosen given her comorbidities. With her history of esophageal varices and upper gastrointestinal bleeding, it would be prudent to avoid using an oral bisphosphonate such as alendronate (Answer A), which could cause esophageal irritation. Since she is planning to have multiple teeth extracted soon, it would also be wise to avoid initiating an intravenous bisphosphonate such as zoledronic acid (Answer B) due to the low risk of osteonecrosis of the jaw. Osteonecrosis of the jaw is defined as exposed necrotic bone in the maxillofacial region, not healing after 8 weeks in patients with no history of craniofacial radiation. It appears as areas of exposed yellow or white hard bone with smooth or ragged borders. Risk factors for developing osteonecrosis of the jaw include dose and duration of exposure to bisphosphonate therapy, intravenous administration of bisphosphonate therapy, glucocorticoids, cancer and anticancer therapy, cigarette smoking, poorly fitting dentures, and preexisting dental disease. As osteonecrosis of the jaw often follows invasive dental procedures (such as extractions or implants), it is recommended that these be performed and that healing be complete before starting bisphosphonate therapy if circumstances allow. After transplant, bisphosphonates are considered the medical therapy of choice for the prevention of bone loss if there are no contraindications.

Denosumab (Answer C) is a fully human monoclonal antibody to the receptor activator of nuclear factor kappaB ligand (RANKL). By blocking the binding of RANKL to RANK, it reduces osteoclast formation, function, and survival, which results in decreased bone resorption and increased bone density. Osteonecrosis of the jaw has also been reported with the use of denosumab, which would eliminate this option as the most appropriate drug for this patient now. Furthermore, there are limited data on the use of this agent after transplant, and a study of kidney transplant recipients revealed an increase in the risk of urinary tract infection (cystitis) in the denosumab group compared with the control group. However, a recent retrospective study evaluating 63 patients who received solid organ transplants (14 of whom were liver transplant recipients) showed promising results without an increase in infectious complications, indicating that denosumab could be a viable therapeutic option for transplant recipients with osteoporosis, especially in those with renal function impairment or bisphosphonate intolerance.

Raloxifene (Answer E) is a selective estrogen receptor modulator approved for the treatment of postmenopausal osteoporosis; however, it is considered a second-line agent because it only decreases the risk of vertebral fractures and has no effect on hip or other nonvertebral fracture risk. This option would not be the best choice in this patient who is at very high risk of future fracture, but it may be reserved as an alternative for women who cannot or choose not to take one of the other osteoporotic agents. Similar to estrogen, safety concerns with raloxifene include an increased risk of venous thromboembolism, another reason why this agent would not be a good choice for this patient who is a current smoker.

Teriparatide (PTH 1-34) (Answer D), which is an anabolic agent used in the treatment of osteoporosis, would be the most appropriate drug to treat her severe osteoporosis, especially given the low bone turnover typically seen before liver transplant. It is administered as a daily subcutaneous injection. Teriparatide has a black box warning of osteosarcoma, and its use is limited to 2 years in a lifetime. Contraindications to its use include history of skeletal irradiation, Paget disease of bone, or unexplained elevation in alkaline phosphatase. It is important to note that although teriparatide has been shown to improve bone mineral density in patients with glucocorticoid-induced osteoporosis, very few studies evaluate its use for the prevention of posttransplant osteoporosis.

Educational Objective
Recommend the most appropriate medical therapy for a liver transplant candidate with severe osteoporosis.

UpToDate Topic Review(s)
Liver transplantation in adults: Patient selection and pretransplantation evaluation
Risks of bisphosphonate therapy in patients with osteoporosis

Reference(s)
Krol CG, Dekkers OM, Kroon HM, Rabelink TJ, van Hoek B, Hamdy NA. Longitudinal changes in BMD and fracture risk in orthotopic liver transplant recipients not using bone-modifying treatment. *J Bone Miner Res.* 2014;29(8):1763-1769. PMID: 24644003

Cohen A, Shane E. Osteoporosis after solid organ and bone marrow transplantation. *Osteoporos Int.* 2003;14(8):617-630. PMID: 12908095

Monegal A, Navasa M, Guañabens N, et al. Bone disease after liver transplantation: a long-term prospective study of bone mass changes, hormonal status and histomorphometric characteristics. *Osteoporos Int.* 2001;12(6):484-492. PMID: 11446565

Vedi S, Greer S, Skingle SJ, et al. Mechanism of bone loss after liver transplantation: a histomorphometric analysis. *J Bone Miner Res.* 1999;14(2):281-287. PMID: 9933483

Bonani M, Frey D, de Rougemont O, et al. Infections in de novo kidney transplant recipients treated with the RANKL inhibitor denosumab. *Transplantation.* 2017;101(9):2139-2145. PMID: 27798510

Brunova J, Kratochvilova S, Stepankova J. Osteoporosis therapy with denosumab in organ transplant recipients. *Front Endocrinol (Lausanne).* 2018;9:162. PMID: 29720961

2 ANSWER: A) Intraarterial calcium stimulation with a selective hepatic venous sampling test

This patient has fulfilled the Whipple triad, strongly suggesting pathologic endogenous hyperinsulinism. Namely, the patient had a glucose level less than 55 mg/dL (<3.1 mmol/L) with neuroglycopenic symptoms that resolved after treatment. When the plasma glucose concentration was 53 mg/dL (2.9 mmol/L), the insulin concentration was greater than 3.0 μIU/mL (>20.8 pmol/L) and the C-peptide concentration was greater than 0.2 ng/mL (>0.07 nmol/L), thus confirming excess endogenous insulin production. Once sulfonylurea ingestion and exogenous insulin use are ruled out, the most likely culprit is an insulinoma, and the Whipple triad is present in more than 90% of such cases. Other rare causes include insulin autoimmune syndrome (Hirata disease) and tumor production of IGF-2. The former is ruled out on the basis of antibody testing, and the latter usually occurs in the setting of large mesenchymal tumors.

Insulinomas are rare neuroendocrine tumors with an annual incidence of 1 to 4 in one million. Insulinomas are usually solitary, small (<2 cm), and benign. Noninvasive imaging techniques are often the first step in localization after biochemical confirmation. Sensitivity for detecting insulinomas by such techniques is relatively poor: 33% for transabdominal ultrasonography, 44% for CT, and 52% for MRI. A Mayo Clinic series suggests a successful detection rate for insulinoma of 75% using transabdominal ultrasonography and/or triple-phase spiral CT. Somatostatin analogue-based imaging (eg, ^{111}In pentetreotide scintigraphy [Answer C] or ^{68}Ga-DOTATATE) can be used as well. However, because insulinomas have poor expression of somatostatin type 2 receptors compared with other neuroendocrine tumors, the sensitivity of such testing is low. If no tumor is localized and ectopic insulinoma is suspected, such scanning may be reasonable.

Invasive techniques are often required for tumor localization. Endoscopic ultrasonography detects insulinomas with a sensitivity of 75% to 83% (not detected by transabdominal ultrasonography or CT). Selective arterial calcium-stimulation testing (Answer A) is useful based on the fact that stimulation of tumor cells by calcium results in insulin release, which is not seen in the case of normal islet cells. In this test, there is selective injection of calcium gluconate into the splenic, gastroduodenal, and superior mesenteric arteries with subsequent sampling of hepatic venous effluent for insulin. A 2-fold rise in insulin levels within 30 to 60 seconds of calcium stimulation as compared to baseline strongly suggests insulinoma with localization as noted in the table. It is important to note that drainage patterns can be aberrant, and this procedure should be done in experienced centers.

Predicted Insulinoma Location	Site of Calcium Gluconate Injection Resulting in Positive Test
Head or neck of pancreas	Gastroduodenal or superior mesenteric artery
Body or tail of pancreas	Proximal splenic or mid-splenic artery
Liver metastases	Proper hepatic artery

Surgical resection is the recommended treatment for patients with insulinoma. For this reason, tumor localization is the key next step, so selective arterial calcium-stimulation testing is the best strategy now. Surgical options include enucleation with preservation of the remainder of the pancreas, distal pancreatectomy, or the Whipple procedure. These choices are based on tumor localization. Selective arterial calcium-stimulation testing localizes tumors accurately in nearly all cases, allowing for better surgical planning. Surgical pancreatic exploration (Answer B) would only be a reasonable next step if selective arterial calcium-stimulation testing were negative.

Medical treatment, such as diazoxide (Answer D) or small frequent meals (Answer E), is considered in cases of unsuccessful surgery, when metastatic disease is not resectable, or when patients are not surgical candidates.

Educational Objective

After establishing a diagnosis of pathologic endogenous hyperinsulinism, recommend invasive diagnostic tests as the best next step despite negative imaging.

UpToDate Topic Review(s)

Insulinoma
Hypoglycemia in adults without diabetes mellitus: Diagnostic approach

Reference(s)

Rosch T, Lightdale CJ, Botet JF, et al. Localization of pancreatic endocrine tumors by endoscopic ultrasonography. *N Engl J Med*. 1992;326(26):1721-1726. PMID: 1317506

Guettier JM, Kam A, Chang R, et al. Localization of insulinomas to regions of the pancreas by intraarterial calcium stimulation: the NIH experience. *J Clin Endocrinol Metab*. 2009;94(4):1074-1080. PMID: 19190102

3 ANSWER: D) Neck ultrasonography in 2 years to monitor thyroid nodule size

This patient has a cystic thyroid nodule. According to the 2015 American Thyroid Association guidelines, the risk of malignancy for a cystic thyroid nodule is less than 1%. Therefore, FNA biopsy (Answer B) is not recommended. This cystic nodule is small, and it can be monitored by performing neck ultrasonography in 2 years to assess for any further interval change in size and/or shape (Answer D). In nodules with a very low-suspicion ultrasonography pattern such as spongiform nodules, if ultrasonography is repeated, it should be done in 24 months. Therefore, in this patient with a small cystic nodule, one could choose no further follow-up. However, this was not offered as an answer choice.

Increasing evidence indicates that the presence of suspicious ultrasonography features is more predictive of malignancy than nodule size. Concerning characteristics are hypoechogenicity or a solid and cystic nodule with 1 or more of the following features: microcalcifications, irregular margins, taller-than-wide shape, rim calcification with a small extrusive soft-tissue component, or evidence of extrathyroidal extension. If a nodule is larger than 1 cm and has 1 of these characteristics, FNA biopsy is indicated. The risk of malignancy based on ultrasonography features is detailed in the 2015 American Thyroid Association guidelines for thyroid nodules and differentiated thyroid cancer:

- Benign pattern on ultrasonography (purely cystic nodule)—FNA biopsy is not indicated, as the risk of malignancy is extremely low (<1%)

- Very low-suspicion pattern on ultrasonography (eg, spongiform and partially cystic with no suspicious features)—FNA biopsy is indicated if the nodule is 2 cm or larger (risk of malignancy <3%)

- Low-suspicion pattern on ultrasonography (eg, hyperechoic solid nodule with regular margins, isoechoic solid nodule with regular margins, partially cystic nodule with eccentric solid areas)—FNA biopsy is indicated if the nodule is 1.5 cm or larger (risk of malignancy 5%-10%)

- Intermediate-suspicion pattern on ultrasonography (eg, hypoechoic solid nodule with smooth margins without microcalcifications, extrathyroidal extension, or taller-than-wide shape)—FNA biopsy is indicated if the nodule is 1 cm or larger (risk of malignancy 10%-20%)

- High-suspicion pattern on ultrasonography (eg, solid hypoechoic nodule or solid hypoechoic component of a partially cystic nodule with irregular margins [infiltrative, microlobulated], microcalcifications, taller-than-wide shape, rim calcifications with small extrusive soft-tissue component, or evidence of extrathyroidal extension)—FNA biopsy is indicated if the nodule is 1 cm or larger (risk of malignancy is >70%-90%).

In addition to the 2015 American Thyroid Association thyroid nodule guidelines, the American College of Radiology has developed the Thyroid Imaging, Reporting, and Data System (TI-RADS), which also provides guidance regarding management of thyroid nodules on the basis of their appearance on ultrasonography.

Thyroid scan (Answer A) is usually obtained in a patient with biochemical findings consistent with hyperthyroidism. In this patient, TSH and free T_4 are normal, so a thyroid scan is not indicated.

Left hemithyroidectomy (Answer C) can be offered to patients with a thyroid nodule confined to the thyroid gland that is proven to be cancerous by FNA biopsy and is smaller than 4 cm. This patient's nodule was cystic and small and confined to the thyroid gland. Lobectomy should not be recommended now.

Suppressing serum TSH with thyroid hormone therapy (Answer E) is no longer recommended to treat thyroid nodules. Randomized controlled trials have failed to show a significant effect on nodule volume. Additionally, the required dose can induce thyrotoxicosis, which is associated with significant risk for cardiovascular complications and osteoporosis.

Educational Objective

Manage thyroid nodules and explain ultrasound characteristics that predict risk of malignancy and indication for fine-needle aspiration biopsy.

UpToDate Topic Review(s)

Diagnostic approach to and treatment of thyroid nodules

Reference(s)

Haugen BR, Alexander EK, Bible KC, et al. 2015 American Thyroid Association management guidelines for adult patients with thyroid nodules and differentiated thyroid cancer: the American Thyroid Association Guidelines Task Force on Thyroid Nodules and Differentiated Thyroid Cancer. *Thyroid.* 2016;26(1):1-133. PMID: 26462967

Gharib H, Papini E, Garber JR, et al; AACE/ACE/AME Task Force on Thyroid Nodules. American Association of Clinical Endocrinologists, American College of Endocrinology, and Associazione Medici Endocrinologi Medical Guidelines for Clinical Practice for the Diagnosis and Management of Thyroid Nodules - 2016 Update. *Endocr Pract.* 2016;22(5):622-639. PMID: 27067915

Tessler FN, Middleton WD, Grant EG, et al. ACR thyroid imaging, reporting and data system (TI-RADS): white paper of the ACR TI-RADS committee. *J Am Coll Radiol.* 2017;14(5):587-595. PMID: 28372962

4 **ANSWER: C) Order a lipid panel**

This patient presents with new-onset diabetes with diabetic ketoacidosis (DKA). In addition, she has symptoms of severe midepigastric pain radiating to her back. Her serum lipase concentration is elevated, and her physical examination findings are remarkable for tenderness in the midepigastric region. These symptoms and signs are suggestive of pancreatitis, which is confirmed by radiographic evidence of stranding in the area surrounding the pancreas, a sign of inflammation. The patient's DKA is improving and her anion gap is closing. Her abdominal pain is controlled with narcotics. Because her clinical status appears to be improving, the clinician is prompted to review whether additional treatment or tests should be pursued.

Acute pancreatitis frequently coexists with DKA. A prospective study of 100 consecutive episodes of DKA at a single hospital revealed that 11% of the patients had coexisting pancreatitis. Of these 11 patients, 4 had hypertriglyceridemia (serum triglycerides ≥1000 mg/dL [≥11.3 mmol/L]). Patients who present to the hospital with hypertriglyceridemia-associated pancreatitis commonly have concurrent DKA. Wang et al performed a retrospective study of 140 patients with hypertriglyceridemia-induced pancreatitis and determined that 26% had concurrent DKA. Hypertriglyceridemia is the third most common cause of pancreatitis (after gallstones and alcohol).

The mechanism for the clustering of DKA, hypertriglyceridemia, and pancreatitis is the overlapping of risk factors for these conditions. Type 2 diabetes in an obese patient is commonly associated with hypertriglyceridemia. As diabetes control worsens, the chronic exposure to hyperglycemia causes a reduction of insulin release from the β cells, which further exacerbates hyperglycemia—a cycle known as glucose toxicity. Insulin is the major regulator of hormone-sensitive lipase, the enzyme responsible for clearing free fatty acids (and triglycerides) from the circulation. As serum insulin levels fall as a result of glucose toxicity, hormone-sensitive lipase activity decreases and triglyceride levels increase. In DKA, lipase activity is very low, causing marked hypertriglyceridemia. Thus, DKA, hypertriglyceridemia, and pancreatitis commonly occur together. Pfeifer et al demonstrated that patients with uncontrolled type 2 diabetes have a defect in lipoprotein lipase activity that is reversed with improved glycemic control.

In this vignette, the clinician is encouraged to reevaluate the current therapy and to look for causes of pancreatitis that are associated with DKA. The serum sodium is appropriately low, as hyperglycemia causes a drop in the serum sodium concentration due to changes in osmolality. If the patient has hypertriglyceridemia, the elevated lipids will also lower the measured serum sodium, a condition called pseudohyponatremia.

Measuring glutamic acid decarboxylase antibodies and C-peptide (Answer A), referring for endoscopic retrograde cholangiopancreatography (Answer B), performing abdominal ultrasonography (Answer D), or measuring serum and ionized calcium (Answer E) are all appropriate components of management for DKA and pancreatitis, but none of these interventions will substitute for determining the cause of the pancreatitis in this particular patient, which can only be accomplished by assessing her lipid profile (Answer C). Importantly, C-peptide levels must be interpreted with caution in renal failure, as approximately half of produced C-peptide is removed by the kidneys. Thus, in the setting of renal impairment, C-peptide may be falsely elevated.

Ideally, a lipid profile should be measured on day 1 of presentation, as serum triglycerides decrease with treatment of DKA. A triglyceride level greater than 1000 mg/dL (>11.3 mmol/L) at the time of diagnosis is consistent with triglyceride-associated pancreatitis.

Educational Objective
Suspect hypertriglyceridemia as the cause of pancreatitis in patients presenting with diabetic ketoacidosis.

UpToDate Topic Review(s)
Diabetic ketoacidosis and hyperosmolar hyperglycemic state in adults: Clinical features, evaluation, and diagnosis

Reference(s)

Nair S, Yadav D, Pitchumoni CS. Association of diabetic ketoacidosis and acute pancreatitis: Observations in 100 consecutive episodes of DKA. *Am J Gastroenterol.* 2000;95(10):2795-2800. PMID: 11051350

Wang Y, Attar BM, Hinami K, et al. Concurrent diabetic ketoacidosis in hypertriglyceridemia-induced pancreatitis: How does it affect the clinical course and severity scores? *Pancreas.* 2017;46(10):1336-1340. PMID: 28984788

Ramachandran V, Vila DM, Cochran JM, Caruso AC, Balchandani R. Acute pancreatitis secondary to hypertriglyceridemia precipitated by diabetic ketoacidosis in a previously undiagnosed ketosis-prone patient with diabetes mellitus. *Proc (Bayl Univ Med Cent).* 2018;31(2):189-191. PMID: 29706815

Leahy JL, Bonner-Weir S, Weir GC. Beta-cell dysfunction induced by chronic hyperglycemia. current ideas on mechanism of impaired glucose-induced insulin secretion. *Diabetes Care.* 1992;15(3):442-455. PMID: 1559411

Pfeifer MA, Brunzell JD, Best JD, Judzewitsch RG, Halter JB, Porte D. The response of plasma triglyceride, cholesterol, and lipoprotein lipase to treatment in non-insulin-dependent diabetic subjects without familial hypertriglyceridemia. *Diabetes.* 1983;32(6):525-531. PMID: 6354782

5 ANSWER: C) Perform a 1-mg dexamethasone suppression test

This patient with hyperandrogenemia and a history of anovulatory cycles was misdiagnosed with polycystic ovary syndrome. Polycystic ovary syndrome is diagnosed only when other conditions have been excluded, including hyperprolactinemia, hypothyroidism, and nonclassic congenital adrenal hyperplasia. Although Cushing syndrome should be in the differential diagnosis of hyperandrogenemia and amenorrhea, further evaluation is dictated by clinical suspicion. It is important to recognize when to suspect Cushing syndrome and when to consider the possibility of misdiagnosis or evolving clinical scenarios that require further evaluation.

In this case, the initial indication that the true diagnosis was not polycystic ovary syndrome was a low day 21 estradiol level. Additional evidence for estrogen deficiency could have been sought by administering 10 days of progesterone to see if she had a withdrawal bleed or by pelvic ultrasonography demonstrating a uterine lining less than 4 mm. Hypercortisolism suppresses hypothalamic-pituitary-ovarian signaling and leads to secondary amenorrhea characterized by estrogen deficiency. She also developed hypertension, weight gain, and a rising DHEA-S. Therefore, further testing for Cushing syndrome is indicated. For a mildly elevated 17-hydroxyprogesterone level, further testing to diagnose nonclassic congenital adrenal hyperplasia could include a cosyntropin-stimulation test (Answer A). However, this patient's progressive clinical symptoms are more suggestive of Cushing syndrome, so this would not be the best next test to consider. In this case, Cushing syndrome was diagnosed with a 1-mg dexamethasone suppression test (Answer C), which demonstrated a cortisol value of 9.8 μg/dL (270.4 nmol/L) (normal <1.8 μg/dL [50 nmol/L]) and urinary free cortisol excretion (not offered as an answer option) of 98 μg/24 h (270.5 nmol/d) (normal <45 μg/24 h [<124.2 nmol/d]).

A common misconception is that an elevated DHEA-S value requires adrenal imaging or abdominal CT (Answer B). Androgen-producing adrenal tumors are rarely diagnosed causes of androgen-excess. Androgens of ovarian origin can be converted to DHEA in local tissues and circulate to the adrenal where the sulfate is added. Most guidelines recommend further evaluation if the DHEA-S concentration is above 700 μg/dL (>19.0 μmol/L). Also, adrenal Cushing syndrome would be associated with a lower-than-normal DHEA-S level. Therefore, the next step should not be an abdominal CT.

Spironolactone (Answer D) is an aldosterone antagonist that also acts as a competitive inhibitor of the androgen receptor. It is considered second-line therapy for the treatment of hirsutism or first-line therapy in a patient who cannot be prescribed combined oral contraceptives. It is also an appropriate addition when symptoms are not controlled with combined oral contraceptives alone. Although combined oral contraceptives would treat the secondary amenorrhea and could be useful when confirming whether hyperandrogenemia is suppressible in the evaluation of hirsutism, it would not be ideal to initiate before evaluating for Cushing syndrome. Combined oral contraceptives would increase hepatic production of cortisol-binding globulin and total cortisol, which would make the evaluation for Cushing syndrome more difficult. A patient with Cushing syndrome is also at higher risk for venous thromboembolic disease. Therefore, restarting combined oral contraceptives (Answer E) is not the best next step.

Educational Objective
Evaluate for Cushing syndrome in a woman with a prior diagnosis of polycystic ovary syndrome.

UpToDate Topic Review(s)
Establishing the diagnosis of Cushing's syndrome

Reference(s)

Legro RS, Arslanian SA, Ehrmann DA, et al; Endocrine Society. Diagnosis and treatment of polycystic ovary syndrome: an Endocrine Society clinical practice guideline. *J Clin Endocrinol Metab.* 2013;98(12):4565-4592. PMID: 24151290

Martin KA, Anderson RR, Chang RJ, et al. Evaluation and treatment of hirsutism in premenopausal women: an Endocrine Society clinical practice guideline. *J Clin Endocrinol Metab.* 2018;103(4):1233-1257. PMID: 29522147

6 ANSWER: B) Essential hypertension (primary hypertension)

Adrenal incidentalomas are common and are identified on 4% to 7% of abdominal CT or MRI scans in patients older than 40 years. While many of these are truly incidental and not associated with endocrine dysfunction, it is important to adopt a systematic approach to assessment. When faced with a patient with an adrenal incidentaloma, the clinician must answer 2 important questions: (1) is there any possibility of a primary (eg, adrenocortical carcinoma) or secondary (eg, metastasis from renal cell carcinoma) malignant tumor? and (2) is the lesion functioning?

With modern imaging techniques (triple-phase CT and in-phase and out-of-phase MRI) most adrenal incidentalomas are readily classified as benign adrenal adenomas. In this vignette, the identification of a 2-cm adrenal mass does not raise concerns on the basis of size alone, but further assessment is required because the Hounsfield unit measurement of 35 is above the threshold of 10 (a value <10 is traditionally used to define a lipid-rich adrenal adenoma).

However, this is a postcontrast measurement and therefore an unenhanced CT of the adrenal glands may be all that is required to provide reassurance. If doubt remains, a washout CT or in-phase and out-of-phase MRI should be performed.

Exclusion of a functioning adrenal lesion (Answer C) typically involves screening for adrenocortical and adrenomedullary causes. Measurement of plasma free metanephrines and 24-hour urinary fractionated metanephrines are the preferred investigations to detect an adrenal pheochromocytoma (although some authors have reasoned that this is not required if the imaging assessment clearly demonstrates features of an adrenocortical adenoma). In this case, the plasma normetanephrine level is only very mildly raised—not in the range typically seen with a catecholamine-secreting tumor—and the plasma metanephrine concentration is normal. Mildly elevated plasma normetanephrine can be observed in patients with essential hypertension or sleep apnea, which is a consideration in this patient with a BMI of 38.6 kg/m^2.

A 1-mg overnight dexamethasone suppression test is usually used to screen for hypercortisolism (Answer A) in a patient with an adrenal incidentaloma. Although this patient's postdexamethasone cortisol value is above the traditional threshold for excluding autonomous hypercortisolism (<1.8 µg/dL [<50 nmol/L]) and merits further investigation (eg, with late-night salivary cortisol, 24-hour urinary free cortisol, and/or low-dose 48-hour dexamethasone suppression test), this is most likely a false-positive result. Several conditions may be associated with false positivity following dexamethasone, including obesity, depression, and alcohol excess. In addition, concomitant use of oral estrogen therapy, which raises cortisol-binding globulin and hence total serum cortisol levels, or enzyme-inducing agents (eg, carbamazepine), which increase dexamethasone clearance, can lead to a false-positive result. Some individuals are also naturally fast metabolizers of dexamethasone.

Primary aldosteronism (Answer D) is important to exclude in any patient with hypertension and hypokalemia (provoked or unprovoked) and requires measurement of paired plasma aldosterone concentration and plasma renin activity (or direct renin concentration). Ideally, these measurements should be conducted in the absence of confounding medications such as β-adrenergic blockers, diuretics, and ACE inhibitors (doxazosin, verapamil, diltiazem, and hydralazine are all considered to be noninterfering). However, performing a first measurement while the patient is on current medications is reasonable, provided that the results are interpreted with caution. In this vignette, the patient's plasma renin activity is low but not fully suppressed as is typically seen with β-adrenergic blockade, and this most likely reflects the counteracting effects of the combination of a diuretic and ACE inhibitor. Although clean measurements would be the only way to be certain that the patient does not have primary aldosteronism, the aldosterone-to-renin ratio of just 7.75 (6.2 ng/dL / 0.8 ng/mL per h) despite low plasma renin activity makes this diagnosis less likely. In this case, the low aldosterone-to-renin ratio reflects an absolute aldosterone concentration less than 7.21 ng/dL [<200 pmol/L]), and indeed some experts recommend that a diagnosis of primary aldosteronism should not be made if the plasma aldosterone concentration is less than 15 ng/dL (<416 pmol/L). The only cautionary note to add is that the patient was mildly hypokalemic at the time of testing and ideally this should be corrected (target serum potassium of 4 mEq/L [4 mmol/L]), as hypokalemia may suppress aldosterone secretion in primary aldosteronism.

The relatively low plasma renin activity and plasma aldosterone levels are also not suggestive of renovascular disease (Answer E).

After considering all the factors, this patient most likely has essential hypertension (Answer B).

Educational Objective
Identify potential confounding factors for interpretation of investigations in the setting of adrenal incidentaloma.

UpToDate Topic Review(s)
The adrenal incidentaloma

Reference(s)

Fassnacht M, Arlt W, Bancos I, et al. Management of adrenal incidentalomas: European Society of Endocrinology clinical practice guideline in collaboration with the European Network for the Study of Adrenal Tumors. *Eur J Endocrinol.* 2016;175(2):G1-G34. PMID: 27390021

Funder JW, Carey RM, Mantero F, et al. The management of primary aldosteronism: case detection, diagnosis, and treatment: an Endocrine Society clinical practice guideline. *J Clin Endocrinol Metab.* 2016;101(5):1889-1916. PMID: 26934393

Nieman LK, Biller BM, Findling JW, et al. The diagnosis of Cushing's syndrome: an Endocrine Society clinical practice guideline. *J Clin Endocrinol Metab.* 2008;93(5):1526-1540. PMID: 18334580

7   ANSWER: A) No further testing needed now

This patient is seeking advice on cardiovascular risk management. His lipid panel is acceptable, and there is no family history of atherosclerotic cardiovascular disease. Standard lipid testing, consisting of total cholesterol, LDL cholesterol, HDL cholesterol, and triglycerides, is a well-established platform for cardiovascular disease risk assessment. Therefore, in this patient, who has no major risk factors and has acceptable triglyceride levels, no further testing is required now (Answer A). Risk should be reassessed annually and therapy should be considered with advancing age.

LDL cholesterol is an estimated number based on the Friedewald formula and is fairly accurate when the plasma triglyceride concentration is less than 400 mg/dL (<4.52 mmol/L). The formula is not valid when triglyceride levels are greater than 400 mg/dL (>4.52 mmol/L) and discrepancies in LDL-cholesterol values have been reported. In such situations, direct LDL-cholesterol measurement (Answer B) can be performed in the laboratory. However, the accuracy of such direct chemical-based LDL-cholesterol assays has not been demonstrated and they incur added expense. Importantly, the Centers for Disease Control and Prevention Lipid Standardization Program standardize assays for total cholesterol, HDL cholesterol, and triglycerides, but do not monitor the accuracy of direct LDL-cholesterol commercial chemical assays. This patient does not have elevated triglyceride levels, so there is no indication for measurement of direct LDL cholesterol.

Apolipoprotein B (Answer C) is the protein signature that is carried by all atherogenic lipoproteins such as VLDL remnants, intermediate-density lipoprotein, and LDL. Most circulating apolipoprotein B is associated with LDL particles, and levels correlate strongly with LDL-cholesterol and non–HDL-cholesterol levels. Apolipoprotein B is an excellent predictor of cardiovascular events. Measurement of apolipoprotein B in addition to traditional risk factors does not significantly alter treatment decisions according to data from several large studies. Therefore, apolipoprotein B measurement would not add helpful information in this case.

C-reactive protein (Answer D) is an acute-phase reactant produced predominantly in hepatocytes and is a nonspecific marker of inflammation. C-reactive protein may be involved in the immunologic process that triggers vascular remodeling and plaque deposition in atherosclerosis. Cardiovascular risk assessment requires measurement of highly sensitive C-reactive protein with a sensitive assay that accurately detects very low levels in healthy individuals. Highly sensitive C-reactive protein levels are variable and are dependent on age, sex, and ethnicity. The association between elevated highly sensitive C-reactive protein levels and cardiovascular disease is well established. However, current data from experimental research, epidemiologic studies, and large clinical trials do not provide conclusive evidence to support the routine measurement of highly sensitive C-reactive protein to predict cardiovascular risk or to use as a tool to determine whether statin therapy should be initiated.

Measuring LDL particle number is an alternative way to quantify LDL burden. There is significant interindividual and intraindividual variability in the amount of cholesterol carried by LDL particles. LDL particle number can be measured directly by nuclear magnetic resonance spectroscopy lipoprotein analysis (Answer E). Several studies have shown that LDL particle number is more strongly associated with atherosclerotic cardiovascular disease than LDL cholesterol. However, in most studies, the predictive strength of LDL particle number is very similar to that of non-HDL cholesterol (part of the standard lipid panel). Measurement is not widely available, is not standardized, and is costly. Also, LDL particle number correlates with apolipoprotein B measurement, which is more widely available. Thus, at this time, there is no evidence that measuring LDL particle number provides a substantial amount of information beyond what is provided by non–HDL-cholesterol and standard risk factor assessment.

Educational Objective

Determine when advanced lipoprotein testing for cardiovascular risk assessment is warranted and when a lipid panel and personal and family history is sufficient.

UpToDate Topic Review(s)

Cardiovascular disease risk assessment for primary prevention: Our approach

Reference(s)

Sniderman AD, Williams K, Contois JH, et al. A meta-analysis of low-density lipoprotein cholesterol, non-high-density lipoprotein cholesterol, and apolipoprotein B as markers of cardiovascular risk. *Circ Cardiovasc Qual Outcomes.* 2011;4(3):337-345. PMID: 21487090

Mora S, Rifai N, Buring JE, Ridker PM. Comparison of LDL cholesterol concentrations by Friedewald calculation and direct measurements in relation to cardiovascular events in 27,331 women. *Clin Chem.* 2009;55(5):888-894. PMID: 19395440

Martin SS, Blaha MJ, Elshazly MB, et al. Friedewald-estimated versus directly measured low-density lipoprotein cholesterol and treatment implications. *J Am Coll Cardiol.* 2013;62(8):732-739. PMID: 23524048

8 ANSWER: C) Teriparatide

Patients with osteoporosis and a history of low-trauma fractures are at a particularly high risk of additional fragility fractures, which generally mandates treatment with an effective antifracture therapy. This is especially true in patients with vertebral fractures, which increases the risk of subsequent vertebral fractures up to 11-fold.

Although adequate intake of calcium and vitamin D (Answer E) is important to maximize the benefits of osteoporosis therapies on bone mineral density, this has a minimal independent impact on fracture risk reduction (5% to 10%) based on available evidence.

Risedronate (Answer B) is proven to reduce the risk of vertebral fractures, but this patient's previous intolerance of alendronate because of musculoskeletal symptoms makes it a less attractive option for her.

The anabolic agent teriparatide (Answer C) is proven to be more effective than risedronate in reducing the risk of vertebral fractures in postmenopausal women at high risk of spine fracture (ie, at least 1 severe [>40%] or 2 moderate [25%-40%] compression fractures), thus making it the most appropriate choice for this patient. Both teriparatide and abaloparatide, the latter of which is a modified form of PTHrP, are subcutaneous injections that stimulate osteoblastic bone formation de novo and are truly anabolic bone agents, as opposed to antiresorptive agents (bisphosphonates, denosumab, selective estrogen-receptor modulators), which inhibit osteoclast-mediated bone resorption. However, both drugs can only be given for 2 years on the basis of toxicology studies that demonstrate an increased risk for osteosarcoma in rats receiving suprapharmacologic dosages of either drug. Therefore, the drugs are contraindicated in patients who have a higher baseline risk for osteosarcoma, including those who have received therapeutic radiotherapy or who have Paget disease of bone.

While zoledronic acid (Answer D) effectively reduces the risk of vertebral fractures and has not been proven to be inferior to teriparatide in this regard, her previous intolerance to alendronate and a higher rate of musculoskeletal symptoms with intravenous bisphosphonates would not make it a wise choice for this patient.

Finally, although proven effective in reducing the risk of vertebral fractures, raloxifene, which is a selective estrogen-receptor modulator (Answer A), is contraindicated in this patient who has a higher risk of fatal stroke given her existing atrial fibrillation. Nonetheless, postmenopausal women with a low risk of stroke according to the Framingham stroke risk calculation (score <13) may still be candidates for raloxifene to reduce the risk of vertebral fracture.

Educational Objective

Recommend the most effective and safe treatment for a postmenopausal woman at high risk of vertebral fracture.

UpToDate Topic Review(s)

Clinical manifestations, diagnosis, and evaluation of osteoporosis in postmenopausal women

Reference(s)

Barrett-Connor E, Cox DA, Song J, Mitlak B, Mosca L, Grady D. Raloxifene and risk for stroke based on the Framingham stroke risk score. *Am J Med.* 2009;122(8):754-761. PMID: 19540454

Kendler DL, Marin F, Zerbini CAF, et al. Effects of teriparatide and risedronate on new fractures in post-menopausal women with severe osteoporosis (VERO): a multicentre, double-blind, double-dummy, randomised controlled trial. *Lancet.* 2018;391(10117):230-240. PMID: 29129436

9 ANSWER: A) Serum prolactin measurement

This man presents with symptoms and signs of hypogonadism, and the clinical diagnosis is confirmed by unequivocally and consistently reduced fasting 8-AM total testosterone concentrations. Therefore, the diagnosis of hypogonadism is clear-cut, and determining free testosterone (Answer B) (usually calculated from total testosterone, SHBG, and albumin) would not add anything to the diagnosis. The Endocrine Society recommends measuring fasting morning total testosterone concentrations using an accurate and reliable assay as the initial diagnostic test. Assessing free testosterone is indicated when total testosterone concentrations are borderline, or if conditions that alter SHBG are suspected, such as increased levels with obesity, diabetes mellitus, use of exogenous androgens, or hypothyroidism or decreased levels with aging, hyperthyroidism, liver disease, anticonvulsant medications, HIV, or use of estrogens.

Once the diagnosis of hypogonadism is established, the next step is to measure gonadotropins to distinguish primary (increased gonadotropins) from secondary hypogonadism (gonadotropins low to low-normal). In this man, the inappropriately low-normal gonadotropins indicate secondary hypogonadism.

Hyperprolactinemia is one of the most common causes of secondary hypogonadism in men. Prolactin excess induces hypogonadism by inhibiting the pulsatile secretion of GnRH and, consequently, gonadotropin secretion. In cases of a pituitary macroadenoma, secondary hypogonadism can also be due to mass effect. Measurement of serum prolactin (Answer A), along with iron saturation to exclude iron overload syndromes, is the first-line investigation in the assessment of secondary hypogonadism recommended by Endocrine Society guidelines.

Pituitary-directed imaging (Answer E) is indicated to exclude pituitary and/or hypothalamic pathology when severe secondary hypogonadism (serum testosterone <150 ng/dL [<5.2 nmol/L]), panhypopituitarism, persistent hyperprolactinemia, or features of tumor mass effects (such as new-onset headache, vision impairment, or visual field defect) are present. However, in this case, alarm features are largely absent, and prolactin should be measured first.

Cushing syndrome can lead to secondary hypogonadism, either due to suppression of GnRH and pituitary gonadotropin secretion by glucocorticoid excess, or due to mass effect of an ACTH-secreting pituitary macroadenoma in the setting of Cushing disease. However, Cushing syndrome severe enough to cause secondary hypogonadism should be clinically obvious, and performing a 1-mg dexamethasone-suppression test (Answer C) would be of very low yield.

Current or previous use of anabolic steroids can cause secondary hypogonadism, but this patient's history and examination are not suggestive of steroid use. Mild anemia would be unlikely given the erythropoietic actions of androgens, and his mild anemia is more consistent with androgen deficiency. Therefore, an anabolic steroid screen (Answer D) is incorrect.

Educational Objective
Assess for microprolactinoma in a man with hypogonadotropic hypogonadism.

UpToDate Topic Review(s)
Causes of secondary hypogonadism in males

Reference(s)

Bhasin S, Brito JP, Cunningham GR, et al. Testosterone therapy in men with hypogonadism: an Endocrine Society clinical practice guideline. *J Clin Endocrinol Metab.* 2018;103(5):1715-1744. PMID: 29562364

De Rosa M, Zarrilli S, Di Sarno A, et al. Hyperprolactinemia in men: clinical and biochemical features and response to treatment. *Endocrine.* 2003;20(1-2):75-82. PMID: 12668871

10

ANSWER: B) Change the insulin-to-carbohydrate ratio to 1 unit per 6 g before each meal

Maintaining glucose levels in the near-normal range is the management goal for women with pregestational diabetes (either type 1 or type 2 diagnosed before pregnancy) to decrease the risk of adverse events in the fetus, newborn, and mother.

Measurement of hemoglobin A_{1c} and glucose levels is used to assess glucose control throughout pregnancy. The American College of Obstetricians and Gynecologists recommends a target hemoglobin A_{1c} level less than 6.0% (<42 mmol/mol) during pregnancy, as long as it is safe. The American Diabetes Association guidelines recommend a target hemoglobin A_{1c} value between 6.0% and 6.5% (42-48 mmol/mol) in early pregnancy, as observational studies have shown that this level of glucose control is associated with the lowest risk of adverse outcomes in early pregnancy. The glycemic targets may need to be relaxed in patients with hypoglycemia unawareness, as in this case.

American College of Obstetricians and Gynecologists and the American Diabetes Association recommend the following glucose targets during pregnancy. Glucose values can be monitored with self-monitoring of blood glucose (capillary measurements) or with continuous glucose monitoring (CGM).

Fasting glucose <95 mg/dL (<5.3 mmol/L)
Premeal glucose <100 mg/dL (<5.6 mmol/L)
1-hour glucose <140 mg/dL (<7.8 mmol/L)
2-hour glucose <120 mg/dL (<6.7 mmol/L)
Nocturnal glucose >60 mg/dL (<3.3 mmol/L)

A large, parallel, open-label, multicenter trial, the CONCEPTT trial, randomly assigned 215 pregnant women with type 1 diabetes on intensive insulin treatment to CGM plus capillary glucose monitoring vs capillary glucose monitoring alone (control group) in early pregnancy (≤13 ± 6 weeks' gestation). The CGM group had a greater reduction in hemoglobin A_{1c} (6.35% [46 mmol/mol]) vs 6.53% [48 mmol/mol] in the control group) (95% confidence interval, –0.34% to –0.03%) at 34 weeks' gestation. The women in the CGM group spent more time in the glucose target range of 63 to 140 mg/dL (3.5-7.8 mmol/L) (68% vs 61% in the control group) and spent less time in the hyperglycemic range (27% vs 32% in the control group). The rates of hypoglycemia in the women were equivalent in both groups. In the CGM group, fewer newborns were treated for hypoglycemia at birth (15% vs 28% in the control group), and fewer newborns were in the large-for-gestational-age category (53% vs 69% in the control group).

The patient in this vignette has hypoglycemia unawareness, so the current hemoglobin A_{1c} level is appropriate. She is using CGM to help monitor her glucose levels. Upon review of the current CGM tracing, the glucose levels are in a good range overnight and before breakfast. Therefore, changing the basal insulin rate, starting at midnight and again at 4 AM (Answers C and D), is not necessary. However, there is evidence of modest glucose excursion after each meal. The patient is appropriately bolusing insulin lispro 15 minutes before meals. Therefore, she should administer a larger insulin bolus before each meal. Changing the insulin-to-carbohydrate ratio from 1:7 to 1:6 (Answer B) is appropriate and is the best recommendation. However, increasing the amount of bolus insulin only before lunch and dinner (Answer A) is not adequate. As she nears the end of the first trimester, the morning sickness should resolve and she will require higher bolus insulin doses before meals. Therefore, decreasing the amount of bolus insulin to a 1:8 ratio (Answer E) is inappropriate. Increasing the basal insulin rate at 7 AM is also not appropriate, as the glucose levels start to trend downward at 9:30 AM.

Educational Objective
Recommend appropriate changes in basal insulin and the insulin-to-carbohydrate ratio to control glucose levels during pregnancy.

UpToDate Topic Review(s)
Pregestational diabetes mellitus: Glycemic control during pregnancy

Reference(s)

American Diabetes Association. 13. Management of diabetes in pregnancy: Standards of Medical Care in Diabetes-2018. *Diabetes Care.* 2018;41(Suppl 1):S137-S143. PMID: 29222384

Nielsen GL, Moller M, Sorensen HT. HbA1c in early pregnancy and pregnancy outcomes: a Danish population-based cohort study of 573 pregnancies in women with type 1 diabetes. *Diabetes Care.* 2006;(12):2612-2616. PMID: 17130193

ACOG Committee on Practice Bulletins. ACOG Practice Bulletin. Clinical management guidelines for obstetrician-gynecologists. Number 60, March 2005. Pregestational diabetes mellitus. *Obstet Gynecol.* 2005;105(3):675-685. PMID: 1578045

Feig DS, Donovan LE, Corcoy R, et al; CONCEPTT Collaborative Group. Continuous glucose monitoring in pregnant women with type 1 diabetes (CONCEPTT): a multicenter international randomized controlled trial. *Lancet.* 2017;390(10110): 2347-2359. PMID: 28923465

11 ANSWER: C) Hyponatremia

Treatment of thyroid cancer with radioactive iodine is effective because of 2 manipulations that increase the activity of the sodium-iodide symporter responsible for transporting iodine into follicular cells. These manipulations are iodine depletion and raising serum TSH. Typically, recombinant human TSH injections are used to raise TSH levels, so that the patient does not have to experience hypothyroidism. However, when a patient has distant metastases from thyroid cancer, some experts believe that preparation using a hypothyroid protocol may result in more effective delivery of radioactive iodine. The combination of following a low-iodine diet and being severely hypothyroid appears to be a "perfect storm" for inducing hyponatremia (Answer C). Typical early symptoms of hyponatremia include headache, fatigue, weakness, lethargy, muscle cramps, nausea, anorexia, and vomiting. This may progress to confusion, focal neurologic deficits, delirium, seizure, and coma.

The number of reported cases of hyponatremia during preparation for radioactive iodine therapy is small and generally associated with fairly severe hyponatremia (serum sodium 107-121 mEq/L [107-121 mmol/L]). However, it is possible that patients with milder degrees of hyponatremia and fewer symptoms are not recognized as having hyponatremia and are therefore not reported. A low-iodine diet may be associated with hyponatremia, partly because while following a low-iodine diet, many patients are actually consuming a low-sodium diet. Although noniodized salt is permitted, not all patients use this product. In addition, because patients are generally avoiding processed foods, dairy products, and sauces, this also contributes to consumption of foods low in sodium. Severe hyponatremia may be associated with hypothyroidism secondary to renal dysfunction and impaired free water clearance. However, the frequency of this association is not generally agreed upon. In one study of hypothyroid patients, only 5 of 128 patients became hyponatremic with sodium values in the range of 132 to 134 mEq/L (132-134 mmol/L). In another study of patients with myxedema, their serum sodium levels increased by about 4 mEq/L (4 mmol/L) after levothyroxine initiation. The hypothyroid state does not appear to be essential for the development of hyponatremia during preparation for radioiodine therapy, as hyponatremia has also been reported in patients prepared using recombinant human TSH.

Additional risk factors for the development of hyponatremia are older age, longer duration of a low-iodine diet, concurrent therapy with thiazide diuretics, and possibly distant metastases. In cases of hyponatremia that are recognized after radioiodine therapy has been administered, there may also be the additional cause of intentional fluid intake beyond normal consumption in order to clear radioisotopes from the patient's body fluids. A serum sodium concentration as low as 98 to 108 mEq/L (98-108 mmol/L) has been reported in these circumstances.

The other answers offer potential, but less likely, causes for the patient's symptoms. Adrenal insufficiency (Answer E) would be expected to have more evidence of progressive hypotension, orthostasis, malaise, and weight loss, particularly if it were primary adrenal insufficiency—for example, due to bilateral metastases to the adrenal glands. There might also be vomiting, in addition to the nausea.

Iodine allergy (Answer D) is uncommon and is more often due to proteins associated with iodine, as in seafood or shellfish allergies. Moreover, the amount of iodine in a diagnostic dose of ^{123}I is small. Many individuals with iodine allergy actually have reactions to contrast media. Symptoms include flushing, urticaria, angioedema, bronchospasm, and hypotension.

If this patient has lung metastases, it is possible that she also has brain metastases (Answer A). However, in addition to headache, neurologic symptoms might be prominent. Also, she had normal findings on brain MRI.

Azotemia (Answer B) due to impaired renal function could be a consideration in this patient. However, there is no loss of appetite, fluid retention, or hypotension described in the vignette.

Educational Objective
Identify the risk factors for hyponatremia during preparation for radioactive iodine treatment in patients with thyroid cancer.

UpToDate Topic Review(s)
Differentiated thyroid cancer: Radioiodine treatment

Reference(s)

Jo HJ, Kim YH, Shin DH, et al. Hyponatremia after thyroid hormone withdrawal in a patient with papillary thyroid carcinoma. *Endocrinol Metab (Seoul)*. 2014;29(1):77-82. PMID: 24741458

Krishnamurthy VR, McDougall IR. Severe hyponatremia: a danger of low-iodine diet. *Thyroid*. 2007;17(9):889-892. PMID: 17822373

Li JH, He ZH, Bansal V, Hennessey JV. Low iodine diet in differentiated thyroid cancer: a review. *Clin Endocrinol (Oxf)*. 2016;84(1):3-12. PMID: 26118628

Shakir MK, Krook LS, Schraml FV, Hays JH, Clyde PW. Symptomatic hyponatremia in association with a low-iodine diet and levothyroxine withdrawal prior to I131 in patients with metastatic thyroid carcinoma. *Thyroid*. 2008;18(7):787-792. PMID: 18631009

12 ANSWER: D) Perform ovarian venous sampling

In this case of abnormal uterine bleeding, several features are concerning for autonomous estradiol secretion from a possible ovarian tumor, including the significantly elevated estradiol, thickened endometrial lining after repeated endometrial ablation, and persistent bleeding despite trials of progesterone and GnRH treatment. Ovarian tumors that can produce estrogen include granulosa cell tumors and thecomas. Granulosa-stromal cell tumors are sex-cord stromal tumors that can produce estrogen through conversion of androstenedione to estradiol. Thecomas are solid, fibromatous, usually benign tumors composed of theca cells derived from the ovarian stroma.

Combined ovarian and adrenal venous sampling (selective venous sampling) is performed in the evaluation of women with hyperandrogenism when clinical suspicion for an androgen-producing tumor is high, pelvic ultrasonography is normal, and adrenal imaging is either normal or identifies a nodule or mass. The procedure includes selective catheterization of the ovarian and adrenal veins to demonstrate a gradient in androgen concentrations and localize the source. This procedure is technically difficult and should only be performed by a highly experienced interventional radiologist. In this patient, there is no evidence of hyperandrogenism, but rather a concern regarding her elevated estradiol. Thus, there is no need to sample the adrenal veins. For diagnostic purposes in this case, the best next step would be to proceed with bilateral ovarian venous sampling (Answer D) to diagnose an ovarian side-to-side gradient. Data suggest that a side-to-side gradient greater than 1.44 in androgen concentrations correctly identifies most androgen-producing tumors.

Initiation of an oral contraceptive (Answer E) is not likely to relieve symptoms and could make bleeding worse. Pelvic ultrasonography did not reveal any masses or enlargement, so pelvic CT (Answer A) is unlikely to be diagnostic. If a pelvic mass is identified, pelvic MRI might be considered because the high-contrast resolution might be able to better distinguish the origin of the mass and better characterize an ovarian lesion.

Tamoxifen (Answer B) is a selective estrogen receptor modulator with mixed antagonist and agonist activity. It is primarily used for adjuvant treatment of estrogen receptor–positive breast cancer or chemoprevention in women at high risk for breast cancer. Tamoxifen can be associated with abnormal uterine bleeding because it has a direct agonist effect on endometrial tissue—stimulating proliferation while also increasing estrogen levels by partial antagonist activity on the hypothalamic-pituitary axis. Tamoxifen would increase gonadotropin and estradiol concentrations, which could worsen abnormal uterine bleeding.

Letrozole (Answer C) is an aromatase inhibitor that decreases conversion of androstenedione and testosterone to estrone and estradiol, and it is used as an adjuvant therapy for postmenopausal women with breast cancer. It is also used off-label for ovulation induction in women with polycystic ovary syndrome, as there is evidence that letrozole, compared with clomiphene, is associated with higher live birth rates. By suppressing ovarian estradiol production and secretion, reduction in the negative feedback of estradiol leads to an increase in FSH, follicular development, and estradiol concentrations. Similar to tamoxifen, letrozole would also increase gonadotropin and estradiol concentrations, which could worsen abnormal uterine bleeding.

Educational Objective
Evaluate elevated estradiol in a perimenopausal woman with irregular menstrual bleeding.

UpToDate Topic Review(s)
Approach to abnormal uterine bleeding in nonpregnant reproductive-age women

Reference(s)

Levens ED, Whitcomb BW, Csokmay JM, Nieman LK. Selective venous sampling for androgen-producing ovarian pathology. *Clin Endocrinol (Oxf)*. 2009;70(4):606-614. PMID: 18721192

13 ANSWER: D) Call her obstetrician and recommend that she be seen immediately

For pregnant women with preexisting diabetes, insulin requirements typically increase steadily with advancing gestation. During the third trimester, a small subgroup of women develops hypoglycemia, which requires a reduction in insulin. This condition is referred to as falling insulin requirement. Falling insulin requirement has been suggested to be a marker of placental insufficiency or compromise. If falling insulin requirement occurs, women with preexisting diabetes are commonly admitted to the hospital for maternal and fetal monitoring.

Padmanabhan et al prospectively studied 158 women with pregestational diabetes (41 with type 1 diabetes, 117 with type 2 diabetes) for falling insulin requirement, which was defined as a 15% or greater decrease in daily insulin requirements from the peak total daily dose after 20 weeks' gestational age. Patients who had falling insulin requirement were the case group (n = 32), while patients who did not have falling insulin requirement were the control group (n = 126). The authors concluded that falling insulin requirement was associated with the following significant adverse effects:

1. Younger gestational age at delivery
2. Higher rate of preterm delivery
3. Higher rate of admission to the intensive care nursery
4. Lower birth weight
5. Higher rate of preeclampsia in the mother

The authors also measured blood biomarkers of placental function and documented that levels of these biomarkers were altered in women with falling insulin requirement. The study authors conclude that clinicians should be watching for falling insulin requirement during the third trimester. Identified women should be evaluated for placental dysfunction (Answer D).

In this vignette, recommending increased dietary carbohydrates (Answer A) and asking the patient to reduce her exercise (Answer C) are useful steps, but these interventions would not help determine the diagnosis. This patient has normal blood pressure and normal levels of serum potassium and sodium, so adrenal insufficiency is unlikely. Therefore, performing a cosyntropin-stimulation test (Answer B) is incorrect. Starting methimazole (Answer E) in a euthyroid patient is not indicated. Pregnancy causes a functional decrease in TSH and an elevation in free T_4, so her thyroid function is normal.

Educational Objective

Recognize falling insulin requirement as a marker of placental insufficiency.

UpToDate Topic Review(s)
Pregestational diabetes mellitus: Obstetrical issues and management

Reference(s)

Padmanabhan S, Lee VW, Mclean M, et al. The association of falling insulin requirements with maternal biomarkers and placental dysfunction: a prospective study of women with preexisting diabetes in pregnancy. *Diabetes Care*. 2017;40(10):1323-1330. PMID: 28798085

14 **ANSWER: E) Obtain a radiograph of the right femur**

The patient described in this vignette sustained a nontraumatic left femur fracture in the setting of osteoporosis. While the most common types of osteoporotic hip fractures are femoral neck and intertrochanteric fractures, review of this patient's left femur radiograph reveals a subtrochanteric midfemur noncomminuted fracture with medial spiking and cortical thickening—all characteristics of an atypical femur fracture. These "chalk-stick" fractures are thought to be stress fractures associated with minimal or no trauma. The fracture line originates at the lateral cortex and is transverse in its orientation, although it may become oblique as it progresses medially across the femur. Affected patients usually present with prodromal pain in the region of the fracture and they exhibit delayed healing. Atypical femur fractures appear to be more common in patients who have been exposed to long-term bisphosphonate or denosumab therapy (although this is not the case with the patient in this vignette). Other risk factors include Asian ethnicity, lateral femoral bowing, varus hip geometry, glucocorticoid use, and genetic predisposition. These fractures can also occur in other types of metabolic bone disease such as hypophosphatasia. Because atypical femur fractures are frequently bilateral, imaging of the contralateral femur is indicated. Conventional radiography (Answer E) is usually the initial imaging procedure of choice because bone scintigraphy (Answer D), MRI, and CT are more costly and less convenient. However, these advanced imaging techniques provide superior sensitivity and specificity for detecting early stages of stress fracture and should be the next step if clinical suspicion is high and conventional radiography is unrevealing. This patient had a radiograph of the contralateral femur, which showed an impending (incomplete) atypical femur fracture, characterized by focal cortical thickening ("beaking or flaring") with central lucency in the midshaft of the right femur (*see image*). Internal fixation with intramedullary nailing is the mainstay of treatment for complete atypical femur fractures, and prophylactic surgical intervention is also recommended for incomplete atypical femur fractures, particularly those with extensive cortical defects and pain and/or marrow edema on MRI. Teriparatide may promote atypical femur fracture healing (off-label use), but limited data support its efficacy. This patient subsequently underwent prophylactic intramedullary nailing on the right side.

Serum protein electrophoresis (Answer A) to test for possible multiple myeloma is unlikely to be diagnostic in this scenario. This patient has a high-normal calcium level in the setting of hydrochlorothiazide use, but she is not frankly hypercalcemic. Furthermore, no "punched out" lytic lesions are noted on her x-ray. Similarly, in the absence of hypercalcemia, measuring serum intact PTH (Answer B) is not indicated. This patient's mildly elevated alkaline phosphatase level is most likely due to her recent femur fracture and surgery. While there are several different etiologies of elevated bone-specific alkaline phosphatase isoenzyme, including Paget disease, metastatic cancer to bone, hyperparathyroidism, and osteomalacia,

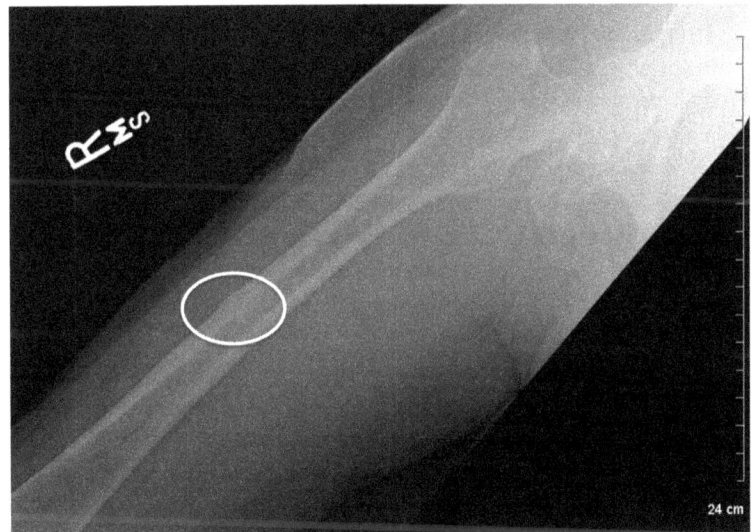

Plain x-ray of the right femur.

there is no reason to suspect any of these etiologies in this patient who has normal calcium, phosphate, and 25-hydroxyvitamin D levels and no evidence of sclerotic or lytic lesions on her imaging.

Finally, while measuring 24-hour urinary calcium excretion (Answer C) is helpful in identifying hypocalciuria or hypercalciuria as a cause of secondary osteoporosis, this would not be the best next step in the evaluation of a patient with an atypical femur fracture. In addition, this patient is taking hydrochlorothiazide, which may affect the result of this test.

Educational Objective

Identify the features of an atypical femur fracture and recommend the appropriate intervention.

Overview of common hip fractures in adults
Risks of bisphosphonate therapy in patients with osteoporosis

Reference(s)

Shane E, Burr D, Abrahamsen B, Adler RA, et al. Atypical subtrochanteric and diaphyseal femoral fractures: second report of a task force of the American Society for Bone and Mineral Research. *J Bone Miner Res.* 2014;29(1):1-23. PMID: 23712442

Starr J, Tay YKD, Shane E. Current understanding of epidemiology, pathophysiology, and management of atypical femur fractures. *Curr Osteoporos Rep.* 2018;16(4):519-529. PMID: 29951870

Watts NB, Aggers D, McCarthy EF, et al. Responses to treatment with teriparatide in patients with atypical femur fractures previously treated with bisphosphonates. *J Bone Miner Res.* 2017;32(5):1027-1033. PMID: 28071822

Greenspan SL, Vujevich K, Britton C, et al. Teriparatide for treatment of patients with bisphosphonate-associated atypical fracture of the femur. *Osteoporos Int.* 2018;29(2):501-506. PMID: 29085957

15 ANSWER: E) *NR0B1* (also known as *DAX1*) (resulting in adrenal hypoplasia congenita)

Although this patient recalls being diagnosed with congenital adrenal hyperplasia, his laboratory values indicate that his diagnosis is more likely to be adrenal hypoplasia congenita (AHC) (or congenital adrenal hypoplasia).

AHC is a rare cause of adrenal insufficiency in children that can present similarly to salt-wasting congenital adrenal hyperplasia due to 21-hydroxylase deficiency (CYP21A2 deficiency caused by pathogenic variants in the *CYP21A2* gene [Answer B]). AHC most commonly results from pathogenic variants in the *NR0B1* gene (Answer E) (also referred to as *DAX1*), located on the X chromosome, which result in failure of fetal adrenal cortical development and consequent deficiency in adrenocortical steroids. Affected patients usually present at birth with a salt-wasting syndrome that can include failure to thrive, hypotension, hyponatremia, hyperkalemia, and hyperpigmentation. This syndrome is due to deficiencies of cortisol and aldosterone and is accompanied by markedly elevated ACTH and plasma renin activity. In contrast to classic 21-hydroxylase deficiency, which is far more common and manifests similarly, 17-hydroxyprogesterone is not elevated in patients with AHC. Rather, all adrenocortical steroids are deficient or low, even after cosyntropin stimulation (as seen in this patient's laboratory values). Neonates with AHC are treated with glucocorticoid and mineralocorticoid therapy, as would be the case with other forms of primary adrenal insufficiency. The terms "adrenal hypoplasia congenita" or "congenital adrenal HYPOplasia" can be synonymous; however, "congenital adrenal HYPERplasia" is not, and this may have resulted in confusion in this patient's care over the years. Retrieval of the patient's prior medical records confirmed that AHC was diagnosed shortly after birth. Over the years, he, his family, and his providing physicians at different institutions incorrectly referred to the diagnosis as "congenital adrenal hyperplasia," resulting in the current confusion.

For reasons that are not clear, patients with AHC due to pathogenic variants in *NR0B1* develop normally during prepubertal years, but develop hypogonadotropic hypogonadism around the time of puberty that may result in failure of normal pubertal development. This patient's physical phenotype and history did not suggest obvious features of pubertal underdevelopment except for his testicular examination, which was remarkable for small testicular size and a biochemical pattern suggestive of hypogonadotropic hypogonadism. Patients with AHC may have successful fertility if treated with exogenous gonadotropins, clomiphene, and/or microsurgical sperm extraction.

All of the other answer choices are genes associated with forms of congenital adrenal HYPERplasia. Pathogenic variants in the *CYP17A1* gene (Answer A) are rare and cause 17-hydroxylase deficiency, which classically presents with impaired cortisol and adrenal androgen synthesis and excessive mineralocorticoid production (deoxycorticosterone and aldosterone). The clinical presentation is typically hypertension and hypokalemia with abnormal pubertal development in girls.

Pathogenic variants in the *CYP11B1* gene (Answer C) are rare and cause 11-hydroxylase deficiency, which usually presents with impaired aldosterone and cortisol synthesis, but excessive deoxycorticosterone, 11-deoxycortisol, and adrenal androgen synthesis. The classic clinical presentation is hypertension, hypokalemia, and ambiguous genitalia in girls.

Pathogenic variants in the *HSD3B2* gene (Answer D) are rare and cause 3β-hydroxysteroid dehydrogenase deficiency, which typically presents with impaired aldosterone and cortisol synthesis, but excessive DHEA synthesis. The classic clinical presentation is salt-wasting with hypotension, hyponatremia, hyperkalemia, and ambiguous genitalia.

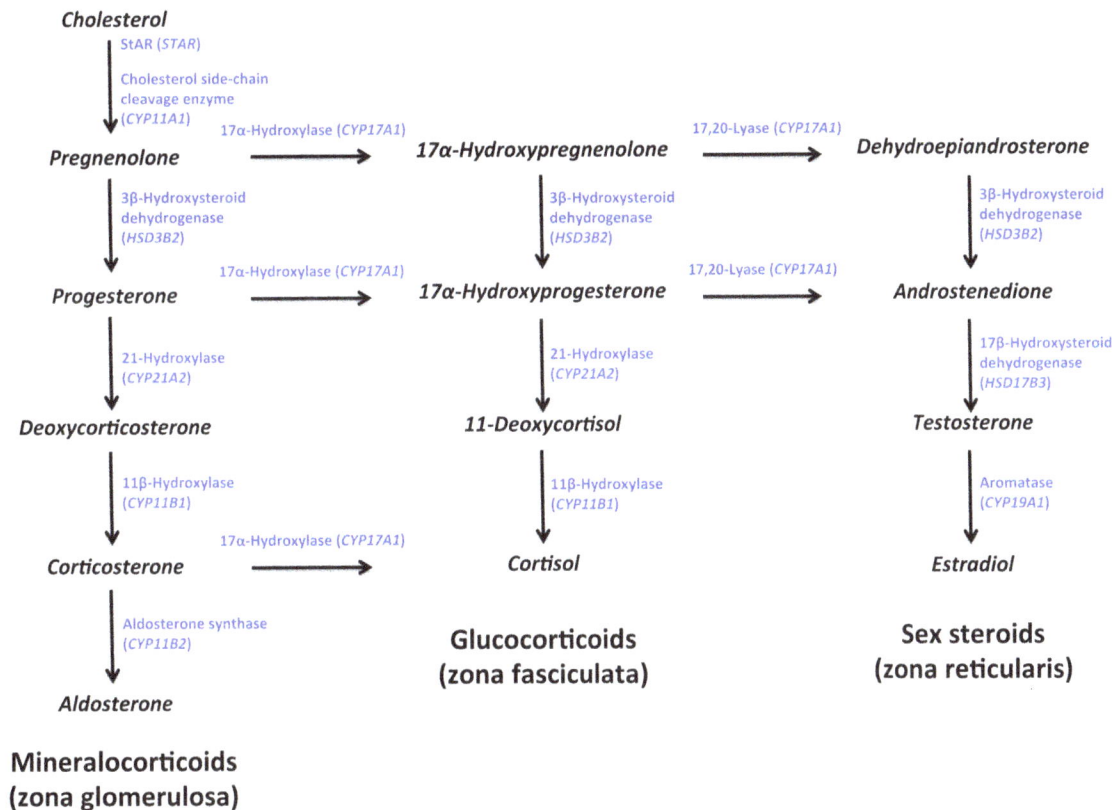

Cholesterol
StAR (*STAR*)
Cholesterol side-chain cleavage enzyme (*CYP11A1*)

Pregnenolone → 17α-Hydroxylase (*CYP17A1*) → **17α-Hydroxypregnenolone** → 17,20-Lyase (*CYP17A1*) → **Dehydroepiandrosterone**

3β-Hydroxysteroid dehydrogenase (*HSD3B2*)   3β-Hydroxysteroid dehydrogenase (*HSD3B2*)   3β-Hydroxysteroid dehydrogenase (*HSD3B2*)

Progesterone → 17α-Hydroxylase (*CYP17A1*) → **17α-Hydroxyprogesterone** → 17,20-Lyase (*CYP17A1*) → **Androstenedione**

21-Hydroxylase (*CYP21A2*)   21-Hydroxylase (*CYP21A2*)   17β-Hydroxysteroid dehydrogenase (*HSD17B3*)

Deoxycorticosterone   **11-Deoxycortisol**   **Testosterone**

11β-Hydroxylase (*CYP11B1*)   11β-Hydroxylase (*CYP11B1*)   Aromatase (*CYP19A1*)

Corticosterone → 17α-Hydroxylase (*CYP17A1*) →   **Cortisol**   **Estradiol**

Aldosterone synthase (*CYP11B2*)

Aldosterone

Mineralocorticoids (zona glomerulosa)   **Glucocorticoids (zona fasciculata)**   **Sex steroids (zona reticularis)**

Educational Objective

Diagnose adrenal hypoplasia congenita on the basis of clinical presentation and laboratory evaluation.

UpToDate Topic Review(s)

Uncommon congenital adrenal hyperplasias
Causes and clinical manifestations of primary adrenal insufficiency in children

Reference(s)

Speiser PW, Arlt W, Auchus RJ, et al. Congenital adrenal hyperplasia due to steroid 21-hydroxylase deficiency: an Endocrine Society clinical practice guideline. *J Clin Endocrinol Metab.* 2018;103(11):4043-4088. PMID: 30272171

16   ANSWER: C) Gonadotropinoma

This patient has a relatively short history of headaches and deteriorating vision, which are explained by the presence of a sella-based mass with suprasellar extension. Her visual acuity is reduced and visual field assessment (perimetry) demonstrates a bitemporal superior quadrantanopia—typical of optic chiasm compression by a lesion arising from within the sella. Consistent with this, the initial endocrine laboratory profile shows a picture of widespread pituitary dysfunction (inappropriate gonadotropin concentrations for a postmenopausal woman; low IGF-1 suggestive, but not diagnostic, of GH deficiency; low-normal 9-AM cortisol concentration; mild central hypothyroidism). This combination most likely explains why the patient is finding it increasingly difficult to cope with the demands of her job.

Her prolactin level is raised, but only modestly for the size of the lesion (<3 times the upper normal limit), which makes it unlikely that the pituitary mass is a prolactinoma (Answer D). This degree of hyperprolactinemia is within the range seen in clinically nonfunctioning pituitary adenomas (most of which originate from the gonadotroph lineage). It is attributable to so-called stalk disconnection (compression) syndrome in which interruption of normal dopaminergic tone allows for increased prolactin secretion from pituitary lactotrophs. Thus, of the options listed in this vignette, a nonsecreting gonadotropinoma (Answer C) is the most likely cause of this patient's clinical presentation and MRI findings. Note that with the advent of new histochemical markers for the pituitary transcription factors SF-1, Pit-1, and Tpit, it is now possible to determine the origin of pituitary adenomas more reliably and to classify tumors as arising from the gonadotroph (SF-1), somatotroph/lactotroph/thyrotroph (Pit-1), or corticotroph (Tpit) lineages. Accordingly, many clinically nonfunctioning tumors that were traditionally considered to be "null cell adenomas" due to lack of immunohistochemical staining for LH or FSH can now be classified as being of gonadotroph origin.

Although intrasellar craniopharyngiomas (Answer B) are recognized and can be mistaken for adenomas, most are suprasellar, with mixed solid and cystic components, and may demonstrate calcification. Diabetes insipidus can also be a presenting feature, which is virtually never the case with pituitary adenomas. Visual field assessment may reveal an unusual pattern in the early stages with bitemporal inferior quadrantanopia, reflecting compression of the optic chiasm from above.

Similarly, Rathke cleft cysts (Answer E) often have a distinct radiologic appearance, arising in the midline at the junction of the anterior and posterior pituitary lobes (originating from the Rathke pouch). The pituitary stalk may be inserted more anteriorly into the gland than is normally observed on sagittal MRI. If the cyst contains proteinaceous fluid, then it will exhibit high signal on noncontrast T1-weighted MRI, which fails to enhance following gadolinium administration.

Autoimmune (lymphocytic) hypophysitis (Answer A) affects both sexes, at all ages, but it is more common in women in later pregnancy or in the early postpartum period. It is characterized by pituitary enlargement due to lymphocytic infiltration, with consequent destruction of normal pituitary tissue. Headaches are a typical presenting feature and can be severe; vision loss may occur due to compression of the optic chiasm. Although some groups have reported an atypical pattern of anterior pituitary hormone loss (with early-onset corticotroph and thyrotroph dysfunction, but preserved gonadotroph and somatotroph function), others have observed anterior pituitary failure involving all axes. Diabetes insipidus is a known complication, which helps to distinguish autoimmune hypophysitis from pituitary adenomas. In this setting, MRI reveals a pituitary mass that can mimic an adenoma, but enhancement is typically diffuse and homogeneous. Other forms of hypophysitis also exist (eg, granulomatous, IgG4-related, xanthomatous), and it can arise as a complication of anticytotoxic T-lymphocyte–associated antigen 4 immunotherapy (eg, ipilimumab).

Educational Objective
Interpret visual fields and pituitary MRI in a patient with a typical presentation of a clinically nonfunctioning macroadenoma.

UpToDate Topic Review(s)
Clinical manifestations and diagnosis of gonadotroph and other clinically nonfunctioning pituitary adenomas

Reference(s)
Karavitaki N, Thanabalasingham G, Shore HC, et al. Do the limits of serum prolactin in disconnection hyperprolactinaemia need re-definition? A study of 226 patients with histologically verified non-functioning pituitary macroadenoma. *Clin Endocrinol (Oxf)*. 2006;65(4):524-529. PMID: 16984247

17 **ANSWER: C) Limited joint mobility syndrome**
Musculoskeletal disorders of the upper limb are common in patients with diabetes mellitus. Diabetic cheiroarthropathy, although derived from a Greek word for hand (*cheiro*), refers to multiple conditions, including adhesive capsulitis or "frozen shoulder," carpal tunnel syndrome, flexor tenosynovitis or "trigger finger," limited joint mobility syndrome with "positive prayer sign," and Dupuytren contractures.

Studies indicate that diabetic cheiroarthropathy is associated with female sex, advanced age, longer duration of diabetes, microvascular complications, and poor glycemic control. Data from the DCCT/EDIC study (Diabetes Control and Complications Trial/Epidemiology of Diabetes Interventions and Complications) suggest that 66% of patients have at least 1 feature of diabetic cheiroarthropathy and 33% have at least 2 musculoskeletal upper limb findings. More recent studies from the T1D Exchange and also from the United Kingdom suggest lower prevalence of diabetic cheiroarthropathy compared with findings in earlier studies, hypothesized to be due to improved glycemic control and/or diabetes care in general.

This patient has limited joint mobility syndrome (Answer C) with positive prayer sign based on the clinical presentation. Limited joint mobility syndrome was first described in 1974 in patients with longstanding type 1 diabetes who had restricted mobility of small and large joints; thick, waxy skin; and short stature. Clinically, affected patients note stiffness and contractures leading to reduced grip strength. Pain is not reported. Flexion contractures involving metacarpophalangeal and proximal interphalangeal joints are most common, but other small and large joints can also be involved. It is classically associated with a positive prayer sign, as described in this patient. Association with type 2 diabetes has also been observed. Some studies do not confirm an association between limited joint mobility syndrome and glycemic control, but rather suggest risk factors including onset of puberty and microalbuminuria. In pediatric and adolescent populations, identification of limited joint mobility syndrome may be important because of an association with microvascular complications. As in this case, limited joint mobility syndrome can coexist with other features of diabetic cheiroarthropathy.

Dupuytren contractures (Answer B) are reported in 16% to 42% of patients with diabetes. Classically, there is flexion contracture of the fourth and fifth digits. Pathologically, there is fibrosis around the palmar fascia, often with nodule formation. Fibrotic bands are often palpable. In this patient, it appears that all the fingers are involved, although fibrotic bands on the palmar surface were not described.

Reflex sympathetic dystrophy (Answer A) is associated with pain or burning in the hand or foot associated with signs or symptoms of vasomotor instability. Often the ipsilateral shoulder shows reduced range of motion. A clear association with diabetes has been suggested but not established.

Stiff-person syndrome (Answer E) is a rare syndrome of stiffness and rigidity presenting most commonly with gait instability or wide-based gait. There is marked rigidity of the axial muscles. Muscle spasms are common and symptoms are progressive. Occasionally, only a single limb is involved. Stiff-person syndrome is associated with high titers of glutamic acid decarboxylase antibodies and can be seen in type 1 diabetes or as a paraneoplastic syndrome not associated with diabetes.

Educational Objective
Diagnose limited joint mobility syndrome in a patient with diabetes mellitus.

UpToDate Topic Review(s)
Limited joint mobility in diabetes mellitus

Reference(s)

Frost D, Beischer W. Limited joint mobility in type 1 diabetic patients: associations with microangiopathy and subclinical macroangiopathy are different in men and women. *Diabetes Care*. 2001;24(1):95-99. PMID: 11194249

Larkin ME, Barnie A, Braffett BH, et al; Diabetes Control and Complications Trial/Epidemiology of Diabetes Interventions and Complications Research Group. Musculoskeletal complications in type 1 diabetes. *Diabetes Care*. 2014;37(7):1863-1869. PMID: 24722493

Lindsay JR, Kennedy L, Atkinson AB, et al. Reduced prevalence of limited joint mobility in type 1 diabetes in a U.K. clinical population over a 20-year period. *Diabetes Care*. 2005;28(3):658-661. PMID: 15735204

18 **ANSWER: B) Increase the levothyroxine dosage to maintain TSH between 0.5 and 2.0 mIU/L**
This patient has papillary thyroid carcinoma; confirmed by histopathologic findings of optically clear nuclei (*orphan Annie nuclei, white arrow*) and psammoma bodies (*calcification, green arrow*). Other findings are nuclear inclusions and grooves and papillary architecture (not shown in these slides).

On the basis of the 2015 American Thyroid Association thyroid cancer guidelines, it is important to assess the patient's risk for recurrence after thyroid surgery and to keep the TSH in the range recommended based on recurrence risk. The TSH goals for long-term follow-up are determined on the basis of treatment response. One study has suggested improved relapse-free survival

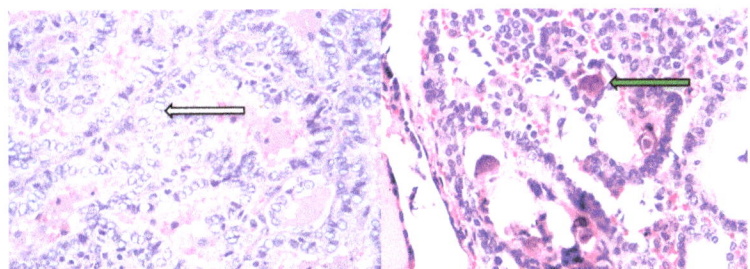

when serum TSH is undetectable during follow-up, but the hypothesis that low serum TSH decreases mortality and morbidity in all patients with differentiated thyroid cancer has not been proven. In accordance with recent American Thyroid Association thyroid cancer guidelines, the TSH goal should be between 0.5 and 2.0 mIU/L for the low-risk group, between 0.1 and 0.5 mIU/L for the intermediate-risk group, and less than 0.1 mIU/L for the high-risk group. Therefore, continuing levothyroxine at the same dosage (Answer A) or increasing the dosage to maintain a TSH level around 0.1 mIU/L (Answer C) is incorrect. This patient has a low risk of thyroid cancer recurrence, and the TSH goal should be between 0.5 and 2.0 mIU/L. Therefore, her levothyroxine dosage should be increased to maintain TSH in this range (Answer B). It is also important to predict the risk from the adverse effects of levothyroxine, taking into account the patient's age, as well as the presence of preexisting cardiovascular and skeletal risk factors that might predispose to the development of long-term adverse cardiovascular or skeletal outcomes, particularly atrial fibrillation and osteoporosis.

The American Thyroid Association low-risk thyroid cancer group is defined as:

- Papillary thyroid cancer with all of the following:

    - No local or distant metastases
    - No tumor invasion of locoregional tissues or structures
    - No aggressive histology (eg, tall cell, hobnail variant, columnar cell carcinoma)
    - No vascular invasion
    - Clinical N0 or ≤5 pathologic N1 micrometastases (<0.2 cm in largest dimension)
    - All macroscopic tumor has been resected
    - If ^{131}I is given, there are no radioiodine-avid metastatic foci outside the thyroid bed on the first posttreatment whole-body radioiodine scan

- Intrathyroidal, encapsulated follicular variant of papillary thyroid cancer

- Intrathyroidal, well-differentiated follicular thyroid cancer with capsular invasion and no or minimal (<4 foci) vascular invasion

- Intrathyroidal, papillary microcarcinoma, unifocal or multifocal, including the *BRAF* V600E pathogenic variant (if known)

In the low-risk thyroid cancer group, the risk of disease-specific mortality is low by definition. The risk of persistent or recurrent disease is around 3%, and there is no evidence that delayed finding and treatment of persistent disease lowers the chance of cure in this patient group.

Prospective data from the National Thyroid Cancer Treatment Cooperative Study Group (NTCTCSG) suggest that overall disease-specific and disease-free survival are not improved by radioiodine treatment in patients with NTCTCSG stage I and II (ie, patients aged <45 years with no distant metastases or patients aged ≥45 years with a primary tumor <4 cm in diameter, no extrathyroidal extension, and no nodal metastases).

In a retrospective study of 1298 patients with differentiated thyroid cancer categorized as being at low risk according to American Thyroid Association categories who had a median follow-up period of 10.3 years, there was no significant effect of adjuvant radioiodine therapy on overall or disease-free survival. Therefore, radioiodine treatment is not routinely recommended in patients with low-risk thyroid cancer. This patient falls in the low-risk group for recurrence and she does not require radioiodine treatment after either thyroid hormone withdrawal whole-body scan or rhTSH injection (Answers D and E).

Educational Objective
Manage the care of a patient with low-risk differentiated thyroid cancer.

UpToDate Topic Review(s)
Differentiated thyroid cancer: Overview of management

Reference(s)

Pujol P, Daures JP, Nsakala N, Baldet L, Bringer J, Jaffiol C. Degree of thyrotropin suppression as a prognostic determinant in differentiated thyroid cancer. *J Clin Endocrinol Metab.* 1996;81(12):4318-4323. PMID: 8954034

Schvartz C, Bonnetain F, Dabakuyo S, et al. Impact on overall survival of radioactive iodine in low-risk differentiated thyroid cancer patients. *J Clin Endocrinol Metab.* 2012;97)5):1526-1535. PMID: 22344193

Jonklaas J, Sarlis NJ, Litofsky D, et al. Outcomes of patients with differentiated thyroid carcinoma following initial therapy. *Thyroid.* 2006;16(12):1229-1242. PMID: 17199433

Jonklaas J, Cooper DS, Ain KB, et al. Radioiodine therapy in patients with stage I differentiated thyroid cancer. *Thyroid.* 2010;20(12):1423-1424. PMID: 21054207

Haugen BR, Alexander EK, Bible KC, et al. 2015 American Thyroid Association management guidelines for adult patients with thyroid nodules and differentiated thyroid cancer: the American Thyroid Association Guidelines Task Force on Thyroid Nodules and Differentiated Thyroid Cancer. *Thyroid.* 2016;26(1):1-133. PMID: 26462967

19 ANSWER: B) Start sitagliptin

Patients with type 2 diabetes mellitus are known to have a higher fracture risk, particularly at sites in the lower extremities. Furthermore, these patients are at a 20% to 30% higher risk of hip fracture. Recognition of this clear association has prompted consideration of type 2 diabetes to be an independent risk factor for fracture in risk prediction tools such as FRAX. Indeed, there is some evidence that one can modify FRAX risk factors (eg, include rheumatoid arthritis, increase age by 10 years, or decrease femoral neck T-score by 0.5) to more accurately define hip and major fracture risk in patients with type 2 diabetes. Furthermore, available evidence suggests that FDA-approved antifracture therapies are equally effective in patients with and without type 2 diabetes. Finally, it is critical to understand that some antihyperglycemic medications have been shown to increase fracture risk. Given these observations, it is very important for health providers to consider both the skeletal and glycemic implications of pharmacotherapy in this patient population.

This patient is not at her target glycemic goal based on currently available evidence. In addition, she has evidence of microvascular disease given the presence of microalbuminuria, which portends a higher risk for future diabetes-related complications if suboptimal glycemic control continues. Therefore, initiation of effective and safe antihyperglycemic therapy is a priority for this patient. Simply maintaining her current therapy with metformin (Answer A) is inappropriate. Of the available choices, both efficacy and safety data support the use of sitagliptin (Answer B). Both rosiglitazone (Answer C) and canagliflozin (Answer D) are associated with increased fracture risk in patients with type 2 diabetes, rendering them inferior options in an older postmenopausal woman with known osteopenia. However, an increase in fracture risk has not been identified to date with the alternative SGLT-2 inhibitors empagliflozin or dapagliflozin. Other type 2 diabetes medications, including metformin, sulfonylureas, DPP-4 inhibitors, GLP-1 receptor agonists, and glinides, have also not been associated with increased fracture risk based on available data. Finally, although oral bisphosphonates such as alendronate (Answer E) effectively reduce fracture risk in such a patient, her relatively low risk of hip fracture and lack of any glycemic benefit would argue against their use in this instance.

Educational Objective

Determine the best antihyperglycemic therapy in a postmenopausal woman with osteopenia and type 2 diabetes mellitus.

UpToDate Topic Review(s)

Bone disease in diabetes mellitus

Reference(s)

Fan Y, Wei F, Lang Y, Liu Y. Diabetes mellitus and risk of hip fractures: a meta-analysis. *Osteoporos Int.* 2016;27(1):219-228. PMID: 26264604

Wolverton D, Blair MM. Fracture risk associated with common medications used in treating type 2 diabetes mellitus. *Am J Health Syst Pharm.* 2017;74(15):1143-1151. PMID: 28743778

Mamza J, Marlin C, Wang C, Chokkalingam K, Idris I. DPP-4 inhibitor therapy and bone fractures in people with type 2 diabetes - a systematic review and meta-analysis. *Diabetes Res Clin Pract.* 2016;116:288-298. PMID: 27321347

Schacter GI, Leslie WD. DXA-based measurements in diabetes: can they predict fracture risk? *Calcif Tissue Int.* 2017;100(2):150-164. PMID: 27591864

20

ANSWER: D) Start a PCSK9 inhibitor

This patient has nephrotic syndrome, one of the most common kidney diseases in children and adults, characterized by massive proteinuria, edema, and hypoalbuminemia. Nephrotic syndrome results in podocyte and glomerular injury, and complications include acute kidney injury, infection, and thromboembolism. Dysregulated lipid metabolism leading to dyslipidemia is an often underrecognized, but nearly universal, complication of persistent nephrotic syndrome. Although long-term cardiovascular consequences of dyslipidemia are unclear, individuals with nephrotic syndrome are at significantly increased risk of cardiovascular disease. Lipid abnormalities in nephrotic syndrome can result in a "lipid nephrotoxicity," although the mechanism is not well understood. Elevated apo B lipoproteins (VLDL, intermediate-density lipoprotein, and LDL) occur due to delayed clearance and, to a lesser extent, increased biosynthesis. These triglyceride-rich lipoproteins can induce further glomerular damage via production of cytotoxic agents, cytokines, and reactive oxygen species. Increased levels of free fatty acids are observed in patients with nephrotic syndrome, with resultant nephrotoxicity and kidney disease progression.

There is compelling evidence that dyslipidemia in nephrotic syndrome can result in progressive kidney injury, and individuals with nephrotic syndrome have an increased risk of myocardial infarction and coronary death. However, little evidence exists to guide the optimal treatment of dyslipidemia in these patients. Statins are effective and are well tolerated, although there is no long-term evidence regarding cardiovascular endpoints in nephrotic syndrome. The patient in this vignette is on high-intensity statin therapy and ezetimibe with persistently elevated LDL-cholesterol levels, necessitating further therapy.

In nephrotic syndrome, hepatic levels of proprotein convertase subtilisin/kexin type 9 (PCSK9) are increased and correlate with proteinuria. PCSK9 degrades the LDL receptor, and it is thus a major therapeutic target for LDL-cholesterol lowering. PCSK9 inhibitors (Answer D) are antibodies that inactivate PCSK9 and decrease LDL-cholesterol levels. Their use is limited to patients with familial hypercholesterolemia and those with atherosclerotic cardiovascular disease who need further risk reduction. There are no studies of PCSK9 inhibitors in individuals with chronic kidney disease and/or nephrotic syndrome. The limited studies that have included individuals with an estimated glomerular filtration rate greater than 30 mL/min per 1.73 m^2 suggest that these medications are safe to use in this population. In this patient who is at very high cardiovascular risk, it is appropriate to attempt PCSK9 inhibitor therapy with the goal of decreasing LDL-cholesterol levels. Hence, prescribing evolocumab is the best next step in this patient, although its use is currently off-label in this setting.

Rosuvastatin (Answer A) is a synthetic selective HMG coA reductase inhibitor with decreased lipophilicity and it is metabolized through CYP2C19 (atorvastatin and simvastatin are metabolized via CYP3A4). Rosuvastatin, 40 mg daily, is slightly more potent than atorvastatin, 80 mg daily, for lowering LDL cholesterol. However, in this patient who has very high LDL cholesterol due to underlying kidney disease, it is unlikely that simply switching to another high-intensity statin will provide the necessary lipid-lowering benefit.

Fibrates, including fenofibrate (Answer B) and gemfibrozil, are agonists of the peroxisome proliferator–activator α receptors. Their principal effects are to lower triglyceride concentrations and raise HDL cholesterol. Fenofibrate can also lower LDL cholesterol. They are widely used for the management of marked hypertriglyceridemia. These drugs are excreted by the kidney and hence must be used with caution. Data on effectiveness of fibrates in nephrotic syndrome are lacking. Fenofibrate can elevate creatinine, so its use in patients with chronic kidney disease is not recommended.

Fish oil (Answer C) can be beneficial in decreasing triglyceride levels. Although published data in patients with chronic kidney disease and/or nephrotic syndrome are limited, omega-3 fatty acids do not have significant interactions with other drugs and do not require dosage reductions in the setting of impaired renal function. However, they do not have any effects on LDL-cholesterol lowering, which is the goal in this individual.

LDL apheresis (Answer E) is a well-established extracorporeal technique that is used to treat patients with homozygous familial hypercholesterolemia. There is promising evidence demonstrating the utility of lipid apheresis in treatment-resistant nephrotic syndrome by enabling partial or complete remission of the condition. The mechanism by which lipid apheresis leads to remission remains unclear, but possible explanations include direct effects associated with improved dyslipidemia, removal of pathogenic vascular permeability factors, and improved response to immunosuppressants. One hypothesis is that LDL apheresis reduces or prevents podocyte damage and reduces proteinuria by lowering the level of free fatty acids. Due to the need for central venous access and the higher cost associated with this procedure, this option could be considered if there is no response to a PCSK9 inhibitor.

Educational Objective
Manage lipid abnormalities in an individual with nephrotic syndrome.

UpToDate Topic Review(s)
Lipid abnormalities in nephrotic syndrome

Reference(s)
Agrawal S, Zaritsky J, Fornoni A, Smoyer WE. Dyslipidaemia in nephrotic syndrome: mechanisms and treatment. *Nat Rev Nephrol*. 2018;14(1):57-70. PMID: 29176657

21 ANSWER: D) Functional hypogonadotropic hypogonadism

Commonly recognized in women as the "athlete triad" of (1) disordered eating (or low energy availability), (2) amenorrhea/oligomenorrhea, and (3) decreased bone mineral density, a similar state of functional hypogonadotropic hypogonadism can occur in men and has been described as the *exercise-hypogonadal male condition*. More recently, the term relative *energy deficiency in sport* (RED-S) has been proposed to denote insufficient caloric intake and/or excessive energy expenditure. RED-S can affect multiple psychobiologic domains and is a diagnosis of exclusion.

In RED-S–associated hypogonadotropic hypogonadism, the history is typically notable for increasing and, at times, excessive exercise, often in conjunction with weight loss due to the relative caloric deficit. The condition overlaps with that of male anorexia, which in itself can cause severe hypogonadism. Approximately 30% of patients diagnosed with the DSM-5 condition *avoidant and restrictive food intake disorder* are male. Findings consistent with the diagnosis of RED-S in this vignette are the elevated serum SHBG level (a stress marker typically increased in excessive exercise/energy-deficient states), the thyroid function tests reflecting a euthyroid sick picture, and the mild anemia consistent with androgen deficiency. Thus, the most likely diagnosis is functional hypogonadotropic hypogonadism (Answer D). Treatment of RED-S consists of correcting the underlying energy deficit by increasing caloric intake and reducing training intensity. If successful, this will lead to gonadal axis recovery.

Covert current or previous anabolic steroid use (Answer A) is an important differential diagnosis, as synthetic anabolic steroids usually do not cross-react with the testosterone assay and mimic laboratory findings of severe central hypogonadism (suppressed gonadotropins, low testosterone). Moreover, high-dosage, long-term anabolic steroid use can lead to persistent gonadal axis suppression for months and occasionally years after cessation. However, covert anabolic use is less likely in this vignette, as such men typically have increased muscle bulk, truncal acne, and, after long-term use, atrophic testes. With anabolic steroid use, hemoglobin would not be expected to be low, given the erythropoietic actions of androgens. Finally, androgens at high dosages reduce SHBG.

This patient's normal prolactin level and the absence of clinical signs of pituitary mass effects make a pituitary adenoma (Answer B) less likely, although pituitary imaging should be considered in this case, as RED-S is a diagnosis of exclusion.

His transferrin saturation is normal and his ferritin concentration is only marginally elevated, possibly reflecting physical stress. These iron studies are not consistent with hemochromatosis (Answer C), which can present as hypogonadotropic hypogonadism in men.

Celiac disease (Answer E) could explain the vague abdominal symptoms, weight loss, and mild anemia, but in that setting, the patient's ferritin would most likely be lower, and celiac disease is not associated with severe hypogonadism.

Educational Objective
Diagnose functional hypogonadotropic hypogonadism due to overtraining/energy deficit (relative energy deficiency of sport).

UpToDate Topic Review(s)
Overtraining syndrome in athletes
Clinical features and diagnosis of male hypogonadism

Reference(s)

Goldman AL, Pope HG Jr, Bhasin S. The health threat posed by the hidden epidemic of anabolic steroid use and body image disorders among young men. *J Clin Endocrinol Metab*. 2019;104(4):1069-1074. PMID: 30239802

Mountjoy M, Sundgot-Borgen J, Burke L, et al. The IOC consensus statement: beyond the female athlete triad--relative energy deficiency in sport (RED-S). *Br J Sports Med*. 2014;48(7):491-497. PMID: 24620037

Wong HK, Hoermann R, Grossmann M. Reversible male hypogonadotropic hypogonadism due to energy deficit. *Clin Endocrinol (Oxf)*. 2019;91(1):3-9. PMID: 30903626

22 ANSWER: A) Call the head nurse at the nursing home to review the patient's medications

Severe hypoglycemia can result in permanent brain injury or death. The etiology of hypoglycemia in patients who present to the emergency department is most commonly iatrogenic and caused by diabetes medications. It is important to inquire whether the patient may have access to insulin or oral diabetes mediations (medications prescribed for the patient or for a family member). In the absence of diabetes medications, new-onset hypoglycemia requires a thorough history, including recent medical problems and, most importantly, a detailed review of all medications, especially any newly started medications. For the endocrinologist, detailed questioning regarding recent exposure to steroid medications (oral, inhaled, and applied to the skin) is useful because steroids can suppress the hypothalamic-pituitary-adrenal axis. In addition, a detailed review of any weight change and complete dietary history is essential, as many elderly patients who are hospitalized have protein or calorie malnutrition.

In this vignette, an elderly nursing home resident has had an episode of severe hypoglycemia while undergoing dialysis. As there is no known exposure to diabetes medications, no recent illness, and no dietary changes, the physician must look for other causes of hypoglycemia. Possible etiologies include organ dysfunction, such as new liver disease, or a change in dialysis schedule, as patients who are underdialyzed may have hypoglycemia. This patient has 19 medications on her medication list. The medication list provided to the emergency department by nursing homes may not be current. A computer inquiry of this patient's listed medications did not flag any possible drug-drug interactions that could cause hypoglycemia. However, a call to the nursing home (Answer A) determined that the patient had recently started oseltamivir as prophylaxis against influenza. Although hypoglycemia is not listed in the adverse events section of oseltamivir's prescribing information, a search in MedWatch (the US FDA Safety Information and Adverse Event Reporting Program) found that hypoglycemia has been reported to occur with similar antiviral medications. Oseltamivir given to pregnant mothers is associated with neonatal hypoglycemia after delivery. A case report of antiviral prophylaxis in a summer camp setting described 2 individuals with diabetes who experienced difficulty maintaining glucose control due to hypoglycemia while receiving oseltamivir. Oseltamivir was stopped in this particular patient, and she did not experience any further episodes of hypoglycemia.

Medication dispensation errors are a common concern, especially in patients with polypharmacy. Thus, even if there were no concerns based on this patient's medication list, asking the nursing home if there are other patients who have diabetes who have similar names, or who are dispensed medications at the same time as the patient in this case, could provide information regarding a potential medication dispensation error. Even in the absence of known risks, measuring insulin secretagogues (sulfonylureas and meglitinides) should be considered.

Stopping other medications that are not associated with hypoglycemia (Answers B and E) will not solve the problem and could be harmful. Performing a cosyntropin-stimulation test (Answer C) is not the best strategy, as she has no other features of adrenal insufficiency. Performing a 48-hour fast (Answer D) is the gold standard to assess for an insulinoma, but stopping the dextrose infusion may be harmful in a patient with profound hypoglycemia. This test can be done, if needed, after other more common causes of hypoglycemia are excluded.

Educational Objective
Obtain accurate information regarding current medications when investigating the cause of hypoglycemia.

UpToDate Topic Review(s)
Hypoglycemia in adults without diabetes mellitus: Diagnostic approach

Reference(s)

Macdonald L. New influenza drugs zanamivir (Relenza) and oseltamivir (Tamiflu): unexpected serious reactions. *CMAJ.* 2000;163(7):879-881. PMID: 11033723

Kimberlin DW, Escude J, Gantner J, et al. Targeted antiviral prophylaxis with oseltamivir in a summer camp setting. *Arch Pediatr Adolesc Med.* 2010;164(4):323-328. PMID: 20124132

23 ANSWER: C) Obtain 2 bedtime salivary cortisol levels

Cushing syndrome often occurs in women of childbearing age. However, because of the high prevalence of ovulatory disturbance caused by hypercortisolism, the presentation of Cushing syndrome during pregnancy is rather rare. Hypercortisolemia not only affects ovarian function, but it can also inhibit the secretion of GnRH from the hypothalamus, which can lead to menstrual disorders, secondary amenorrhea, and infertility.

Changes in the hypothalamic-pituitary-adrenal axis during normal pregnancy may mislead the diagnosis of Cushing syndrome during this period. Many laboratory assessments suggestive of Cushing syndrome can be present in normal pregnancy, and pregnancy is associated with clinical features mimicking those seen in patients with Cushing syndrome (weight gain, fatigue, worsening glucose metabolism).

Contrary to the etiology of Cushing syndrome in nonpregnant young patients (in whom the most frequent cause is Cushing disease), Cushing syndrome in pregnancy is equally caused by adrenal and pituitary adenomas. Twenty-four–hour urinary free cortisol is considered to be a good screening test for hypercortisolism in nonpregnant patients. However, during normal pregnancy, urinary free cortisol increases progressively, and in the second and third trimesters it is suggestive of Cushing syndrome only when it is 3 times greater than the upper normal limit. Therefore, repeating the urinary free cortisol measurement in this case (Answer A) would not be informative. Because the circadian rhythm of cortisol is preserved during normal pregnancy, bedtime salivary cortisol (Answer C) is best tool to detect Cushing syndrome in this setting. This test reflects free serum cortisol, and it is not influenced by changes in cortisol-binding globulin. Nevertheless, to date, threshold values for the diagnosis of Cushing syndrome during pregnancy are not well validated.

During pregnancy, high estrogen levels cause a progressive increase in cortisol-binding globulin. This causes an increase in total serum cortisol, making serum cortisol measurement after dexamethasone (Answer B) an unreliable test to diagnose hypercortisolism in pregnancy.

During pregnancy, there is a progressive increase in plasma ACTH levels, most likely due to an increase in corticotropin-releasing factor secretion by the placenta. Therefore, measurement of ACTH (Answer D) is an unreliable indicator of hypercortisolism.

Performing pituitary MRI (Answer E) is not indicated in the absence of an established diagnosis of ACTH-dependent Cushing syndrome.

When Cushing syndrome is diagnosed in a pregnant woman, management is challenging. Hypercortisolism increases the risk of diabetes, hypertension, preeclampsia, infection, prematurity, intrauterine growth retardation, and stillbirth. Mild cases can be managed conservatively, by controlling comorbidities. Medications used to treat hypercortisolism are not approved during pregnancy, but are used in severe cases. Pituitary or adrenal surgery can be performed in the second or third trimester.

Educational Objective
Evaluate for Cushing syndrome in a pregnant woman.

UpToDate Topic Review(s)
Cushing's syndrome in pregnancy

Reference(s)

Jung C, Ho JT, Torpy DJ, et al. A longitudinal study of plasma and urinary cortisol in pregnancy and postpartum. *J Clin Endocrinol Metab.* 2011;96(5):1533-1540. PMID: 25872515

Bronstein MD, Machado MC, Fragoso MC. Management of endocrine disease: management of pregnant patients with Cushing's syndrome. *Eur J Endocrinol.* 2015;173(2):R85-R91. PMID: 25872515

Brue T, Amodru V, Castinetti F. Management of endocrine disease: management of Cushing's syndrome during pregnancy: solved and unsolved questions. *Eur J Endocrinol.* 2018;178(6):R259-R266. PMID: 29523633

24 ANSWER: D) Switch to burosumab therapy

The patient described in this vignette has X-linked hypophosphatemia (XLH). The gene responsible for XLH, *PHEX* (phosphate-regulating endopeptidase on the X chromosome), is expressed predominantly in bone and teeth. Inactivating pathogenic variants in *PHEX* cause XLH by increasing production of fibroblast growth factor 23 (FGF-23), a phosphatonin. It has an X-linked dominant pattern of inheritance. Clinical features of XLH in adults include fatigue, muscle weakness, stiffness, bone pain, and gait abnormalities. The major clinical findings are leg deformities, teeth defects, and osteomalacia. Most affected adults also have short stature due to limitations in growth during childhood. Accelerated osteoarthritis and enthesopathy (calcification of tendons and ligaments) are very common, usually beginning in the second or third decade of life. Typical biochemical findings are hypophosphatemia and low-normal circulating 1,25-dihydroxyvitamin D levels thought to be due to decreased expression of 1α-hydroxylase, as well as increased catabolism of 1,25-dihydroxyvitamin D.

XLH is currently treated with phosphate and active vitamin D supplementation. In adult patients with XLH, the goals of therapy are to relieve symptoms, reduce the extent of osteomalacia, and/or improve fracture healing or surgical recovery. Although available data support the use of phosphate and calcitriol in selected adults with XLH, the benefits of treatment need to be balanced with the complicated monitoring and potential risks of such therapy. The frequent follow-up visits and required laboratory testing may be burdensome to patients, compromising compliance. The most important complications of the treatment of XLH using calcitriol and phosphate are hypercalcemia, hypercalciuria, nephrolithiasis, nephrocalcinosis, and hyperparathyroidism. If significant secondary or tertiary hyperparathyroidism develops and persists during therapy despite optimal calcitriol dosage, cinacalcet can be used to attempt to normalize PTH values, although it would be off-label use for this indication.

Since this patient's calcium level is already high-normal, increasing the calcitriol dosage (Answer B) would not be appropriate, as this would precipitate hypercalcemia by increasing intestinal calcium absorption. Similarly, because this patient already has evidence of preexisting secondary hyperparathyroidism, increasing her oral phosphate intake (Answer A) would not be the best option. This may worsen her hyperparathyroidism, mainly due to transient lowering of the ionized calcium concentration, and result in an increase in urinary phosphate excretion that may aggravate the bone disease and thereby defeat the purpose of oral therapy. Intravenous phosphate therapy (Answer E) is typically reserved for patients with severe, symptomatic hypophosphatemia (serum phosphate <1.0 mg/dL [<0.3 mmol/L]) or an inability to take oral therapy. Intravenous phosphate is potentially dangerous because it can precipitate with calcium and cause hypocalcemia, renal failure, and/or arrhythmias. Teriparatide or PTH (1-34) therapy (Answer C) has no role in the treatment of XLH.

In 2018, the US FDA approved burosumab (Answer D), a monoclonal antibody to FGF-23, as a new option for the treatment of XLH in children and adults. In a trial of adults with XLH, anti-FGF-23 monoclonal antibody therapy improved symptoms and enhanced healing of XLH-associated fractures. There were no treatment-related serious adverse events or significant changes from baseline in serum or urine calcium or intact PTH levels. This treatment is recommended for patients who cannot achieve good control on conventional therapy, including adults who are symptomatic or have fractures. For adults, burosumab is administered as a subcutaneous injection every 4 weeks. It is available in 10 mg/mL, 20 mg/mL, and 30 mg/mL single-dose vials. The dosing regimen is 1 mg/kg body weight rounded to the nearest 10 mg, up to a maximum dosage of 90 mg administered every 4 weeks. The dosage of burosumab is adjusted based on blood phosphate levels. Fasting blood phosphate levels are initially assessed at weeks 4, 6, or 8, and 10 or 12. Beyond week 12, phosphate levels are assessed as deemed clinically appropriate and 2 weeks after any dosage change.

There are cost concerns with the use of this medication—the price of the 10-mg vial is about $3400 to $4000, with the higher-dose vials priced linearly. The estimated treatment cost after rebates is approximately $200,000 per patient per year for adults, depending on body weight. Finally, there are no data on the use of burosumab in pregnant women.

Educational Objective
Recommend anti-FGF-23 monoclonal antibody therapy in a patient with X-linked hypophosphatemia not responding to conventional therapy.

UpToDate Topic Review(s)
Hereditary hypophosphatemic rickets and tumor-induced osteomalacia

Reference(s)

Insogna KL, Briot K, Imel EA, et al. A randomized, double-blind, placebo-controlled, phase 3 trial evaluating the efficacy of burosumab, an anti-FGF23 antibody, in adults with X-linked hypophosphatemia: week 24 primary analysis. *J Bone Miner Res.* 2018;33(8):1383-1393. PMID: 29947083

Carpenter TO, Imel EA, Holm IA, Jan de Beur SM, Insogna KL. A clinician's guide to X-linked hypophosphatemia. *J Bone Miner Res.* 2011;26(7):1381-1388. PMID: 21538511

25   ANSWER: C) Switch to transdermal testosterone

For both cisgender and transgender men, the most common adverse effect or complication of testosterone hormone therapy is erythrocytosis or polycythemia (hemoglobin above the male reference range for cisgender men). The exact mechanisms are not known, but this phenomenon might be mediated by a combination of observed factors, including increased production of erythropoietin by the kidneys, a new erythropoietin to hemoglobin set point, decrease in hepcidin and subsequent increase in iron turnover, or direct bone marrow stimulation by dihydrotestosterone or estradiol derived from testosterone. Other secondary causes of polycythemia should be considered, including cardiopulmonary disease, obesity-related obstructive sleep apnea, and tobacco use. Transgender men with erythrocytosis or polycythemia should first have their peak testosterone levels measured and dosages adjusted accordingly. An initial strategy can be to lower the injected testosterone dose with a more frequent schedule, as in this vignette.

Because there are data showing that transdermal testosterone is less likely to cause erythrocytosis than injections, it would be reasonable to switch to transdermal testosterone (Answer C). This patient was switched to transdermal testosterone, and after 3 months, his hemoglobin level decreased to 15.4 g/dL (154 g/L) and total testosterone was maintained in the range of 400 to 500 ng/dL (13.9-17.4 nmol/L).

Although discontinuing testosterone therapy (Answer E) would lead to earlier resolution of the erythrocytosis, this is not the best option because it could worsen gender dysphoria, especially if menstrual bleeding resumes.

Phlebotomy or blood donation (Answer D) might be a short-term strategy, but it should not be a long-term management plan. Especially in light of data demonstrating lower rates of erythrocytosis with transdermal administration than with short-acting intramuscular injections, alternative forms and routes of testosterone should be considered first. Other routes such as longer-acting intramuscular injections (eg, testosterone undecanoate or subcutaneous testosterone pellets) could also be considered.

Because this patient's erythropoietin is not suppressed below normal, he has secondary erythrocytosis, so testing for primary causes of polycythemia, myeloproliferative disorders, and polycythemia vera with genetic testing for the *JAK2* pathogenic variant (Answer B) is not indicated.

Educational Objective

Evaluate and treat polycythemia in a transgender man on testosterone therapy.

UpToDate Topic Review(s)

Transgender men: Evaluation and management

Reference(s)

Center of Excellence for Transgender Health, Department of Family and Community Medicine, University of California San Francisco. Guidelines for the Primary and Gender-Affirming Care of Transgender and Gender Nonbinary People. 2nd edition. Deutsch MB, ed. June 2016. Available at: www.transhealth.ucsf.edu/guidelines. Accessed for verification March 2019.

Hembree WC, Cohen-Kettenis PT, et al. Endocrine treatment of gender-dysphoric/gender-incongruent persons: an Endocrine Society clinical practice guideline. *J Clin Endocrinol Metab.* 2017;102(11):3869-3903. PMID: 28945902

Ohlander SJ, Varghese B, Pastuszak AW. Erythrocytosis following testosterone therapy. *Sex Med Rev.* 2018;6(1):77-85. PMID: 28526632

26   ANSWER: B) Start pioglitazone

Lipodystrophy refers to a group of metabolic disorders characterized by complete or partial loss of adiposity in some areas with abnormal accumulation of adiposity in other areas in some cases. Lipodystrophy can be inherited or acquired and also classified as partial or generalized. A common form of lipodystrophy is acquired as a consequence of HIV therapy (highly active antiretroviral therapy [HAART]). A number of metabolic complications are associated with lipodystrophy, including diabetes, hypertriglyceridemia, low HDL-cholesterol levels, and liver disease (due to fatty infiltration). Affected women can have a phenotype of functional hyperandrogenism and gestational diabetes as well.

This patient has congenital partial lipodystrophy that is associated with a pathogenic variant in the *LMNA* gene. This is classified as type 2 (Dunnigan type) partial lipodystrophy, and it is inherited in an autosomal dominant manner. The *LMNA* gene, located on chromosome 1q21-q22, encodes nuclear envelope protein lamins A and C, which serve as nuclear architectural proteins. Another form of partial congenital lipodystrophy (type 3) is associated with pathogenic variants in the *PPARG* gene, which has a role in the differentiation of adipocytes. Serum leptin and adiponectin levels are low in patients with lipodystrophy, but the levels vary based on the precise etiology. The metabolic derangements are thought to be associated with low levels of these adipokines.

Besides diet and exercise, medications that improve insulin resistance are often used in the management of lipodystrophy. This patient is already on metformin. Thiazolidinediones are also used in patients with lipodystrophy. In addition to better glycemic control, case reports describe improved triglyceride and liver enzyme levels in patients treated with pioglitazone. Animal studies suggest that pioglitazone improves insulin resistance at least partly via its affect on serum adiponectin levels. The IRIS trial (Pioglitazone After Ischemic Stroke or Transient Ischemic Attack) also showed that pioglitazone reduced the development of type 2 diabetes in patients with insulin resistance. Rosiglitazone may not have the same effect on lipid levels. In this case, pioglitazone (Answer B) is the right choice, as it will help the patient with achieving both glycemic and triglyceride control.

Insulin (Answer A) might be a reasonable option in a patient with more severe hyperglycemia. Sometimes U500 insulin is required. Insulin should not be the next choice in this patient, as her hemoglobin A_{1c} level is 7.6% (60 mmol/mol) on a single glucose-lowering agent.

In the United States, metreleptin (Answer C) is approved for treatment of patients with congenital generalized lipodystrophy if other therapeutic modalities fail (eg, lifestyle, oral diabetes medications). It is not approved for use in patients with partial or acquired lipodystrophy.

Closely monitoring this patient and not providing glucose-lowering therapy (Answer E) is incorrect because the addition of a thiazolidinedione to metformin therapy will most likely help bring her hemoglobin A_{1c} level to goal.

There are no data on adiponectin infusion (Answer D) for the management of partial lipodystrophy.

Educational Objective
Manage a patient with an inherited partial lipodystrophy.

UpToDate Topic Review(s)
Lipodystrophic syndromes

Reference(s)
Fiorenza CG, Chou SH, Mantzoros CS. Lipodystrophy: pathophysiology and advances in treatment. *Nat Rev Endocrinol.* 2011;7(3):137-150. PMID: 21079616

Park JY, Javor ED, Cochran EK, DePaoli AM, Gorden P. Long-term efficacy of leptin replacement in patients with Dunnigan-type familial partial lipodystrophy. *Metabolism.* 2007;56(4):508-516. PMID: 17379009

Kernan WN, Viscoli CM, Furie KL, et al; IRIS Trial Investigators. Pioglitazone after ischemic stroke or transient ischemic attack. *N Engl J Med.* 2016;374(14):1321-1331. PMID: 26886418

27 **ANSWER: B) The patient has unilateral primary aldosteronism due to a left aldosterone-producing adenoma**

This patient has confirmed primary aldosteronism, and the single representative slice from the CT scan shows a well-defined, 10-mm lesion projecting from the posterior aspect of the left adrenal gland. The right adrenal gland is well visualized on the same slice and appears normal. However, current guidelines continue to recommend the use of a separate lateralizing procedure to address the possibility that the lesion is an adrenal incidentaloma or to detect possible small (subcentimeter) nodules in the contralateral gland.

Various criteria have been proposed to define successful cannulation and demonstration of lateralization after adrenal venous sampling, and they are summarized in the expert consensus statement of Rossi and colleagues (2014).

Adequacy of cannulation: in the absence of cosyntropin stimulation, the ratio of adrenal vein to low inferior vena cava cortisol concentration is above the threshold (≥2) for both the right and left adrenal veins, indicating satisfactory cannulation bilaterally (thus, Answers D and E are incorrect).

Lateralization: the aldosterone-to-cortisol ratio on the left is 6.2 times greater than that on the right, and it comfortably exceeds even the most stringent criteria for defining unilateral disease (>4:1), suggesting that the left-sided lesion seen on CT is indeed an aldosterone- producing adenoma (thus, Answer B is correct and Answer A is incorrect). In addition, the aldosterone-to-cortisol ratio in the right adrenal vein is actually lower than that observed in the low inferior vena cava, which suggests there is not excess aldosterone production from the right adrenal gland. However, this finding in isolation (ie, if the left adrenal vein had not been successfully cannulated) would need to be interpreted with caution, as it is not less than 50% of the inferior vena cava ratio.

The presence of cortisol cosecretion (which has been estimated to occur in up to 14% of aldosterone-producing adenomas) is not reliably diagnosed using samples taken at adrenal venous sampling (thus, Answer C is incorrect). Conventional screening methods (eg, overnight dexamethasone suppression test [1 mg]) should be performed to exclude hypercortisolism.

Educational Objective
Interpret adrenal CT and adrenal venous sampling results to distinguish unilateral from bilateral primary aldosteronism.

UpToDate Topic Review(s)
Diagnosis of primary aldosteronism

Reference(s)
Funder JW, Carey RM, Mantero F, et al. The management of primary aldosteronism: case detection, diagnosis, and treatment: an Endocrine Society clinical practice guideline. *J Clin Endocrinol Metab.* 2016;101(5):1889-1916. PMID: 26934393

Rossi GP, Auchus RJ, Brown M, et al. An expert consensus statement on use of adrenal vein sampling for the subtyping of primary aldosteronism. *Hypertension.* 2014;63(1):151-160. PMID: 24218436

28 ANSWER: D) Prednisone

Hypercalcemia is quite common in the general population and it is a frequent reason for referral to an endocrine specialist. Aside from careful elicitation of a pertinent history (medical, family, and medications), the single most important laboratory test after biochemical confirmation of hypercalcemia is a concomitant serum PTH level. The PTH result will, with very few exceptions, define whether the hypercalcemic disorder is PTH dependent or independent, thereby guiding the rest of the clinical workup. In this patient, the PTH level is borderline suppressed, which is compatible with a PTH-independent process. PTH levels in the mid-range of normal (30-40 pg/mL) may present some diagnostic difficulty that requires broader testing to address both PTH-dependent and independent processes. However, PTH concentrations above 40 pg/mL in the context of an elevated calcium level are most consistent with primary hyperparathyroidism, as a PTH value in this range is considered inappropriate for the level of serum calcium.

This particular patient has clinical evidence of sarcoidosis (hilar prominence) and would be best served by a course of prednisone (Answer D). Sarcoidosis is the most common cause of granulomatous disease–related hypercalcemia, which is due to the unregulated overproduction of calcitriol (1,25-dihydroxyvitamin D) from epithelioid cells within noncaseating granulomas. High calcitriol levels enhance both intestinal absorption of calcium, as well as skeletal resorption to a lesser extent, leading to hypercalcemia. Affected patients almost universally have quite high urinary calcium excretion due to enhanced calcitriol-mediated intestinal calcium absorption and resultant increased urinary calcium excretion, coupled with concomitant reduced renal calcium absorption caused by low PTH levels.

Other causes of granulomatous disease–related hypercalcemia include—but are not limited to—fungal disease (histoplasmosis) and mycobacterial disease (typical and atypical). Neoplastic disease, including various forms of lymphoma, can also overproduce calcitriol and cause hypercalcemia. Glucocorticoids rapidly reduce the production of calcitriol from cellular sources through transcriptional suppression, usually resulting in a marked reduction in serum calcium within a few days. Targeted treatment of the underlying disorder (antifungals or chemotherapy) is also recommended when indicated, and will permit the gradual tapering of glucocorticoid therapy.

Zoledronic acid (Answer C) is useful in hypercalcemia due to accelerated osteoclast resorption from bone, but it has limited utility in granulomatous-related hypercalcemia because of the mechanism of the disease. Alendronate (Answer A) is a less potent bisphosphonate than zoledronic acid and has no established utility in patients with hypercalcemia. Cinacalcet (Answer B), a calcium-sensing receptor agonist that has utility in patients with hypercalcemia due to PTH elevation, would not be helpful in this patient with a PTH-independent process. Finally, although hydrochlorothiazide treatment (Answer E) could possibly benefit this patient's hypercalciuria, it would not lower and, in fact, could worsen hypercalcemia based on the known mechanism of action.

Educational Objective
Recommend appropriate therapy in a patient with 1,25-dihydroxyvitamin D–mediated hypercalcemia due to sarcoidosis.

UpToDate Topic Review(s)
Hypercalcemia in granulomatous diseases

Reference(s)

Tebben PJ, Singh RJ, Kumar R. Vitamin D-mediated hypercalcemia: mechanisms, diagnosis, and treatment. *Endocr Rev.* 2016;37(5):521-547. PMID: 27588937

29 ANSWER: B) Phentermine/topiramate

Weight-loss treatment options for adults include lifestyle modification alone or in combination with weight-loss medications or bariatric surgery. According to established criteria, candidates for a weight-loss medication are adults with a BMI of 27 kg/m^2 or greater who have an obesity-related comorbidity or adults with a BMI greater than 30 kg/m^2. Candidates for surgical therapy are adults with a BMI of 40 kg/m^2 or greater or adults with a BMI between 35 kg/m^2 and 40 kg/m^2 who have at least 1 obesity-related comorbidity. According to these criteria, this patient is a candidate for bariatric surgery (either Roux-en-Y gastric bypass [Answer A] or sleeve gastrectomy [Answer C]). However, his HIV status is a relative contraindication to surgery.

Obesity and its comorbidities are a problem in patients with HIV. Data from the 2015 National Health and Nutrition Examination Survey (NHANES) show that obesity affects 2 in 5 HIV-infected women and 1 in 5 HIV-infected men. HIV-infected patients who are obese have greater morbidity than those who are not obese. The use of bariatric surgery in this setting is controversial. Questions that have not been answered by clinical studies include determining the effects of the surgery on HIV viral load and on CD$_4$ cell count, whether absorption of antiretroviral therapy is decreased or unchanged, whether one type surgery is better for this population, and whether there is a percentage weight loss that would be detrimental for these patients.

Few studies have been published regarding the outcomes of obese individuals with HIV who undergo bariatric surgery. Available studies show that weight loss is comparable to that in patients without HIV. The mean follow-up for 9 studies (25 patients who underwent Roux-en-Y gastric bypass) was 19 months; at 1 year, the BMI reduction ranged from 4% to 47%.

Importantly, most antiretroviral agents are primarily absorbed in the proximal intestine. There are conflicting data regarding antiretroviral absorption following bariatric surgery. One study reported that extremely rapid weight loss leads to decreased and subtherapeutic serum antiretroviral levels. However, some case reports show that antiretroviral levels are lower than before surgery, but are still within an expected range to achieve viral suppression. There is still debate on which procedure is safer in this population and how big the pouch must be to reduce absorption difficulties.

A retrospective analysis using the United States Nationwide Inpatient Sample database from 2004 to 2014 identified 346 obese patients with HIV who underwent bariatric surgery. Patients who had surgery were younger than those who did not have surgery and more women had surgery than men. The number of surgeries increased from 2004 (n = 12) to 2014 (n = 76). No difference in in-hospital mortality was observed between patients who had surgery vs those who did not. Despite the rising trends of obesity in this patient group, only 4.4% had bariatric surgery. To date, there is no standard or approved approach for addressing obesity in patients with HIV. When surgery was performed, each case was discussed in a multidisciplinary team, including an HIV specialist.

For this patient, it would be reasonable to start a weight-loss medication that can be used long term and to consider starting a discussion with the surgery and infectious disease teams about the possibility of bariatric surgery. Before prescribing a weight-loss medication, it is important to rule out drug-drug interactions. None of the medications listed have a drug-drug interaction with his antiretroviral therapy. Lorcaserin (Answer E) is not the first choice because he is taking fluoxetine. The use of 2 serotoninergic agents is discouraged because it increases the risk of serotonin syndrome. Naltrexone/bupropion (Answer D) is contraindicated for this patient because he has a seizure disorder. His best option is to start phentermine/topiramate (Answer B). At one year, when taking the regular phentermine/topiramate dosage (7.5/46 mg), patients lost 9.3% of their weight compared with 2.2% in the placebo group. Contraindications to use of phentermine/topiramate include coronary artery disease, uncontrolled hypertension, pregnancy, glaucoma, hyperthyroidism, and use of a monoamine oxidase inhibitor within 14 days. Common adverse effects of phentermine/topiramate include tachycardia, paresthesias, headache, insomnia, decreased serum bicarbonate, dry mouth, constipation, and upper respiratory tract infection.

Educational Objective
Identify patients who are not candidates for Roux-en-Y gastric bypass given their comorbidities and recommend alternative treatment options.

UpToDate Topic Review(s)
Bariatric procedures for the management of severe obesity: Descriptions

Reference(s)

Kassir R, Huart E, Tiffet O, et al. Feasibility of bariatric surgery in the HIV-infected patients. *Obes Surg.* 2017;27(3):818-819. PMID: 28054292

Thompson-Paul AM, Wei SC, Mattson CL, et al. Obesity among HIV-infected adults receiving medical care in the United States: data from the cross-sectional medical monitoring project and National Health and Nutrition Examination Survey. *Medicine (Baltimore).* 2015;94(27):e1081. PMID: 26166086

Sharma P, McCarty TR, Ngu JN, O'Donnell M, Njei B. Impact of bariatric surgery in patients with HIV infection: a nationwide inpatient sample analysis, 2004-2014. *AIDS.* 2018;32(14):1959-1965. PMID: 30157083

Akbari K, Som R, Sampson M, Abbas SH, Ramus J, Jones G. The effect of bariatric surgery on patients with HIV infection: a literature review. *Obes Surg.* 2018;28(8):2550-2559. PMID: 29948874

30 **ANSWER: D) Elevated thyroid-stimulating immunoglobulin titer**
On the basis of her tumor size, gross extrathyroidal extension, and lymph node metastases, this patient with thyroid cancer is at high risk of structural disease recurrence. Such a patient would definitely benefit from radioactive iodine therapy. Thyroid cancer prognosis is usually worse in older individuals. There is controversy about whether prognosis gradually worsens with advancing age or whether there is an age cutoff above which prognosis worsens. An age cutoff of 55 years is used in the eighth edition of the American Joint Commission on Cancer thyroid cancer staging system, such that for the same histopathologic features, stage is higher and expected survival is less for a patient diagnosed when they are older than 55 years. This patient's young age (Answer A) will positively affect her survival, not negatively affect it.

Total thyroidectomy is the best surgical approach for a patient such as this with extensive thyroid cancer. If surgery is the option chosen to treat Graves disease, total thyroidectomy is generally pursued, rather than subtotal thyroidectomy because of the recurrence risk of hyperthyroidism if sufficient thyroid tissue is left behind. In this particular patient, thyroidectomy was undertaken with the knowledge that the patient has thyroid cancer, and there is no reason to suspect that a thorough resection was not undertaken. Surgery can be more difficult in the setting of Graves disease because of the vascularity of the gland, but this should not preclude a thorough surgery in the hands of an experienced surgeon. Therefore, surgery being performed for dual diagnoses of Graves disease and thyroid cancer (Answer B) is incorrect.

Thyroglobulin antibodies are present in approximately 15% of patients with differentiated thyroid cancer. When present, these antibodies confound the accurate measurement of thyroglobulin itself by causing falsely high or low readings, depending on the thyroglobulin assay being used. The trend in thyroglobulin antibodies over time is useful as a surrogate marker of thyroglobulin itself, and thus an increasing titer of thyroglobulin antibodies can be indicative of thyroid cancer recurrence or progression. However, a baseline presence of thyroglobulin antibodies

(Answer C) is not a negative prognosticator, and often these antibodies trend down over time. In this patient, the thyroglobulin antibodies may be an indicator of her autoimmune thyroid disease.

In patients who have no residual thyroid cancer after thyroidectomy, thyroglobulin levels are quite low (<0.1-5.0 ng/mL) 6 weeks or more after surgery. The interpretation of this patient's thyroglobulin is clouded by the fact that her laboratory evaluation was performed 2 weeks after surgery, so this concentration may reflect the damage to and manipulation of her thyroid gland during surgery, and the trajectory of the thyroglobulin concentration may still be downwards. The coexistence of Graves disease might also lead to a thyroglobulin value that is higher than would be seen if Graves disease were not also present. Therefore, the baseline thyroglobulin level of 14.5 ng/mL (14.5 μg/L) (Answer E) will not necessarily negatively affect her prognosis.

In addition to a beneficial effect of radioiodine therapy to reduce the recurrence and increase the survival after thyroidectomy for intermediate- or high-risk thyroid cancer, TSH suppression is also a beneficial manipulation. This benefit does not seem to extend to patients with low-risk thyroid cancer who have undergone surgery, but it may extend to patients with papillary microcarcinomas who are undergoing active surveillance. The advantage of TSH suppression is believed to be due to the lowering of one of several growth factors that stimulate thyroid tissue, including thyroid cancer tissue itself. As thyroid-stimulating immunoglobulin, which is the causative agent for Graves disease, is also a stimulator of thyroid tissue and has a longer duration of action than TSH, it would be theoretically predicted to adversely affect thyroid cancer outcomes and, in fact, may antagonize the effects of TSH suppression. Despite this logical prediction, the various case series examining the association between Graves disease and thyroid cancer outcomes have not provided consistent results. However, there is a sufficient body of evidence to suggest that differentiated thyroid cancer may be more aggressive in some patients with Graves disease. Therefore, of the listed options, elevated thyroid-stimulating immunoglobulin titer (Answer D) is the best choice. One study suggested that elevated interleukin-4 levels in Graves disease may protect thyroid cancer cells from apoptosis.

Educational Objective
Explain the potential effect of thyroid-stimulating immunoglobulin on differentiated thyroid cancer prognosis.

UpToDate Topic Review(s)
Differentiated thyroid cancer: Overview of management

Reference(s)

Belfiore A, Garofalo MR, Giuffrida D, et al. Increased aggressiveness of thyroid cancer in patients with Graves' disease. *J Clin Endocrinol Metab.* 1990;70(4):830-835. PMID: 2180978

Medas F, Erdas E, Canu GL, et al. Does hyperthyroidism worsen prognosis of thyroid carcinoma? A retrospective analysis on 2820 consecutive thyroidectomies. *J Otolaryngol Head Neck Surg.* 2018;47(1):6. PMID: 29357932

Menon R, Nair CG, Babu M, Jacob P, Krishna GP. The outcome of papillary thyroid cancer associated with Graves' disease: a case control study. *J Thyroid Res.* 2018;2018:8253094. PMID: 29854383

Pellegriti G, Mannarino C, Russo M, et al. Increased mortality in patients with differentiated thyroid cancer associated with Graves' disease. *J Clin Endocrinol Metab.* 2013;98(3):1014-1021. PMID: 23348395

Vella V, Mineo R, Frasca F, et al. Interleukin-4 stimulates papillary thyroid cancer cell survival: implications in patients with thyroid cancer and concomitant Graves' disease. *J Clin Endocrinol Metab.* 2004;89(6):2880-2889. PMID: 15181072

31 ANSWER: B) Type 1 diabetes mellitus
Cancer treatment has been revolutionized by the use of immune checkpoint inhibitors to overcome antitumor immunity and evasion. Cytotoxic T-lymphocyte–associated protein 4 (CTLA-4) inhibitors (eg, ipilimumab), programmed cell death protein 1 (PD-1) inhibitors (eg, nivolumab and pembrolizumab), and programmed cell death ligand 1 (3 PD-L1) inhibitors (eg, atezolizumab, avelumab, and durvalumab) have been used to treat numerous solid-organ malignancies, including multiple myeloma.

Immune checkpoint inhibitors activate T lymphocytes and thereby have the potential to induce endocrine autoimmune diseases, including hypophysitis, thyroid dysfunction, primary adrenal insufficiency, and autoimmune diabetes. The frequency of these autoimmune adverse reactions is approximately 10% as reported in a recent meta-analysis. The risk of developing autoimmune endocrine disorders is even higher when checkpoint inhibitors are combined as in this vignette. In the meta-analysis, patients treated with ipilimumab had an incidence of developing hypothyroidism of 3.8% (95% confidence interval [CI], 1.9%- 7.8%) vs an incidence of 13.2% (95% CI, 6.9%-23.8%) with use of combination checkpoint inhibitors. The incidence of hyperthyroidism was 0.6% (95% CI, 0.2%-1.8%) with the 3 PD-L1 inhibitor compared with an incidence of 8.0% (95% CI, 4.1%-15.3%) with combination therapy. Using meta-regression modeling, patients treated with CTLA-4 inhibitors, including ipilimumab, had an incidence of developing hypophysitis of 3.8% (95% CI, 2.7%-5.2%) compared with an incidence of 8.0% (95% CI, 5.9%-10.8%) with combination therapy. Primary adrenal insufficiency and insulin-deficient diabetes were uncommonly diagnosed.

The development of diabetic ketoacidosis 9 weeks after the patient was started on ipilimumab and nivolumab is consistent with precipitation of autoimmune diabetes mellitus (Answer B), even though glutamic acid decarboxylase antibodies were undetectable. If glutamic acid decarboxylase antibodies are negative, it is often useful to obtain additional autoimmune diabetes markers to determine the etiology of the diabetes. In this case, the insulin-antigen (IA-2A) titer was ordered after glutamic acid decarboxylase antibodies were documented to be undetectable, and it was elevated, thus confirming the presence of autoimmune diabetes.

Diabetes that develops following a single bout of pancreatitis (Answer A) is possible, but this is an unlikely etiology of diabetes in this vignette. Diabetes does not usually develop in association with malignant melanoma (Answer D) unless glucocorticoids are used in the treatment, which was not the case here. The abrupt onset of diabetes and presentation with diabetic ketoacidosis is not typical of type 2 diabetes (Answer E). Finally, latent autoimmune diabetes in adults (LADA) (Answer C) by definition is typified by onset after age 30 years, with at least a 6-month initial treatment period without insulin and elevation in autoimmune markers such as glutamic acid decarboxylase antibodies.

Educational Objective
Identify immune checkpoint inhibitors as a potential cause of autoimmune disorders such as type 1 diabetes mellitus.

UpToDate Topic Review(s)
Patient selection criteria and toxicities associated with checkpoint inhibitor immunotherapy

Reference(s)
Hughes J, Vudattu N, Sznol M, et al. Precipitation of autoimmune diabetes with Anti-PD-1 immunotherapy. *Diabetes Care*. 2015;38(4):e55-e57. PMID: 25805871

Barroso-Sousa R, Barry WT, Garrido-Castro AC, et al. Incidence of endocrine dysfunction following the use of different checkpoint inhibitor regimens: a systematic review and meta-analysis. *JAMA Oncol*. 2017;4(2):173-182. PMID: 28973656

Naik RG, Brooks-Worrell BM, Palmer JP. Latent autoimmune diabetes in adults. *J Clin Endocrinol Metab*. 2009;94(12):4635-4644. PMID: 19837918

32   ANSWER: A) Relax carbohydrate restriction and recheck lipids
Ketogenic diets restrict carbohydrate intake, typically to 20 to 50 g daily, to induce nutritional ketosis. Restricting carbohydrates to less than 50 g induces glycogen depletion and ketone production due to fat mobilization from adipose tissue. Nutritional ketosis produces ketone bodies (acetone, acetoacetate and β-hydroxybutyrate) that are measurable as serum or urinary ketones. Serum ketones in nutritional ketosis ranges from 1 to 7 mmol/L, but do not produce metabolic acidosis. In contrast, diabetic ketoacidosis includes metabolic acidosis, hyperglycemia, and serum ketones generally greater than 10 mmol/L.

Ketogenic diets are often prescribed for individuals with intractable seizures and have demonstrated great benefit in this setting. Ketogenic diets are also effective in the management of obesity, metabolic syndrome, and type 2 diabetes. As dietary carbohydrate is replaced by fat, postprandial spikes in blood concentrations of glucose and insulin decrease, glucagon secretion increases, and metabolism shifts to a greater reliance on fat oxidation. In obese patients, ketogenic diets have shown greater weight loss when compared with other balanced diets. Mechanisms of enhanced weight loss with ketogenic diets despite intake of calorie-dense fats may be related to increased satiety, allowing a lower energy intake without hunger, as well as increased protein intake and resultant increased thermogenesis.

Carbohydrate restriction improves atherogenic dyslipidemia of high triglycerides, low HDL cholesterol, and small, dense LDL cholesterol. A reduction in serum triglycerides is a hallmark response to ketogenic diets. However, effects on LDL-cholesterol levels are less predictable. Several studies suggest that ketogenic diets have a neutral or lowering effect on total cholesterol and LDL cholesterol. However, there is increasing evidence of a unique subset of patients following ketogenic diets who develop a lipid profile characterized by very high LDL cholesterol and HDL cholesterol and less small, dense LDL cholesterol. In the "ketogenic diet world," these individuals are referred to as "lean mass hyperresponders." The hypercholesterolemia can be related to greater intake of saturated fat and cholesterol and lower fiber intake. From a cardiovascular risk aspect, the levels of total and LDL cholesterol observed in patients on these diets suggest high risk of cardiovascular disease; however, there are no long-term studies of the effects of ketogenic diets on cardiovascular morbidity and mortality. This patient's lipid elevations are most likely due to her dietary modification, especially since her lipid panel before starting the ketogenic diet was quite different. Relaxing the intense carbohydrate restriction and rechecking lipids (Answer A) is the best next step.

A diet rich in unsaturated fat and protein (Answer B) does not cause such profound changes in cholesterol levels. Current evidence does not suggest that these diets have any specific benefit on cardiovascular risk reduction. Adding a statin (Answer C) or a PCSK9 inhibitor (Answer D) is not necessary now, as her cardiovascular risk before intense carbohydrate restriction is known. Her current lipid panel is quite alarming. At age 57 years, although long-term cardiovascular disease data for patients following these diets are unavailable, recommending no intervention (Answer E) is incorrect. However, it should be noted that many individuals are hesitant to alter dietary habits after significant success. Due to the varied and individualized response, obtaining a baseline fasting lipid profile, adhering to periodic monitoring, and engaging in shared decision-making should be considered. A decision to continue on such an intense and restrictive diet should be based on patient-clinician discussion.

Educational Objective
Describe the effects of very low-carbohydrate diets on the lipid profile.

UpToDate Topic Review(s)
Obesity in adults: Dietary therapy

Reference(s)

Ludwig DS, Willett WC, Volek JS, Neuhouser ML. Dietary fat: from foe to friend? *Science*. 2018;362(6416):764-770. PMID: 30442800

Paoli A, Rubini A, Volek JS, Grimaldi KA. Beyond weight loss: a review of the therapeutic uses of very-low-carbohydrate (ketogenic) diets. *Eur J Clin Nutr*. 2013;67(8):789-796. PMID: 23801097

33   ANSWER: B) Secondary hyperparathyroidism

The patient described in this vignette has osteoporosis in the setting of stage 4 chronic kidney disease (CKD). She has completed 2 years of teriparatide therapy, which has been shown to be effective and safe in patients with an estimated glomerular filtration rate as low as 30 mL/min per 1.73 m^2, but it is important to mention that there are very limited data on the use of teriparatide in patients with more advanced kidney disease and no data on its use with coexisting hyperparathyroidism since the teriparatide clinical trials excluded patients with elevated baseline serum PTH levels. Denosumab, a fully human monoclonal antibody to the receptor activator of nuclear factor kappaB ligand (RANKL), would be the most appropriate agent to treat her osteoporosis at this time because it is not excreted by the kidneys. Although denosumab has no glomerular filtration rate restrictions since it is not cleared by the kidneys, a fracture benefit in advanced CKD, especially stage 5, is lacking. Denosumab should be avoided in stages 4 and 5 CKD if there is concern for preexisting adynamic bone disease. Denosumab is administered by subcutaneous injection once every 6 months. It may induce significant hypocalcemia in patients with renal impairment and should not be given to patients with preexisting hypocalcemia until it is corrected. Other conditions that predispose to symptomatic hypocalcemia following denosumab injection include high bone turnover and malabsorption syndromes. Patients with vitamin D deficiency should receive vitamin D replacement before denosumab is administered. In advanced CKD, a decline in calcitriol synthesis occurs due to increased FGF-23 levels, hyperphosphatemia, and loss of renal mass. Calcitriol or synthetic vitamin D analogues may be used in patients with severe and progressive hyperparathyroidism. Monitoring serum calcium is required in patients with risk factors for hypocalcemia. In such patients, serum calcium should be measured approximately 10 days after denosumab administration, as this is when the nadir in serum calcium typically occurs.

This patient's baseline laboratory abnormalities include hyperphosphatemia and secondary hyperparathyroidism in the context of stage 4 CKD. She was normocalcemic with a low-normal 25-hydroxyvitamin D level before receiving denosumab, but her serum calcium decreased to 6.1 mg/dL (8.2-10.2 mg/dL)

(SI: 1.5 mmol/L [2.1-2.6 mmol/L]) after the denosumab injection despite taking calcium and vitamin D supplementation. Her serum intact PTH level increased significantly albeit appropriately in the setting of hypocalcemia, consistent with a diagnosis of severe secondary hyperparathyroidism (Answer B). Primary hyperparathyroidism (Answer A), tertiary hyperparathyroidism (Answer C), and parathyroid carcinoma (Answer D) are all characterized by hypercalcemia, which is not the case here. Tertiary hyperparathyroidism specifically refers to the development of autonomous parathyroid function and excessive PTH secretion after longstanding secondary hyperparathyroidism; it typically occurs in patients with end-stage renal disease and after kidney transplant. Parathyroid carcinoma should be suspected in patients with primary hyperparathyroidism who present with marked hypercalcemia, very high PTH levels, and a neck mass.

Hungry bone syndrome (Answer E) refers to the hypocalcemia that typically occurs after parathyroidectomy in patients who had developed bone disease preoperatively due to a chronic increase in bone resorption induced by high PTH levels. In addition to reduced serum calcium, reduced serum phosphate and increased serum potassium levels may also be observed in this phenomenon, most likely reflecting increased bone influx and efflux, respectively. This postoperative hypocalcemia tends to be severe and prolonged despite normal or even elevated PTH levels.

Educational Objective
Explain how denosumab therapy can induce significant hypocalcemia in patients with renal impairment, resulting in severe secondary hyperparathyroidism.

UpToDate Topic Review(s)
Denosumab for osteoporosis

Reference(s)

Ungprasert P, Cheungpasitporn W, Srivali N, Kittanamongkolchai W, Bischof EF. Life-threatening hypocalcemia associated with denosumab in a patient with moderate renal insufficiency. *Am J Emerg Med.* 2013;31(4):756.e1-2. PMID: 23399342

Ishikawa K, Nagai T, Sakamoto K, et al. High bone turnover elevates the risk of denosumab-induced hypocalcemia in women with postmenopausal osteoporosis. *Ther Clin Risk Manag.* 2016;12:1831-1840. PMID: 27980413

Jamal SA, Miller PD. Secondary and tertiary hyperparathyroidism. *J Clin Densitom.* 2013;16(1):64-68. PMID: 23267748

Miller PD, Schwartz EN, Chen P, Misurski DA, Krege JH. Teriparatide in postmenopausal women with osteoporosis and mild or moderate renal impairment. *Osteoporos Int.* 2007;18(1):59-68. PMID: 17013567

Jamal SA, Ljunggren O, Stehman-Breen C, et al. Effects of denosumab on fracture and bone mineral density by level of kidney function. *J Bone Miner Res.* 2011;26(8):1829-1835. PMID: 21491487

34 ANSWER: E) TSH dilution study

This patient has numerous clinical features that suggest she is genuinely thyrotoxic, although she does not display pathognomonic eye signs to confirm underlying Graves disease. The serum free T_4 and free T_3 levels are both clearly elevated, which is consistent with the clinical picture.

However, serum TSH is not suppressed (<0.1 mIU/L and typically <0.01 mIU/L) as should be the case in primary hyperthyroidism. At this point, it is necessary to consider the possible causes of hyperthyroxinemia with nonsuppressed TSH (*see box*).

- Increased thyroid hormone-binding capacity (leading to increased total T_4 and total T_3, but typically normal free hormone levels (eg, due to oral oestrogen therapy, pregnancy)

- Laboratory assays interference

  Falsely elevated free thyroid hormones:
  Heterophilic antibodies
  Antiiodothyronine antibodies
  Familial dysalbuminemic hyperthyroxinemia

  Falsely nonsuppressed TSH:
  Heterophilic or human antianimal antibodies
  Macro-TSH

- Thyroxine replacement therapy (including poor adherence)

- Medications (eg, amiodarone, heparin, biotin)

- Nonthyroidal illness (including acute psychiatric disorders or in the neonatal period)

- TSH-secreting pituitary adenoma

- Resistance to thyroid hormone

- Disorders of thyroid hormone transport or metabolism

In the absence of confounding medications or intercurrent illness, the next step is to exclude assay interference. In this case, as the free thyroid hormone levels are consistent with the clinical presentation, attention turns to the nonsuppressed TSH value—is this genuine or erroneous? To answer this question, it is crucial to involve the clinical biochemistry laboratory at an early stage. Specifically, they should be asked to exclude interference in the TSH assay, for example, due to heterophilic or human antianimal immunoglobulins. This can be readily achieved through one of several approaches: TSH dilution studies (Answer E), polyethylene glycol precipitation of interfering immunoglobulins (with measurement of TSH in the supernatant), or gel filtration chromatography.

Investigation	Thyrotropinoma	Resistance to Thyroid Hormone
Serum SHBG	Increased (but may be normal if cosecretion of GH)	Normal
Serum α-subunit (Answer C)	Increased/normal	Normal
Thyrotropin-releasing hormone stimulation test (Answer B)	Absent/attenuated	Preserved/exaggerated
Pituitary MRI (Answer A)	Adenoma (although some microadenomas may not be visualized on standard clinical MR sequences)	Normal (but incidentalomas in 10%-15%)

Only when assay interference has been excluded should more rare causes be considered, such as a TSH-secreting pituitary adenoma (thyrotropinoma) or resistance to thyroid hormone (due to a loss-of-function pathogenic variant in the human thyroid hormone receptor β gene [*THRB*] [Answer D]).

Three of the other investigations offered as answer choices, together with SHBG measurement, are of potential use in distinguishing a thyrotropinoma from resistance to thyroid hormone (*see table*).

Educational Objective

Explain how laboratory assay interference can confound the interpretation of thyroid function test results and lead to inappropriate investigation and management.

UpToDate Topic Review(s)

Laboratory assessment of thyroid function

Reference(s)

Koulouri O, Moran C, Halsall DJ, Chatterjee K, Gurnell M. Pitfalls in the measurement and interpretation of thyroid function tests. *Best Pract Res Clin Endocrinol Metab.* 2013;27(6):745-762. PMID: 24275187

Koulouri O, Gurnell M. How to interpret thyroid function tests. *Clin Med.* 2013;13(3):282-286. PMID: 23760704

35 ANSWER: E) Elevated D-lactic acid

Lactic acid levels that are typically measured are L-lactate. L-lactate is the major enantiomer of lactic acid in the body and is formed from pyruvic acid during anaerobic glycolysis. Studies suggest that elevated lactate is present in patients with diabetic ketoacidosis (DKA) but clinically significant lactate levels (>45 mg/dL [>5 mmol/L]) are rare. This patient had mildly elevated lactate levels, but they were not high enough to account for the persistent anion gap. However, the D-enantiomer is also present under physiologic conditions, although at low levels, accounting for 1% to 5% of L-lactate. D-lactate (Answer E) is formed by the glyoxylate pathway from methylglyoxal. During periods of normoglycemia, methylglyoxal is typically only produced in small amounts. However, during periods of sustained hyperglycemia, methylglyoxal is produced in much larger quantities and has been associated with diabetes complications. Elevated D-lactate has been well described in DKA, and one study documented a 5- to 8-fold increase in D-lactate in patients with DKA compared with levels in patients with diabetes who did not have DKA. In the same study, L-lactate levels in patients with DKA were twice those of levels in patients with diabetes who did not have DKA. Mildly elevated D-lactate levels are most commonly seen in patients with short-bowel syndrome and are not associated with symptoms. However, after carbohydrate loading, D-lactate levels can rise dramatically and cause a metabolic acidosis associated with substantial neurologic symptoms, including memory loss, slurred speech, ataxia, and confusion—often described as feeling drunk. Most clinicians do not believe it is necessary to measure D-lactate under these conditions unless there is a reason to investigate why anion gap acidosis persists. The long-term clinical consequences of elevated D-lactate are not well described.

In patients with DKA, there are rare occasions when the nitroprusside reaction, which detects acetoacetate and acetone but not β-hydroxybutyrate, can be falsely negative because the ratio of β-hydroxybutyrate to acetoacetate can be as high as 10:1. However, with insulin treatment, β-hydroxybutyrate levels decrease substantially within the first 24 hours, so persistent β-hydroxybutyrate (Answer A) is unlikely. In such cases, serum β-hydroxybutyrate can be measured, although there are no guidelines about how to use such data. Also, some centers do not have rapid turnaround of the serum β-hydroxybutyrate assay.

This patient does not have diabetic nephropathy or hyperkalemia to suggest hyporeninemic hypoaldosteronism or renal tubular acidosis type 4 (Answer B).

Patients with ethylene glycol poisoning (Answer C) often have both an anion gap and osmolal gap along with acute renal insufficiency.

Patients with mitochondrial DNA defects may have diabetes. The most common cause is a tRNA A to G mutation at position 3243. Patients with this condition often present in their 30s and 40s with hearing loss and diabetes that may resemble type 1 or type 2 diabetes. The diabetes is often progressive. There is overlap between this syndrome and MELAS (mitochondrial encephalopathy, lactic acidosis, and stroke-like syndromes). However, this patient does not present with findings consistent with diabetes due to a mitochondrial DNA defect (Answer D).

Educational Objective

Identify D-lactic acidosis as a cause of persistent anion gap acidosis in the setting of diabetic ketoacidosis.

UpToDate Topic Review(s)

D-lactic acidosis

Reference(s)

Lu J, Zello GA, Randell E, Adeli K, Krahn J, Meng QH. Closing the anion gap: contribution of D-lactate to diabetic ketoacidosis. *Clin Chim Acta*. 2011;412(3-4):286-291. PMID: 21036159

Feenstra RA, Kiewiet MK, Boerma EC, ter Avest E. Lactic acidosis in diabetic ketoacidosis. *BMJ Case Rep*. 2014;2014:bcr2014203594. PMID: 24654253

36 ANSWER: B) Initiate levothyroxine

This 32-year-old woman has a history of 3 miscarriages since the birth of her son 4 years ago. She has tried to conceive for 1 year while off oral contraceptive pills and has not been successful. Laboratory tests reveal a TSH value of 3.0 mIU/L with elevated TPO antibodies, which is consistent with Hashimoto thyroiditis. The best next step is to initiate levothyroxine therapy (Answer B) to improve her TSH level, increase her chance of conception, and potentially reduce the risk of miscarriage.

Women with positive TPO antibodies have an increased risk of pregnancy complications, including miscarriage and preterm labor. Some studies report a benefit from thyroid hormone replacement, which can reduce the risk of miscarriage and preterm labor. In a randomized controlled trial, administration of levothyroxine in early pregnancy (mean dosage of 50 mcg daily) to euthyroid woman with TPO antibodies decreased the risk of miscarriage from 13.8% to 3.5% (relative risk, 1.72; 95% confidence interval, 1.13-2.25).

TPO antibody measurement should be considered when evaluating patients with recurrent miscarriage, with or without infertility. In accordance with guidelines for hypothyroidism in adults, levothyroxine treatment should be considered for women of childbearing age with normal serum TSH levels when they are pregnant or planning a pregnancy (including assisted reproduction in the immediate future) if they have or have had positive serum TPO antibodies, particularly when there is a history of miscarriage or hypothyroidism. Also, levothyroxine therapy is recommended for women of childbearing age who are pregnant or planning a pregnancy (including assisted reproduction in the immediate future) if they have or have had positive serum TPO antibodies and their TSH level is greater than 2.5 mIU/L. Population-based trimester-specific reference ranges for serum TSH should be used during pregnancy. Reference range determinations should only include pregnant women with no known thyroid disease, optimal iodine intake, and negative TPO antibodies. In early pregnancy, this corresponds to a TSH upper reference limit of 4.0 mIU/L. This reference limit should generally be applied beginning with the late first trimester (weeks 7-12). In the second and third trimester, there should be a gradual return of TSH towards the nonpregnant normal range.

However, the recent TABLET trial (Thyroid Antibodies and levothyroxine study) was a double-blind, placebo-controlled trial of 952 euthyroid women with TPO antibodies, a history of miscarriage or infertility, and a TSH level of 2.5 mIU/L or greater who were randomly assigned to receive either levothyroxine, 50 mcg once daily, (476 women) or placebo (476 women) before conception through the end of pregnancy. The primary outcome was live birth after at least 34 weeks of gestation. This study showed that levothyroxine use, compared with placebo, in euthyroid women with TPO antibodies did not result in a higher live birth rate. Importantly, there is a lag before study results affect clinical practice. Depending on results of future studies in the next few years, it is possible that the next pregnancy guidelines may have a different recommendation that reflects the results of the TABLET trial.

Although this patient has a palpable thyroid gland, this by itself should not cause difficulty with conception. Therefore, performing thyroid ultrasonography (Answer A) would not help her achieve pregnancy.

In addition to Hashimoto thyroiditis, she has vitiligo and a family history of lupus systemic erythematosus. She does not exhibit any signs or symptoms of celiac disease (no gastrointestinal symptoms or weight loss), so there is no reason to start a gluten-free diet (Answer C). Such intervention is recommended if esophagogastroduodenoscopy with duodenal biopsy confirms celiac disease.

She does not have any symptoms consistent with primary adrenal insufficiency such as hypotension, abdominal pain, weight loss, or electrolyte abnormalities. Thus, there is no indication to perform a cosyntropin-stimulation test (Answer D), which is usually ordered to confirm or rule out adrenal insufficiency.

In this patient with recurrent miscarriage, one can think of causes such as Lupus anticoagulant and cardiolipin antibodies. However, she has been evaluated by her obstetrician/gynecologist and all workups have been negative. Therefore, repeating these tests (Answer E) is unnecessary.

Educational Objective

Explain the role of thyroid antibodies in women who desire pregnancy and have a history of miscarriage.

Reference(s)

Garber JR, Cobin RH, Gharib H, et al; American Association of Clinical Endocrinologists and American Thyroid Association Taskforce on Hypothyroidism in Adults. Clinical practice guidelines for hypothyroidism in adults: cosponsored by the American Association of Clinical Endocrinologists and the American Thyroid Association [published correction appears in *Endocr Pract*. 2013;19(1):175]. *Endocr Pract.* 2012;18(6):989-1028. PMID: 23246686

Negro R, Formoso G, Mangieri T, Pezzarossa A, Dazzi D, Hassan H. Levothyroxine treatment in euthyroid pregnant women with autoimmune thyroid disease: effects on obstetrical complications. *J Clin Endocrinol Metab.* 2006;91(7):2587-2591. PMID: 16621910

Alexander EK, Pearce EN, Brent GA, et al. 2017 Guidelines of the American Thyroid Association for the diagnosis and management of thyroid disease during pregnancy and the postpartum. *Thyroid.* 2017;27(3):315-389. PMID: 28056690

Dhillon-Smith RK, Middleton LJ, Sunner KK, et al. Levothyroxine in women with thyroid peroxidase antibodies before conception. *N Engl J Med.* 2019;380(14):1316-1325. PMID: 30907987

37 ANSWER: D) IGF-2-to-IGF-1 ratio

With this patient's history of gastrointestinal stromal tumor, he could have multiple etiologies of non–insulin-mediated hypoglycemia. Adrenal insufficiency was excluded by normal results on a cosyntropin-stimulation test. He might have low hepatic glucose production either from low glycogen stores due to malnutrition or from large metastases to the liver. Low hepatic glucose output should be ruled out in patients who present with malignancy and hypoglycemia. The patient's glucose level rose by more than 25 mg/dL (1.4 mmol/L) following glucagon administration, which suggests hepatic glycogen stores are adequate.

This patient was thought to have non–islet-cell hypoglycemia (NICTH). This is a rare paraneoplastic process that is associated with tumor release of high–molecular weight IGF-2. Although insulin antibodies (Answer A) or insulin receptor antibodies can also be found in NICTH, they are less common than IGF-2 production. In NICTH, the IGF-2 released is not the normal 7.5-kDa form, but rather a higher–molecular weight form that is a result of abnormal processing of the IGF-2 precursor. It is referred to as "big IGF-2." Normal IGF-2 is usually bound to IGFBP-3 and then complexed to acid-labile subunit. About 80% of IGF-2 is in tertiary complexes and 20% is in binary complexes. About 80% of big IGF-2 is in binary complexes and 20% is in tertiary complexes. Binary complexes are able to cross the endothelial barrier and cause hypoglycemia. IGF-2 (similar to insulin) reduces glucose production by the liver and increases glucose uptake by the skeletal muscles. IGF-2 also suppresses the production of counterregulatory hormones such as glucagon.

Typical laboratory findings associated with NICTH are low glucose (serum glucose <55 mg/dL [<3.1 mmol/L]) with simultaneously low insulin, proinsulin, C-peptide, and β-hydroxybutyrate levels and a negative oral hypoglycemic agent screen. Low β-hydroxybutyrate levels are due to insulinlike activity of IGF-2. IGF-2 levels may or may not be elevated based on the assay used, and normal levels do not rule out NICTH. Thus, measuring IGF-2 (Answer C) would not help determine the etiology of this patient's hypoglycemia. There are no commercial assays for big IGF-2, so routine testing is not feasible in clinical practice. In the setting of NICTH, IGF-1 levels are often low. Measuring IGF-1 (Answer B) would not help with the diagnosis. The IGF-2-to-IGF-1 ratio is typically higher than the usual molar ratio of 3:1. The ratio is most likely the best screening test for NICTH (Answer D). Glucagon will most likely be suppressed in this patient, but its measurement (Answer E) is not a screening test for NICTH.

When evaluating a patient with malignancy and hypoglycemia, a reasonable approach is to rule out insulin-mediated/medication-induced hypoglycemia. One must also exclude adrenal insufficiency and reduced hepatic glucose output. Some advocate for making a presumptive diagnosis of NICTH in patients with malignancy and low insulin levels in whom adrenal insufficiency is ruled out and hepatic glucose production is appropriate. This might be particularly useful in situations when testing for IGF-1 and IGF-2 is not feasible.

Treatment of hypoglycemia related to NICTH should be considered in the following ways: (1) management of acute hypoglycemia, (2) management of the underlying tumor, and (3) long-term medical management if needed. Acute management includes administration of dextrose. If hypoglycemia is severe, one can use 25 g of 50% dextrose intravenously. In addition, 0.5 to 1 mg of glucagon can be administered. This is followed by continuous glucose infusion. Management of the underlying tumor includes surgical resection. If resection is incomplete, long-term medical management is required. This includes increased caloric intake and the addition of glucocorticoids. If hypoglycemia persists, glucagon infusion might be required. Although use of recombinant human GH in this setting is described in the literature, there is concern about tumor growth, so GH is not routinely used.

Educational Objective
Investigate the etiology of hypoglycemia in patients with non–islet-cell tumors.

UpToDate Topic Review(s)
Hypoglycemia in adults without diabetes mellitus: diagnostic approach

Reference(s)

Bodnar TW, Acevedo MJ, Pietropaolo M. Management of non-islet-cell tumor hypoglycemia: a clinical review. *J Clin Endocrinol Metab.* 2014;99(3):713-722. PMID: 24423303

Zapf J, Futo E, Peter M, Froesch ER. Can "big" insulin-like growth factor II in serum of tumor patients account for the development of extrapancreatic tumor hypoglycemia? *J Clin Invest.* 1992;90(6):2574-2584. PMID: 1281841

38 ANSWER: D) Exposure to husband's testosterone gel

In this woman with postmenopausal hyperandrogenism, exposure to her husband's testosterone gel (Answer D) is the most probable explanation for her increased and fluctuating serum testosterone concentrations. Alternative diagnoses are much less likely.

In women with androgen excess, a careful drug history is important to exclude exposure to exogenous androgens, including anabolic steroid use or transfer from a partner's testosterone gel. Hyperandrogenization after transfer of topical testosterone gel has been reported in exposed women and prepubertal children, at times leading to significant virilization and, in prepubertal boys, precocious puberty. Patients should be routinely warned of this potential adverse effect if topical testosterone gels are prescribed. In many countries, including the United States, topical testosterone has a black box warning regarding inadvertent secondary exposure due to passive testosterone transfer via skin-to-skin contact. Patients must be counseled to strictly adhere to precautions to minimize the potential for secondary exposure, including washing hands immediately after applying testosterone gel and covering the application site(s) with clothing.

The premenopausal absence of hyperandrogenic symptoms, menstrual disturbances, or infertility is not consistent with a diagnosis of polycystic ovary syndrome (Answer A) or late-onset congenital adrenal hyperplasia (Answer B), as these conditions typically present after puberty. Moreover, 17-hydroxyprogesterone is expected to be increased in the setting of congenital adrenal hyperplasia, especially with cosyntropin stimulation.

Adrenal androgen-secreting tumors (Answer C) are rare, usually large, and typically present with rapidly progressive virilization, features of Cushing syndrome, and increased DHEA-S (which is normal in this vignette). The prevalence of small, lipid-rich adrenal adenomas is approximately 5% in this age group, and the adenoma in this case almost certainly represents an incidental finding. Given that adrenal imaging can be misleading, it is not indicated in the evaluation of postmenopausal androgen excess unless the patient's serum testosterone is markedly elevated or the serum DHEA-S concentration is greater than 700 μg/dL (>18.9 μmol/L).

While normal transvaginal imaging does not rule out an ovarian source, in ovarian hyperthecosis (Answer E), ovarian volume is usually, but not always, increased. Moreover, if the increased serum testosterone is due to an ovarian source, serum testosterone concentrations typically decrease by more than 50% after GnRH analogue administration.

Educational Objective
Explain the risk of inadvertent testosterone exposure from prescribed testosterone gel.

UpToDate Topic Review(s)
Testosterone treatment of male hypogonadism

Reference(s)

de Ronde W. Hyperandrogenism after transfer of topical testosterone gel: case report and review of published and unpublished studies. *Hum Reprod*. 2009;24(2):425-428. PMID: 18948313

Kunz GJ, Klein KO, Clemons RD, Gottschalk ME, Jones KL. Virilization of young children after topical androgen use by their parents. *Pediatrics*. 2004;114(1):282-284. PMID: 15231947

Rothman MS, Wierman ME. How should postmenopausal androgen excess be evaluated? *Clin Endocrinol (Oxf)*. 2011;75(2):160-164. PMID: 21521309

39 ANSWER: D) Combined oral contraceptive pill

This patient has nonclassic 21-hydroxylase deficiency diagnosed by an elevated 17-hydroxyprogesterone level at baseline and following cosyntropin stimulation. A 17-hydroxyprogesterone level greater than 1500 ng/dL (>45.4 nmol/L), when measured before 8 AM and during the early follicular phase, is diagnostic. Levels between 200 and 1500 ng/dL (6.1-45.4 nmol/L) are suggestive and can be confirmed with a cosyntropin-stimulation test. An increase in 17-hydroxyprogesterone to greater than 1500 ng/dL (>45.4 nmol/L) is confirmatory. In situations where these thresholds are not definitively met but clinical suspicion remains high, genetic testing of the *CYP21A2* gene can be also be used to support the diagnosis.

The clinical presentation of nonclassic 21-hydroxylase deficiency can occur at any time after infancy, and it may manifest as premature puberty, amenorrhea, irregular menses after menarche or oligomenorrhea, and/or signs of hyperandrogenism (hirsutism, clitoromegaly, acne, oily skin). It is important to note that these presenting signs and symptoms in women can be similar to those of polycystic ovary syndrome, which should not be diagnosed until 21-hydroxylase deficiency has been excluded.

The treatment goals for nonclassic 21-hydroxylase deficiency are (1) to treat adrenal insufficiency by replacing deficiencies in cortisol and/or aldosterone and (2) to address excess ACTH secretion, which can result in hyperandrogenism in females (causing oligomenorrhea and virilization) and increased risk for testicular rest tumors in males. This patient has no signs or symptoms of adrenal insufficiency and has a normal morning cortisol level. As with most patients who present with 21-hydroxylase deficiency in the teenage years, this patient most likely has only a mild deficiency in 21-hydroxylase activity and is able to produce sufficient cortisol and aldosterone. Therefore, the primary treatment focus for this patient is addressing the hyperandrogenism and oligomenorrhea. A combined oral contraceptive pill (Answer D) would be the most effective treatment for her, as it would normalize estrogen status and menses, increase SHBG, and consequently decrease free androgen bioavailability. The use of spironolactone (Answer E), in addition to a combined oral contraceptive pill, could also be considered if there is insufficient improvement in symptoms of hyperandrogenism.

Because this patient does not have any signs or symptoms of adrenal insufficiency, it is not necessary to treat with glucocorticoids (Answers A, B, and C) as first-line therapy. The use of glucocorticoids in this patient would certainly lower ACTH effectively and consequently lower androgens; however, this approach increases the risk for Cushing syndrome (particularly weight gain, mood disorder, low bone density) and secondary adrenal insufficiency. Glucocorticoid therapy to normalize or fully suppress 17-hydroxyprogesterone is usually an indicator of overtreatment. In particular, nocturnal glucocorticoids are especially effective at lowering morning rises in ACTH and adrenal androgen production, but impart a greater nonphysiologic effect and higher risk for Cushing syndrome and mood disorders. If this patient continued to have persistent and undesired clinical signs of hyperandrogenism after 6 to 12 months of treatment with an oral contraceptive and spironolactone (often in addition to other methods to treat hirsutism), a discussion regarding the pros and cons of using a low-dosage glucocorticoid could be considered. In addition, if the patient could not tolerate oral contraceptive pill therapy, or was seeking to become pregnant in the near future, then low-dosage glucocorticoid therapy could also be considered.

When glucocorticoids are used, dexamethasone may be the most effective, but given its long half-life and high potency, it can impart the greatest cushingoid effects. Dexamethasone is also not inactivated by placental 11β-hydroxysteroid dehydrogenase type 2, and therefore, in pregnant women, it will expose the fetus. Thus, when needed, hydrocortisone, prednisone, or prednisolone are preferred, as they have shorter half-lives and are metabolized by placental 11β-hydroxysteroid dehydrogenase.

Educational Objective

Recommend treatment approaches for a woman with nonclassic 21-hydroxylase deficiency.

Diagnosis and treatment of nonclassic (late-onset) congenital adrenal hyperplasia due to 21-hydroxylase deficiency

Reference(s)

Speiser PW, Arlt W, Auchus RJ, et al. Congenital adrenal hyperplasia due to steroid 21-hydroxylase deficiency: an Endocrine Society clinical practice guideline. *J Clin Endocrinol Metab.* 2018;103(11):4043-4088. PMID: 30272171

40 ANSWER: A) *MEN1*

The patient in this vignette presents with hypercalcemia, hyperparathyroidism, hypercalciuria, and a history of kidney stones, all of which are consistent with a diagnosis of primary hyperparathyroidism (PHPT). Most patients with PHPT do not require genetic testing. However, genetic testing should be performed in selected patients in whom a familial form of PHPT is suspected: young patients (<30 years of age); patients with a family history of PHPT; patients with clinical findings suspicious for familial syndromes such as multiple endocrine neoplasia (MEN); and patients with multiglandular disease, parathyroid carcinoma, or atypical adenoma. Inactivating pathogenic variants in the *MEN1* gene (Answer A), which is a tumor suppressor gene, lead to an autosomal dominant predisposition to tumors of the parathyroid glands, anterior pituitary, and enteropancreatic endocrine cells. The fact that this young man's brother has peptic ulcer disease should raise suspicion for Zollinger-Ellison syndrome (gastrinoma) and therefore MEN type 1.

Activating pathogenic variants in the *RET* proto-oncogene (Answer C) lead to MEN type 2A, which is also inherited in an autosomal dominant pattern. MEN type 2A is characterized by medullary thyroid cancer, pheochromocytoma, and primary parathyroid hyperplasia. The hyperparathyroidism in MEN type 2A is often mild and asymptomatic.

The *CASR* gene (Answer B) encodes the calcium-sensing receptor, which is expressed in multiple tissues, including the parathyroid glands and the kidneys. Loss-of-function mutations in this gene have been shown to cause a rare disorder called familial hypocalciuric hypercalcemia, which in most cases is a benign cause of mild hypercalcemia that is inherited in an autosomal dominant fashion. Conversely, gain-of-function mutations in this gene cause autosomal dominant hypocalcemia. About 20% of patients with familial hypocalciuric hypercalcemia may have a mildly elevated PTH concentration, and the major feature that distinguishes familial hypocalciuric hypercalcemia from PHPT is low urinary calcium excretion and calcium-to-creatinine clearance ratio. Individuals with familial hypocalciuric hypercalcemia tend to develop hypercalcemia at a younger age than the typical patient with primary hyperparathyroidism (usually present in childhood), and there is usually a family history of asymptomatic hypercalcemia.

The *CDC73* gene (formerly *HRPT2*) (Answer D) encodes a protein called parafibromin, which functions as a tumor suppressor. Inactivating *CDC73* pathogenic variants have been described in a type of familial hyperparathyroidism called hyperparathyroidism–jaw tumor syndrome, a condition characterized by tumors of the jaw and parathyroid glands. Hyperparathyroidism–jaw tumor syndrome is associated with an increased risk of parathyroid cancer.

Finally, the *VDR* gene (Answer E) encodes the vitamin D receptor. Inactivating pathogenic variants in this gene lead to vitamin D resistance, but they do not seem to have a primary role in parathyroid gland tumorigenesis.

Educational Objective

Identify the clinical manifestations of multiple endocrine neoplasia type 1 in a patient presenting for evaluation of hypercalcemia and recall the gene associated with this condition.

Multiple endocrine neoplasia type 1: Clinical manifestations and diagnosis

Reference(s)

Bilezikian JP, Cusano NE, Khan AA, Liu JM, Marcocci C, Bandeira F. Primary hyperparathyroidism. *Nat Rev Dis Primers.* 2016;2:16033. PMID: 27194212

Eastell R, Brandi ML, Costa AG, D'Amour P, Shoback DM, Thakker RV. Diagnosis of asymptomatic primary hyperparathyroidism: proceedings of the Fourth International Workshop. *J Clin Endocrinol Metab.* 2014;99(10):3570-3579. PMID: 25162666

Falchetti A, Marini F, Giusti F, Cavalli L, Cavalli T, Brandi ML. DNA-based test: when and why to apply it to primary hyperparathyroidism clinical phenotypes. *J Intern Med.* 2009;266(1):69-83. PMID: 19522827

Samander EH, Arnold A. Mutational analysis of the vitamin D receptor does not support its candidacy as a tumor suppressor gene in parathyroid adenomas. *J Clin Endocrinol Metab.* 2006;91(12):5019-5021. PMID: 17003089

41 ANSWER: B) Discontinuation of antithyroidal drugs

The patient described in this vignette exhibits a classic presentation of thyroid storm. Given the rarity of thyroid storm, objective analysis of the published cases series is difficult. However, there are 2 analyses from Japan that have focused on a larger number of patients and have thus shed light on its epidemiology, precipitating factors, clinical manifestations, diagnosis, treatment, and prognosis. The incidence of thyroid storm is estimated to be very low at 0.2 persons per 100,000 in Japan, or 0.22% of all thyrotoxic patients. In the analyses, the average age of patients with thyroid storm was 44 years and the female-to-male ratio was 3 to 1. The overwhelming cause of the thyroid storm was Graves disease, although destructive thyroiditis was reported in a handful of cases. About 20% of patients were diagnosed with thyroid storm before antithyroidal medication was initiated. Surprisingly, the death rate from thyroid storm in Japan remains high, and during the period of 2004 to 2008 it was 10%, with deaths mostly being due to multiorgan failure and congestive heart failure. A recent analysis from the United States showed an incidence of thyroid storm of between 0.57 to 0.76 cases per 100,000 persons per year and a mortality rate of 1.2% to 3.6% compared with 0.1% to 0.4%, (P <.01) in patients with thyrotoxicosis without thyroid storm.

As expected, clinical manifestations are hyperthermia, tachycardia, neurologic manifestations (including abnormal Glasgow Coma Score values), gastrointestinal abnormalities, and cardiac manifestations (including congestive heart failure and atrial fibrillation). Diagnosis hinges not on the actual thyroid hormone levels, as these can be comparable in thyrotoxic patients with and without thyroid storm, but on the systemic decompensation that occurs in response to these levels. Scoring systems for judging whether thyroid storm is present can be helpful in confirming a practitioner's clinical suspicion. Scoring systems developed in the United States and Japan exist. Perhaps the best known is the Burch-Wartofsky score, which assigns points based on the severity of involvement of each organ system, and the points are added to provide a total score, with higher scores making thyroid storm more likely. For example, the scoring system assigns points for the cardiovascular system based on the degree of heart rate elevation, the severity of congestive heart failure, and the presence or absence of atrial fibrillation. A score of 45 or greater is consider highly suggestive of thyroid storm. This patient's Burch-Wartofsky score is 80.

Both the thyroid emergencies, thyroid storm and myxedema coma, are often associated with precipitating events, and in fact, a precipitant is included in the scoring systems used to aid in the diagnosis of these conditions. In the United States' analysis of thyroid storm, reported precipitants were noncompliance with medications and surgery, including thyroid and parathyroid surgery. In the Japanese analyses of thyroid storm, about 70% of patients had one of the triggers considered to be classic. On the basis of 282 patients studied in Japan, the 2 most common triggers were irregular use or discontinuation of antithyroidal drugs (43% of cases) and infection (31% of cases). Diabetic ketoacidosis, severe emotional stress, trauma, and thyroid surgery accounted for approximately 3% to 4% of cases each. Radioiodine therapy, administration of iodinated contrast medium, pregnancy or delivery, adrenal insufficiency, tooth extraction, and exercise are triggers that accounted for less than 2.1% of cases. Another potential trigger not mentioned in these series is substance abuse.

Included in this vignette are several circumstances that could potentially have precipitated the presentation of thyroid storm in this patient. He participated in strenuous exercise (Answer D) and recently had a tooth extraction (Answer E). Although these precipitants are possibilities, they occurred 1 day and 28 days ago, respectively, thus making them less likely factors. No history of trauma (Answer C) is provided, so this is an unlikely precipitant as well. He also has a family history of autoimmune disease and therefore an additional autoimmune disease, such as adrenal insufficiency or type 1 diabetes, should be considered. On the basis of the Japanese experience, diabetic ketoacidosis is more common than adrenal insufficiency (Answer A), but both of these seem unlikely in a patient with normal concentrations of serum sodium, potassium, and bicarbonate.

Considering the Japanese analysis and the patient's age, failure to adhere to his medical regimen (Answer B) appears to be the most likely precipitant. Additional history, when the patient is able to provide it, would be helpful. For example, he might describe not having filled his methimazole prescription because he was feeling asymptomatic, or having forgotten to refill his prescription when coming home for the holidays. A review of pharmacy records might also clarify the situation. This case highlights the need to educate patients and their families about the nature and course of hyperthyroidism as an important means of preventing thyroid storm.

Educational Objective
List the precipitants of thyroid storm and be aware of their relative frequency.

UpToDate Topic Review(s)
Thyroid storm

Reference(s)

Akamizu T. Thyroid storm: a Japanese perspective. *Thyroid*. 2018;28(1):32-40. PMID: 28899229

Akamizu T, Satoh T, Isozaki O, et al; Japan Thyroid Association. Diagnostic criteria, clinical features, and incidence of thyroid storm based on nationwide surveys [published correction appears in *Thyroid*. 2012;22(9):979]. *Thyroid*. 2012;22(7):661-679. PMID: 22690898

Burch HB, Wartofsky L. Life-threatening thyrotoxicosis. Thyroid storm. *Endocrinol Metab Clin North Am*. 1993;22(2):263-277. PMID: 8325286

Galindo RJ, Hurtado CR, Pasquel FJ, et al. National trends in incidence, mortality, and clinical outcomes of patients hospitalized for thyrotoxicosis with and without thyroid storm in the United States, 2004-2013. *Thyroid*. 2019;29(1):36-43. PMID: 30382003

42 ANSWER: D) Melanocortin 4 receptor gene (*MC4R*)

A small percentage of obese individuals have a monogenic cause for their obesity. In most cases, weight gain is due to the interactions between environmental factors and genetic susceptibility. Genome-wide association studies have found several genetic variants that predispose individuals to gain weight in response to an obesogenic environment.

The gene encoding the melanocortin 4 receptor (*MC4R*) (Answer D) is located on chromosome 18. Loss-of-function pathogenic variants are the most common cause of monogenic obesity. These variants can be inherited in both dominant and recessive forms. MC4R is a G protein–coupled receptor that has an important role in the regulation of food intake and energy homeostasis. Individuals with a mutation in the *MC4R* gene become hyperphagic during infancy, have increased lean body mass, and have increased linear growth and final height. The linear growth acceleration is thought to result from hyperinsulinism. The patient in this vignette had early-onset obesity and increased linear growth during childhood. The most likely cause of her obesity is a pathogenic variant in the *MC4R* gene.

The fat mass and obesity-associated gene (*FTO*) (Answer A) is located on chromosome 16 and it is expressed in the arcuate nucleus of the hypothalamus. Population-based studies have found that variants residing in the first intron of this gene are associated with increased BMI in adults (BMI is increased by 0.36 kg/m^2 per allele, range 0.34 to 0.46 kg/m^2) and children (BMI is increased by 0.08 Z-score units). In children, the association starts at age 7 years and persists through adulthood. This variant is not associated with fetal growth. The presence of this genetic variant would not explain the weight gain described by the patient, as her weight gain started at age 1.

The arcuate nucleus of the hypothalamus has neurons that express the proopiomelanocortin gene (*POMC*) (Answer B), which makes the POMC protein. This gene is located on the short arm of chromosome 2. POMC is a prohormone; after posttranslational processing by prohormone convertases, it generates the following peptides: ACTH; α, β, and γ melanocyte-stimulating hormone (MSH); and β endorphin. Melanocyte-stimulating hormone binds to its receptor, melanocortin receptor 4, which induces anorexia. POMC deficiency gives rise to adrenal insufficiency (present in newborns), pigmentation abnormalities (usually red hair and pale skin due to lack of melanocyte-stimulating hormone action on the melanocortin 1 receptor), and early-onset, severe hyperphagia that results in severe obesity. Such patients have a normal birth weight, but start gaining weight shortly after birth. Weight usually exceeds 33 lb (15 kg) by age 1 and 55 lb (25 kg) by age 3. This patient does not have a history of adrenal insufficiency, hypopigmentation, or red hair, so it is unlikely that she has a pathogenic variant in the *POMC* gene.

Leptin is a hormone synthesized by adipose tissue that has an important role in regulating food intake and energy expenditure. Leptin is anorexigenic and its levels are directly related to the amount of adipose tissue present. Leptin binds to its receptor in the arcuate nucleus in the hypothalamus and its signaling is via the JAK-STAT pathway. Congenital leptin deficiency is a rare cause of early-onset obesity and it is due to pathogenic variants in the *LEP* gene (Answer C). The *LEP* gene is located on the long arm of chromosome 7. Eleven different pathogenic variants in the *LEP* gene have been described. Persons affected with this condition have rapid weight gain in the first few months of life leading to severe obesity. They have severe hyperphagia, hypogonadotropic hypogonadism, hyperinsulinemia, and an advanced bone age. Their hyperphagia is more severe than that of patients with *MC4R*-related obesity. Leptin deficiency is treated with subcutaneous administration of leptin. Individuals who receive leptin replacement therapy begin losing weight 2 weeks after starting therapy. Leptin's main therapeutic effect is to reduce hyperphagia. The patient described in this vignette has an elevated leptin level; therefore, she does not have leptin deficiency.

Prader-Willi syndrome is the most common syndromic form of obesity. It is caused by the absence of expression of the paternal alleles in the Prader-Willi critical region on chromosome 15 (Answer E). Affected patients have a lower birth weight than their siblings. During their first year of life, they have hypotonia with difficulty feeding and decreased appetite. From age 2 to 4 their appetite improves, and they start gaining weight appropriately. Around age 5 they start to gain excessive weight due to hyperphagia. These patients have global developmental delay, cognitive impairment, and behavioral problems. In addition, this condition is associated with hypogonadism. This patient's clinical presentation is not consistent with Prader-Willi syndrome.

Educational Objective
Identify patients with monogenic forms of obesity.

UpToDate Topic Review(s)
Genetic contribution and pathophysiology of obesity

Reference(s)

Frayling TM, Timpson NJ, Weedon MN, et al. A common variant in the FTO gene is associated with body mass index and predisposes to childhood and adult obesity. *Science.* 2007;316(5826):889-894. PMID: 17434869

Farooqi IS, Matarese G, Lord GM, et al. Beneficial effects of leptin on obesity, T cell hyporesponsiveness, and neuroendocrine/metabolic dysfunction of human congenital leptin deficiency. *J Clin Invest.* 2002;110(8):1093-1103. PMID: 12393845

Fairbrother U, Kidd E, Malagamuwa T, Walley A. Genetics of severe obesity. *Curr Diab Rep.* 2018;18:85. PMID: 30121879

Ranadive SA, Vaisse C. Lessons from extreme human obesity: monogenic disorders. *Endocrinol Metab Clin North Am.* 2008;37(3):733-751, x. PMID: 18775361

Angulo MA, Butler MG, Cataletto ME. Prader-Willi syndrome: a review of clinical, genetic, and endocrine findings. *J Endocrinol Invest.* 2015;38(12):1249-1263. PMID: 26062517

Farooqi IS, O'Rahilly S. Monogenic obesity in humans. *Annu Rev Med.* 2005;56:443-458. PMID: 15660521

43 ANSWER: A) Supervised fast in the hospital

Hypoglycemia that occurs in patients without a history of diabetes mellitus is unusual. Hypoglycemia can occur in the fasting state in some individuals, exclusively in the postprandial state in others, or, in a subset of patients, in both the fasting and postprandial state. The critical point is that the Whipple triad must be fulfilled to establish that a hypoglycemic disorder is present. The patient must have symptoms of hypoglycemia, with documentation of true hypoglycemia, and resolution of symptoms once the hypoglycemia has been appropriately treated.

The Whipple triad has not been confirmed in this case. The point-of-care glucose value was 57 mg/dL (3.2 mmol/L) in the emergency department, but the plasma glucose value from a sample drawn several minutes later, before treatment of hypoglycemia, was 63 mg/dL (3.2 mmol/L). Point-of-care or capillary glucose values cannot be used for diagnostic purposes in the setting of hypoglycemia, as glucose meters are often inaccurate at low glucose readings. A laboratory plasma or serum glucose measurement must be used to confirm true hypoglycemia. In this vignette, the plasma glucose does not reach the cutpoint of 55 mg/dL (3.1 mmol/L) necessary for the diagnosis of hypoglycemia.

In the setting of insulin-mediated hypoglycemia, plasma insulin, C-peptide, and proinsulin levels are high-normal or frankly elevated. Therefore, even though there is suspicion that the patient has insulin-mediated hypoglycemia, this has not been confirmed with laboratory testing.

The episode of hypoglycemia in this case occurred after the patient missed breakfast. Confirmation of hypoglycemia with a supervised fast, preferably in the hospital setting (Answer A), is the best step in the diagnostic cascade. There is nothing in this patient's history that would suggest the presence of postprandial hypoglycemia, so a mixed-meal test (Answer B) is not necessary. During the fast, if the patient has symptoms of hypoglycemia and has a point-of-care glucose measurement less than 55 mg/dL (<3.1 mmol/L), blood must be drawn for the following laboratory tests to determine whether she has insulin- or non–insulin-mediated hypoglycemia: plasma glucose, insulin, C-peptide, proinsulin, β-hydroxybutyrate and insulin antibodies. A plasma screen for insulin secretogogues should also be done to rule out surreptitious use of a secretogogue such as glyburide or a glinide.

Although the patient has had significant weight loss, performing abdominal CT (Answer C) is not the best next test in this case. Similarly, PET-CT (Answer E) should not be ordered now. Ordering an imaging study may be helpful once a diagnosis of hypoglycemia has been confirmed.

Ruling out adrenal insufficiency in a patient with hypoglycemia that is not associated with diabetes is important. However, a cosyntropin-stimulation test (Answer D) is not the best next diagnostic test.

Educational Objective
Define the diagnostic criteria for hypoglycemia in patients without diabetes mellitus.

UpToDate Topic Review(s)
Hypoglycemia in adults without diabetes: diagnostic approach

Reference(s)

Cryer PE, Axelrod L, Grossman AB, et al; Endocrine Society. Evaluation and management of adult hypoglycemic disorders: an Endocrine Society clinical practice guideline. *J Clin Endocrinol Metab.*2009;94(3):709-728. PMID: 19088155

Service, FJ. Diagnostic approach to adults with hypoglycemic disorders. *Endocrinol Metab Clin North Am.* 1999;28(3):519-532, vi. PMID: 10500929

Dynkevich Y, Rother KI, Whitford I, et al. Tumors, IGF-2, and hypoglycemia: insights from the clinic, the laboratory, and the historical archive. *Endocr Rev.* 2013;34(6):798-826. PMID: 2361135

44   ANSWER: B) Restart cabergoline

Hyperprolactinemia is often seen in end-stage renal disease. This is thought to be secondary to increased secretion and, to a lesser extent, reduced renal clearance of prolactin. Prolactin levels are mildly to moderately elevated in most patients with end-stage renal disease (81%). In a recent study, the median serum prolactin concentration was 65 ng/mL (2.8 nmol/L) (the 25th-75th percentiles, 48-195 ng/mL [2.1-8.5 nmol/L]).

However, this patient had a markedly elevated prolactin level (273.8 ng/mL [11.9 nmol/L]), which is unlikely to be solely related to end-stage renal disease. While his MRI is normal, it was done without gadolinium (due to his kidney disease), therefore greatly reducing the ability to detect a small adenoma. Despite the absence of radiologic evidence, the most likely diagnosis is a prolactin-secreting microadenoma. His prolactin elevation responded very well to cabergoline, with full normalization of both prolactin and testosterone. Therefore, cabergoline should be restarted (Answer B), with no negative effect on his transplant outcome. Because of this patient's end-stage renal disease and his good response to cabergoline, obtaining an MRI with contrast and referring him to neurosurgery (Answer A) is incorrect.

Interestingly, he had a mildly elevated serum IGF-1 level. This occurs in 2.5% of the normal population. He has no signs or symptoms of acromegaly. Normal GH suppression after a glucose load is 1.0 or 0.4 ng/mL, depending on the source. In this patient, cabergoline was stopped before the GH suppression test, as it can reduce the GH level in the setting of acromegaly. Regardless of which cutoff is used, his GH did not suppress after glucose. This has been reported in end-stage renal disease. The lack of acromegalic features suggests that the inability to fully suppress serum GH is due to renal failure, which leads to an increase in peripheral tissue resistance to GH, possibly due to decreased GH receptor numbers. Therefore, there is no indication to start any acromegaly-specific therapy, such as pegvisomant (Answer C) or a somatostatin receptor ligand (Answer D). Recommending no therapy (Answer E) is wrong, as it would most likely result in recurrence of hyperprolactinemia and hypogonadism.

Educational Objective
Explain the observation of hyperprolactinemia in patients with end-stage renal disease and the limitations of GH-suppression testing in this setting.

UpToDate Topic Review(s)
Clinical manifestations and evaluation of hyperprolactinemia

Reference(s)

Lo JC, Beck GJ, Kaysen GA, et al; FHN Study. Hyperprolactinemia in end-stage renal disease and effects of frequent hemodialysis. *Hemodial Int.* 2017;21(2):190-196. PMID: 27774730

García-Mayor RV, Pérez AJ, Gandara A, Andrade A, Mallo F, Casanueva FF. Metabolic clearance rate of biosynthetic growth hormone after endogenous growth hormone suppression with a somatostatin analogue in chronic renal failure patients and control subjects. *Clin Endocrinol (Oxf).* 1993;39(3):337-343. PMID: 8222296

Müssig K, Gallwitz B, Ranke MB, Horger M, Häring HU, Quabbe HJ. Acromegaly and end-stage renal disease: a diagnostic challenge. *J Endocrinol Invest.* 2006;29(8):745-749. PMID: 17033266

Wong NA, Ahlquist JA, Camacho-Hübner C, et al. Acromegaly or chronic renal failure: a diagnostic dilemma. *Clin Endocrinol (Oxf).* 1997;46(2):221-226. PMID: 9135706

45   ANSWER: B) Lipoprotein lipase

This patient has marked hypertriglyceridemia and chylomicronemia syndrome. Marked hypertriglyceridemia occurs when there is a pathogenic variant in a gene resulting in delayed clearance of chylomicrons, lipoproteins that carry dietary triglycerides in the circulation. These conditions typically present in children (almost always by adolescence or early adulthood) and are referred to as familial chylomicronemia syndrome. Familial chylomicronemia syndrome is caused by pathogenic variants in 1 of 5 genes that are involved in the functionality of lipoprotein lipase, the key enzyme that hydrolyzes triglycerides in lipoproteins. These mutations are inherited in an autosomal recessive fashion and lead to abnormal persistence of chylomicrons after a 12-hour fast. Of these, lipoprotein lipase deficiency due to pathogenic variants in the *LPL* gene (Answer B) is the most common, with an estimated prevalence of 1 in 1 million. Currently, full gene sequencing of *LPL* and 4 cofactor genes is the preferred method of establishing the diagnosis in patients with suspected familial chylomicronemia syndrome.

Affected patients have an increased lifetime risk of recurrent pancreatitis. This risk increases when the triglyceride concentration is greater than 1000 mg/dL (>11.30 mmol/L) and is greatest when the triglyceride concentration is higher than 2000 mg/dL (>22.60 mmol/L). Hypertriglyceridemia-induced pancreatitis develops possibly due to increased exocrine pancreatic lipase activity and resultant hydrolysis of circulating triglycerides within the pancreatic vasculature. Partial hydrolysis of fatty acids leads to acinar cell injury, activation of trypsinogen, and local autodigestion of pancreatic tissue. Increased chylomicrons in pancreatic capillaries might contribute by causing capillary plugging and local ischemia. Treatment of patients with familial chylomicronemia syndrome includes dietary and lifestyle interventions—primarily dramatic restriction of fat intake—and control of secondary factors. Pharmacologic therapies such as fibrates are ineffective for familial chylomicronemia and are not recommended. Identifying and treating secondary causes of hypertriglyceridemia (eg, controlling weight, eliminating alcohol intake, and avoiding use of triglyceride-raising medications) is important. Pregnancy, hypothyroidism, diabetes, and chronic renal failure can also worsen hypertriglyceridemia and increase the risk of pancreatitis. Plasmapheresis rarely has a role in this setting.

Pathogenic variants in the gene encoding apolipoprotein A-1 (Answer A) result in very low HDL-cholesterol levels and do not affect triglycerides. Pathogenic variants in the gene encoding the LDL receptor (Answer C) cause LDL-cholesterol elevation (but not triglyceride elevation). Truncating mutations in the apolipoprotein B gene (Answer D) cause hypolipidemias or elevated LDL cholesterol. Pathogenic variants in the gene encoding apolipoprotein E (Answer E) can cause remnant removal disease or dysbetalipoproteinemia. Affected individuals are largely asymptomatic well into adulthood until a secondary factor is present (see above), and marked hypertriglyceridemia can occur with resultant pancreatitis. Management involves treatment with statin and fibrates.

Educational Objective

Identify the underlying etiology of very high triglyceride levels.

UpToDate Topic Review(s)

Hypertriglyceridemia

Reference(s)

Brahm AJ, Hegele RA. Chylomicronaemia—current diagnosis and future therapies. *Nat Rev Endocrinol.* 2015;11(6):352-362. PMID: 25732519

46 ANSWER: A) Increase the spironolactone dosage

Primary aldosteronism is a common disorder that can induce hypertension, hypokalemia, and metabolic alkalosis, and it increases the risk for incident cardiovascular and kidney disease. Importantly, patients with primary aldosteronism have a higher risk for cardiovascular and kidney disease than do blood pressure–matched patients with essential hypertension, highlighting the adverse consequences of aldosterone on extrarenal mineralocorticoid receptors in primary aldosteronism that are independent of blood pressure. Consequently, early diagnosis and treatment of primary aldosteronism is important to mitigate adverse outcomes. The classic dogma is that patients with unilateral primary aldosteronism should be advised to undergo curative adrenalectomy, whereas patients with bilateral primary aldosteronism should be advised to take lifelong mineralocorticoid receptor antagonists. Whether these 2 approaches are equally effective at lowering cardiovascular risk is not clear.

This patient was diagnosed with bilateral primary aldosteronism and started on a mineralocorticoid receptor (MR) antagonist (spironolactone, 50 mg daily). Before initiating spironolactone, his laboratory values demonstrated substantial aldosterone production in the context of suppressed renin activity (autonomous and renin-independent aldosteronism), as well as hypokalemia and uncontrolled blood pressure despite the use of 3 antihypertensive agents. Three months after treatment with spironolactone was initiated, his blood pressure was lower, although still greater than the target of 130/80 mm Hg, and serum potassium was improved, but still lower than 4.0 mEq/L (4.0 mmol/L). Notably, his plasma renin activity remained suppressed and serum creatinine had increased, resulting in a decline in the estimated glomerular filtration rate to 60 mL/min per 1.73 m^2 (chronic kidney disease 3A is defined as an estimated glomerular filtration rate less than 60 mL/min per 1.73 m^2).

What are the goals of MR antagonist therapy in primary aldosteronism? Beyond normalization of hypertension and hypokalemia, adequate blockade of the MR may be an important factor in lowering cardiovascular risk. Treatment with an MR antagonist blocks the MR in the principal cell of the distal nephron, thereby decreasing sodium reabsorption by epithelial sodium channels and limiting potassium excretion. Decreasing sodium reabsorption decreases water reabsorption and consequently limits the volume expansion that characterizes primary aldosteronism. Effective MR antagonist therapy should therefore contract intravascular volume to lower blood pressure, decrease glomerular hyperfiltration, and minimize urinary potassium excretion. If this is done effectively to substantially contract intravascular volume, renin secretion from juxtaglomerular cells will increase. Thus, biomarkers suggestive of adequate renal MR blockade in primary aldosteronism include decreased blood pressure, increased serum potassium, increased renin activity from suppressed to unsuppressed, and decreased estimated glomerular filtration rate. Because the MR expressed in cardiovascular tissues can impart cardiovascular risk in primary aldosteronism, these biomarkers may serve as an indirect proxy of cardiovascular tissue aldosterone-MR interactions as well.

Recent retrospective cohort studies have shown that when patients with primary aldosteronism were treated with MR antagonists such that their renin activity remained suppressed, they had a substantially higher risk for incident cardiovascular events (myocardial infarction, stroke, heart failure) and death than patients with primary aldosteronism whose renin activity substantially increased with MR antagonists, as well as matched patients with essential hypertension and patients with primary aldosteronism who underwent curative adrenalectomy.

Thus, MR antagonist therapy in primary aldosteronism should be titrated, when possible, to normalize blood pressure, normalize potassium, and increase renin from a suppressed to an unsuppressed level, all as proxies of adequate MR blockade and cardiovascular risk reduction. It is anticipated that the estimated glomerular filtration rate will decrease with this approach, but this decline should not be mistaken for a medication adverse effect or induction of kidney disease. Rather, this decline in the estimated glomerular filtration rate represents an unmasking of the underlying chronic kidney disease that was not evident in untreated primary aldosteronism where there is hyperfiltration of serum creatinine. MR antagonist therapy can be continued in these patients, even when the estimated glomerular filtration rate declines, as long as recurrent or severe hyperkalemia is not a problem (usually a bigger issue when the estimated glomerular filtration rate decreases below 30-35 mL/min per 1.73 m^2). Since this patient still has elevated blood pressure, a serum potassium concentration less than 4.0 mEq/L (<4.0 mmol/L), and suppressed renin activity, increasing the spironolactone dosage (eg, to 75 or 100 mg daily) (Answer A) should be attempted to achieve better control and possibly improve long-term cardiovascular risk.

Eplerenone is another mineralocorticoid antagonist that can be used in lieu of spironolactone. Eplerenone is less potent than spironolactone, but it has the benefit of not having antiandrogenic effects and therefore is sometimes preferred in male patients.

Lisinopril should not be stopped (Answers D and E). ACE inhibitors are preferred antihypertensive medications whose use in lowering cardiovascular and kidney disease risk has been established. Spironolactone should not be stopped (Answer B) despite the reduction in the estimated glomerular filtration rate, because it is likely to still be effective and safe. Amiloride (Answers C and E) is an excellent antihypertensive agent, but its mechanisms of action are similar to those of spironolactone. As an epithelial sodium-channel inhibitor, amiloride treats the excessive renal sodium reabsorption and potassium excretion in the same manner as spironolactone. However, amiloride does not block the MR. Whether this difference could decrease its ability to prevent cardiovascular disease attributable to extrarenal MR activation is not known.

Figure 7. Optimal medical treatment with MR antagonists in primary aldosteronism. The action of MR antagonists in the principal cell results in decreased ENaC-mediated urinary sodium reabsorption, and consequently decreased volume expansion and potassium and hydrogen ion excretion. If the effect of this action is sufficient, the contraction of the intravascular volume may result in a relative renal hypoperfusion and increased secretion of renin by juxtaglomerular cells. Thus, the rise in renin, from suppressed to unsuppressed, may serve as a biomarker of optimal MR antagonism in primary aldosteronism. AngII, angiotensin II. [© 2018 Illustration ENDOCRINE SOCIETY]

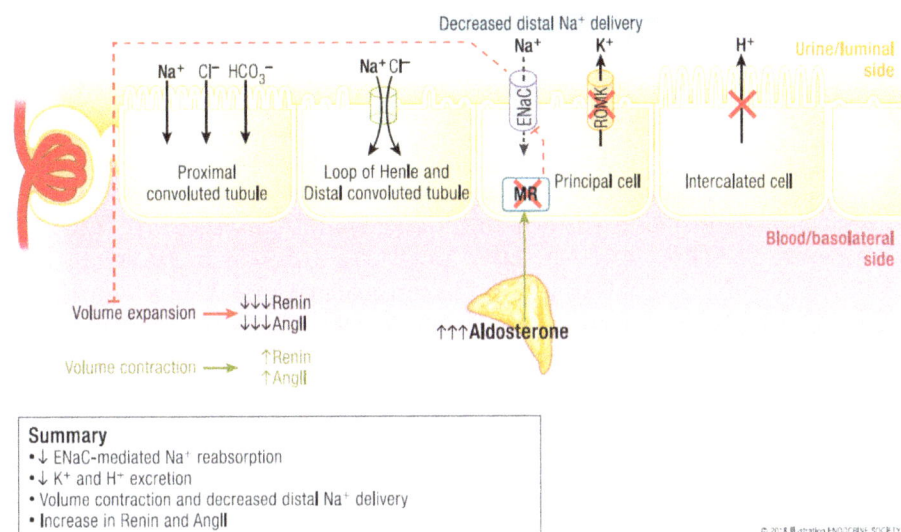

Reprinted from Vaidya A, Mulatero P, Baudrand R, Adler GK. The expanding spectrum of primary aldosteronism: implications for diagnosis, pathogenesis, and treatment. *Endocr Rev.* 2018;39(6):1057-1088.

Educational Objective
Guide the medical treatment of primary aldosteronism.

UpToDate Topic Review(s)
Treatment of primary aldosteronism

Reference(s)

Hundemer GL, Curhan GC, Yozamp N, Wang M, Vaidya A. Cardiometabolic outcomes and mortality in medically treated primary aldosteronism: a retrospective cohort study. *Lancet Diabetes Endocrinol.* 2018;6(1):51-59. PMID: 29129576

Hundemer GL, Curhan GC, Yozamp N, Wang M, Vaidya A. Incidence of atrial fibrillation and mineralocorticoid receptor antagonist activity in patients with medically and surgically treated primary aldosteronism. *JAMA Cardiol.* 2018;3(8):768-774. PMID: 30027227

Vaidya A, Mulatero P, Baudrand R, Adler GK. The expanding spectrum of primary aldosteronism: implications for diagnosis, pathogenesis, and treatment. *Endocr Rev.* 2018;39(6):1057-1088. PMID: 30124805

47   ANSWER: D) Perform contrast-enhanced liver MRI

This patient has known medullary thyroid carcinoma (MTC) with elevated calcitonin and carcinoembryonic antigen (CEA) levels and abnormal findings on CT of the neck and chest, but normal findings on abdominal CT. However, the elevated calcitonin and CEA levels raise suspicion for distant metastases. Over the last 2 years, repeated CT of the neck, chest, and abdomen have shown several cervical neck adenopathies and 2 small lung nodules—findings that have been stable over this period. Because her calcitonin and CEA levels have been rising, the clinician should search for distant metastases in addition to following up on current abnormal findings on neck and chest CT. Therefore, contrast-enhanced liver MRI (Answer D) should be performed to check for liver metastases. This patient might also need bone scintigraphy to assess for bone metastases.

MTC is a neuroendocrine tumor of the parafollicular C cells of the thyroid. The C cells originate from the embryonic neural crest. MTC accounts for 1% to 2% of thyroid cancers. Most cases are sporadic. Serum calcitonin and CEA concentrations are both used as markers of MTC, and these values have prognostic value postoperatively. Assessment of calcitonin and CEA doubling times postoperatively provides sensitive markers for progression and aggressiveness of metastatic MTC. MTC can spread by local invasion and can also metastasize within the neck or distantly. Radiologic evaluation should be obtained in patients with rising serum calcitonin and CEA levels (usually calcitonin ≥150 pg/mL [≥43.8 pmol/L] per MTC clinical guidelines). Imaging modalities are neck ultrasonography, neck CT, chest CT, 3-phase contrast-enhanced liver CT or contrast-enhanced liver MRI, axial MRI, and bone scintigraphy. MRI of spine may be superior to other imaging modalities for skeletal metastases. Neither fluorodeoxyglucose PET imaging or somatostatin receptor imaging is recommended as a routine initial screening test for metastases. Fluorodeoxyglucose PET scanning has higher sensitivity when the serum calcitonin concentration is 1000 pg/mL or greater (≥292 pmol/L). Three-phase contrast-enhanced multidetector liver CT and contrast-enhanced MRI (Answer D) are the most sensitive methods to detect liver metastases. This patient underwent a regular abdominal CT, which is not the best test for detecting liver metastases. If standard imaging procedures fail to detect MTC metastases in the liver, laparoscopic or open evaluation of the liver is an option. Liver metastases occur in 45% of patients with advanced MTC. Treatment is considered in patients with liver metastases that are large, increasing in size, or associated with symptoms such as diarrhea or pain. A single large metastasis should be resected if possible. Liver metastases, however, are often multiple and disseminated throughout the parenchyma and are usually not amenable to surgery, percutaneous ethanol ablation, or radiofrequency ablation. The best treatment may be either chemoembolization or systemic therapy.

Recently, ^{68}Ga-DOTATATE PET-CT (Answer C) became available for surveillance of neuroendocrine tumors, but a clear indication in the case of MTC has not been established. This imaging modality has also been proven to be useful in the management of neuroendocrine cancer, indicating an important role in the clinical care of somatostatin-avid malignancies. Medullary thyroid cancer expresses somatostatin receptors in only 20% of cases.

All patients with MTC should undergo germline *RET* genetic testing, given the association with multiple endocrine neoplasia type 2. If test results are unknown or not available, preoperative testing should include measurement of serum calcium and plasma free metanephrines to screen for primary hyperparathyroidism and pheochromocytoma, respectively. Total thyroidectomy with central neck dissection remains the standard therapy for a patient with recent diagnosis of MTC.

Tyrosine kinase inhibitors (Answer B) can be initiated in patients with MTC and significant tumor burden and symptomatic or progressive metastatic disease according to RECIST (Response Evaluation Criteria in Solid Tumors). Vandetanib or cabozantinib (FDA-approved tyrosine kinase inhibitors to treat MTC) can be used in patients with advanced progressive MTC. Octreotide (Answer A) can be initiated in patients with severe diarrhea, but this patient has only occasional diarrhea. This patient has not yet had a complete workup for metastases. Starting a tyrosine kinase inhibitor or octreotide would be premature. MTC does not respond to suppressive levothyroxine therapy (Answer E) because it derives from parafollicular cells, which are different from follicular cells.

Educational Objective
Determine the appropriate imaging in patients with medullary thyroid cancer and elevated calcitonin levels.

UpToDate Topic Review(s)
Medullary thyroid cancer: surgical treatment and prognosis

Reference(s)

Wells SA Jr, Asa SL, Dralle H, et al; American Thyroid Association Guidelines Task Force on Medullary Thyroid Carcinoma. Revised American Thyroid Association guidelines for the management of medullary thyroid carcinoma. *Thyroid*. 2015;25(6):567-610. PMID: 25810047

Ong SC, Schoder H, Patel SG, et al. Diagnostic accuracy of 18F-FDG PET in restaging patients with medullary thyroid carcinoma and elevated calcitonin levels. *J Nucl Med*. 2007;48(4):501-507. PMID: 17401085.

Mojtahedi A, Thamake S, Tworowska I, Ranganathan D, Delpassand ES. The value of (68)Ga-DOTATATE PET/CT in diagnosis and management of neuroendocrine tumors compared to current FDA approved imaging modalities: a review of literature. *Am J Nucl Med Mol Imaging*. 2014;4(5):426-434. PMID: 25143861

48

ANSWER: A) Recommend no changes

This case reviews the role of antiplatelet and statin therapy in the primary prevention of cardiovascular disease in patients with diabetes mellitus. Although the use of aspirin in secondary prevention offers clear benefit, its role in primary prevention in patients with diabetes is unclear. The 2019 American Diabetes Association Standards of Care recommend that daily aspirin (75-162 mg) for primary prevention be considered in patients with type 1 or type 2 diabetes who have an increased risk of atherosclerotic cardiovascular disease (ASCVD) and no increased risk of bleeding. The guideline states that this group includes men and women older than 50 years who have at least 1 major risk factor for ASCVD and no increased bleeding risk. In patients older than 70 years, the bleeding risk appears to be greater, and aspirin use for primary prevention of ASCVD should be carefully considered. In patients younger than 50 years who have a higher risk of ASCVD, management should be individualized, as there are limited data to guide clinical practice. In the recent ASCEND trial (A Study of Cardiovascular Events in Diabetes), the use of aspirin, 100 mg daily, in patients with diabetes and no known history of ASCVD was studied. Although vascular events (nonfatal myocardial infarction, nonfatal stroke, death from any vascular event) were reduced by 12%, the risk of a major bleeding event rose by 29%. The investigators conclude that the benefit does not justify the risk. There are no data on the use of aspirin with sucralfate in the primary prevention of cardiovascular disease in patients with diabetes. This patient is younger than 50 years and is not at very high risk for cardiovascular disease in 10 years. Therefore, aspirin use (Answers B and C) is not indicated now.

Diabetes mellitus is considered a coronary heart disease risk equivalent. The 2018 American Heart Association/American College of Cardiology guideline on treatment of blood cholesterol to reduce atherosclerotic cardiovascular risk in adults continues to treat it as such. The recommendations are to treat patients between ages 40 and 75 years who have an LDL-cholesterol level between 70 and 189 mg/dL (1.81-4.90 mmol/L). All adults with LDL-cholesterol levels greater than 190 mg/dL (>4.92 mmol/L) need evaluation for secondary causes and appropriate treatment. The guidance is to use moderate-intensity statin therapy, which this patient already takes (atorvastatin, 20 mg daily). Higher-intensity statin therapy would be indicated for primary prevention in patients with a 10-year risk of cardiovascular disease greater than 7.5%. This patient's pretreatment 10-year risk was 1.1%, so increasing the statin dosage (Answer D) is not required. The addition of nonstatin therapy is recommended in patients at high risk who have an insufficient response to or are intolerant of statin therapy. Neither is the case with this patient, so adding ezetimibe (Answer E) is incorrect.

At this time, no change in lipid management or addition of an antiplatelet agent is indicated for this patient (Answer A).

Educational Objective
Manage antiplatelet and statin therapy in the primary prevention of cardiovascular disease in patients with diabetes mellitus.

UpToDate Topic Review(s)
Overview of primary prevention of coronary heart disease and stroke
Overview of medical care in adults with diabetes mellitus

Reference(s)

American Diabetes Association. 9. Cardiovascular disease and risk management: Standards of Medical Care in Diabetes-2018. *Diabetes Care.* 2018;41(Suppl 1):S86-S104. PMID: 29222380

Capodanno D, Angiolillo DJ. Aspirin for primary cardiovascular risk prevention and beyond in diabetes mellitus. *Circulation.* 2016;134(20):1579-1594. PMID: 27729421

ASCEND Study Collaborative Group, Bowman L, Mafham M, et al. The effects of aspirin for primary prevention in persons with diabetes mellitus. *N Engl J Med.* 2018;379(16):1529-1539. PMID: 30146931

49

ANSWER: E) Maintain current regimen

Hypoparathyroidism, which most commonly occurs following thyroid or parathyroid surgery, represents a challenging disorder to manage. This challenge is even more amplified in pregnancy, which superimposes significant physiologic changes in calciotropic hormones under normal conditions. Specifically, serum calcium is typically lower in pregnancy, although ionized calcium and calcium corrected for albumin are usually still within the normal range. Serum calcitriol, however, which is derived from renal and placental sources, typically increases throughout pregnancy. Indeed, calcitriol levels in the third trimester are elevated in up to 80% of patients, although hypercalcemia is rare. This increase is thought to be due to higher levels of vitamin D–binding protein, as well as stimulated production by factors such as PTHrP and prolactin. Given these physiologic changes, management of hypoparathyroidism in these patients requires close follow-up and a solid understanding of the potential impact of pregnancy-related changes in calcium physiology.

Although there are no specific guidelines for managing these patients, the continued use of calcium and vitamin D analogues such as calcitriol to target a serum calcium level in the lower range of normal is reasonable. Measurement of serum calcium and albumin every 6 to 8 weeks during pregnancy is advisable, given the potential for serious fetal consequences if calcium is not well maintained (ie, fetal hypoparathyroidism if the mother is hypercalcemic for a prolonged period during pregnancy). This patient's current serum and urine calcium levels are at goal. As such, no changes in her regimen are necessary now (Answer E), including no need for increased supplemental calcium (Answer B).

Although current evidence suggests that adequate maternal 25-hydroxyvitamin D is important for fetal outcomes, this patient's vitamin D level is sufficient and does not require supplementation now (Answer A). Given the expected increase in 1,25-dihydroxyvitamin D during pregnancy, as well as the potential contribution of oral calcitriol to the observed measurement, this patient's calcitriol dosage should not be decreased (Answer C). Of note, due to these confounding factors, serum 1,25-dihydroxyvitamin D should not be routinely measured in pregnancy, as it was in this particular patient. Indeed, this patient's oral calcitriol dosage was initially reduced based on an elevated serum 1,25-dihydroxyvitamin D level, which resulted in symptomatic hypocalcemia. Finally, although acceptable for use in pregnancy, hydrochlorothiazide (Answer D) is not indicated as an adjunct, off-label therapy to improve her serum calcium, as it is within the preferred range.

Educational Objective
Recommend the optimal approach to monitoring and managing a patient with preexisting hypoparathyroidism during pregnancy.

UpToDate Topic Review(s)
Hypoparathyroidism

Reference(s)

Souberbielle JC, Cavalier E, Delanaye P, et al. Serum calcitriol concentrations measured with a new direct automated assay in a large population of adult healthy subjects and in various clinical situations. *Clin Chim Acta.* 2015;451(Pt B):149-153. PMID: 26409159

Hatswell BL, Allan CA, Teng J, et al. Management of hypoparathyroidism in pregnancy and lactation - a report of 10 cases. *Bone Rep.* 2015;3:15-19. PMID: 28377963

50 **ANSWER: C) Initiate estrogen replacement therapy**
In this perimenopausal patient, the main clinical question is whether her symptoms of estrogen deficiency are due to hyperprolactinemia or menopause. The elevated FSH value is more consistent with perimenopause or menopausal estrogen deficiency. If the prolactin elevation were causing significant estrogen deficiency, one would expect the FSH concentration to be low or falsely normal with a low estradiol concentration. Therefore, this patient's estrogen deficiency is due to perimenopause/menopause, not hyperprolactinemia.

In the management of a prolactin-producing pituitary adenoma, cabergoline treatment could be withdrawn as early as 2 years after starting treatment, with the best remission rates observed when prolactin has normalized and the pituitary adenoma is no longer visible. In premenopausal women, additional considerations are whether an elevated prolactin level is associated with symptoms of galactorrhea or hypogonadism in view of fertility concerns or long-term effects of premature estrogen deficiency. In perimenopausal or postmenopausal women, even if hyperprolactinemia is present, a prolactinoma can be monitored (off dopamine agonist therapy) to assess for growth that could affect pituitary function or threaten the optic chiasm or vision. This perimenopausal patient could be monitored off dopamine agonist therapy because the pituitary adenoma is no longer visible and she has been treated with cabergoline for many years. Restarting cabergoline (Answers A and B) is not indicated.

However, this patient is having significant estrogen deficiency symptoms with hot flashes that are causing poor sleep and are affecting her work. Therefore, simply monitoring off therapy (Answer E) is not the best option.

Although vaginal estrogen (Answer D) is a good treatment for genitourinary syndrome of menopause, it is not the best option to treat vasomotor hot flashes. These symptoms are best treated with systemic estrogen (Answer C).

In the past, concern about prolactinoma growth induced by estrogen therapy was raised by case reports of prolactinomas developing in men on high-dosage estrogen therapy or progression of microadenoma to macroadenoma and early reports of an increase in prolactinomas in women taking oral contraceptives. Data from autopsy series did not find an increase in prolactinomas in men who were given high-dosage diethylstilbestrol. Similarly, data from case-control studies in women on oral contraceptives did not show an increase in prolactinomas either. In a few small prospective studies, menopausal hormone replacement therapy or oral contraceptives did not increase the risk for worsening previously diagnosed and treated hyperprolactinemia. It is important to be aware of the potential for estrogen therapy to increase prolactin concentrations or to stimulate prolactinoma growth, and repeated imaging would be appropriate for a rising prolactin level in this setting. However, estrogen therapy or oral contraceptives are not contraindicated in premenopausal or postmenopausal women with a prolactinoma and should not be withheld in symptomatic women.

Educational Objective
Counsel a menopausal woman about treatment options for prolactinoma and determine whether estrogen deficiency symptoms are due to hyperprolactinemia or menopause.

UpToDate Topic Review(s)
Management of hyperprolactinemia

Reference(s)

Melmed S, Casanueva FF, Hoffman AR, et al; Endocrine Society. Diagnosis and treatment of hyperprolactinemia: an Endocrine Society clinical practice guideline. *J Clin Endocrinol Metab.* 2011;96(2):273-288. PMID: 21296991

Gooren LJ, Assies J, Asscheman H, de Slegte R, van Kessel H. Estrogen-induced prolactinoma in a man. *J Clin Endocrinol Metab.* 1988;66(2):444-446. PMID: 3339116

Garcia MM, Kapcala LP. Growth of a microprolactinoma to a macroprolactinoma during estrogen therapy. *J Endocrinol Invest.* 1995;18(6):450-455. PMID: 7594240

Scheithauer BW, Kovacs KT, Randall RV, Ryan N. Effects of estrogen on the human pituitary: a clinicopathologic study. *Mayo Clin Proceedings.* 1989;64(9):1077-1084. PMID: 2811485

Pituitary Adenoma Study Group. Pituitary adenomas and oral contraceptives: a multicenter case-control study. *Fertil Steril.* 1983;39(6):753-760. PMID: 6682810

Touraine P, Deneux C, Plu-Bureau G, Mauvais-Jarvis P, Kuttenn F. Hormonal replacement therapy in menopausal women with a history of hyperprolactinemia. *J Endocrinol Invest.* 1998;21(11):732-736. PMID: 9972671

Testa G, Vegetti W, Motta T, et al. Two-year treatment with oral contraceptives in hyperprolactinemic patients. *Contraception.* 1998;58(2):69-73. PMID: 9773260

Christin-Maître S, Delemer B, Touraine P, Young J. Prolactinoma and estrogens: pregnancy, contraception and hormonal replacement therapy. *Ann Endocrinol (Paris).* 2007;68(2-3):106-112. PMID: 17540335

51 ANSWER: D) Increased conversion of T_4 to T_3

This patient has a diagnosis of panhypopituitarism with deficits in both his anterior and posterior pituitary hormones. Several interactions can occur between the various end-organ hormones when more than one is being replaced. For example, initiation of gonadal hormones can change the requirement for thyroid hormones, and estrogen therapy can increase the requirement for GH. The Endocrine Society's guidelines for GH replacement state the following about the interaction between GH and thyroid hormone: "We suggest that thyroid and adrenal function be monitored during growth hormone therapy of adults with growth hormone deficiency" and "hypopituitary patients on thyroid hormone replacement may need dose adjustments after starting growth hormone replacement."

A number of studies have evaluated thyroid parameters when GH is initiated in individuals with hypopituitarism. Several studies have noted a decline in free T_4 concentrations in such patients. In one study of those who were not already taking levothyroxine, 36% were started on levothyroxine as a result of decreases in serum free T_4 following GH treatment. In those already taking levothyroxine, 16% had their dosage increased in response to the lowering of free T_4 after GH had been started. The authors hypothesized that GH unmasked central hypothyroidism. Another study found that free T_4 levels declined below the reference range in 47% of those who were not taking levothyroxine before GH was commenced and in 18% of those already taking levothyroxine. In another placebo-controlled study of levothyroxine-untreated and levothyroxine-treated groups, GH, but not placebo, was associated with a decline in free T_4. In another study, the largest decline in free T_4 occurred within 6 months of starting GH.

In the studies that examined either free T_3 or total T_3 levels after initiation of GH, most showed an increase in their concentrations, suggesting an acceleration of the metabolism of T_4 to T_3. Human cell lines treated in vitro with GH were found to have an increase in the expression of type 2 deiodinase RNA, as well as increased type 2 deiodinase protein levels and activity, again suggesting accelerated T_4 metabolism. Thus, increased conversion of T_4 to T_3 (Answer D) is the best choice.

Nonadherence to levothyroxine therapy (Answer A) is always a possibility. However, this is perhaps made less likely by the fact that the patient appears to being taking both his GH and testosterone (on the basis of their normalized serum concentrations). Similarly, although impaired levothyroxine absorption (Answer B) is not an uncommon occurrence, there is nothing in this patient's history to suggest it. A decreased thyroxine-binding globulin concentration (Answer C), as occurs with initiation of testosterone therapy, is associated with increased free T_4 and, if anything, a decreased levothyroxine requirement. Increased body weight (Answer E) can be associated with an increased levothyroxine requirement. However, no weight alterations are suggested in the vignette, and the body weight changes associated with the favorable body composition changes seen with GH repletion are usually relatively weight neutral.

Educational Objective
Describe the relationship between growth hormone initiation and free T_4 concentrations.

UpToDate Topic Review(s)
Growth hormone deficiency in adults
Treatment of hypopituitarism

Reference(s)

Agha A, Walker D, Perry L, et al. Unmasking of central hypothyroidism following growth hormone replacement in adult hypopituitary patients. *Clin Endocrinol (Oxf)*. 2007;66(1):72-77. PMID: 17201804

Jorgensen JO, Pedersen SA, Laurberg P, et al. Effects of growth hormone therapy on thyroid function of growth hormone-deficient adults with and without concomitant thyroxine-substituted central hypothyroidism. *J Clin Endocrinol Metab*. 1989;69(6):1127-1132. PMID: 2685007

Molitch ME, Clemmons DR, Malozowski S, Merriam GR, Vance ML; Endocrine S. Evaluation and treatment of adult growth hormone deficiency: an Endocrine Society clinical practice guideline. *J Clin Endocrinol Metab*. 2011;96(6):1587-1609. PMID: 21602453

Porretti S, Giavoli C, Ronchi C, et al. Recombinant human GH replacement therapy and thyroid function in a large group of adult GH-deficient patients: when does L-T(4) therapy become mandatory? *J Clin Endocrinol Metab*. 2002;87(5):2042-2045. PMID: 11994338

Yamauchi I, Sakane Y, Yamashita T, et al. Effects of growth hormone on thyroid function are mediated by type 2 iodothyronine deiodinase in humans. *Endocrine*. 2018;59(2):353-363. PMID: 29274063

52 ANSWER: E) Change his evening basal insulin to 30 units of NPH

The purpose of this vignette is to highlight the effect of peritoneal dialysis on daily blood glucose excursions. Hemodialysis is the most common method of renal replacement therapy when a patient is not a candidate for renal transplant. Peritoneal dialysis is used in 5% to 7% of patients. One potential advantage of peritoneal dialysis is that the patient is not burdened by travel to a dialysis center. He or she can freely travel, although the large amounts of fluid in bags can be cumbersome. For a patient with diabetes, peritoneal dialysis has less risk for severe hypoglycemia, but, as this vignette highlights, it can be associated with episodes of hyperglycemia during the time that the peritoneal dialysis fluid is in the abdomen. Peritoneal dialysis is most effective when the patient has good glucose control, as the method depends on a near-normal glucose level. Glucose is the preferred osmotic agent for peritoneal dialysis solution and patients can absorb up to 200 g of glucose per day, depending on the glucose concentration in the fluid and the frequency of exchanges. This patient was experiencing a 150 to 200 mg/dL (8.3-11.1 mmol/L) increase in glucose overnight (documented by continuous glucose monitoring); this interval coincides with the timing of when he has a large dextrose load in his abdomen.

To address his overnight hyperglycemia, his insulin prescription should be altered. Increasing either the nighttime insulin glargine dose (Answer A) or changing to insulin degludec (Answer B) may cause daytime hypoglycemia once the peritoneal dialysis is completed at 8 AM, as these insulins have approximately 24-hour activity; his current daytime glucose control is reasonable. Encouraging the patient to switch to insulin pump therapy (Answer C) could improve nocturnal glucose control, but this is not necessary and has significant cost and patient education is required for effective use. Adding an extra dose of insulin lispro at the start of dialysis (Answer D) is not likely to help, as the duration of lispro action is significantly shorter than the duration of his dialysis and glucose exposure. While extra lispro at the start of dialysis would be expected to improve his glucose readings at 10 PM, he would most likely still be hyperglycemic at 3 AM and 6 AM. Of the available choices, changing the evening basal insulin to NPH (Answer E) is the best strategy for controlling the nocturnal hyperglycemia in this patient, as the action of NPH is similar to the duration of dialysis and glucose exposure. However, it is critical that the patient be educated about the timing of insulins—if he takes NPH insulin and changes his peritoneal dialysis routine, he may be at risk for hypoglycemia. In addition, this patient should be counseled to decrease his morning lispro dose. With use of NPH at the start of dialysis, his 8-AM glucose readings should be much lower and he would be at risk of hypoglycemia if this morning dose is not adjusted.

Educational Objective
Explain the role of peritoneal dialysis fluid in causing hyperglycemia.

UpToDate Topic Review(s)
Dialysis in diabetic nephropathy

Reference(s)
Burkart J. Metabolic consequences of peritoneal dialysis. *Semin Dial.* 2004;17(6):498-504. PMID: 15660581

53 ANSWER: A) Serum thyroglobulin measurement
Although this patient's clinical presentation is complicated by overlapping symptoms and signs from several different disease processes (malignancy, sepsis, and thyrotoxicosis), he does meet thyroid storm criteria. Thyroid storm appears to have been caused by destructive thyroiditis. By far the most common underlying cause of thyroid storm is Graves disease. However, destructive thyroiditis has also been reported as an etiology. In a Japanese study, 4.8% of thyroid storm cases were thought to have this etiology. Thyroiditis presenting in thyroid storm has also been reported by Sherman et al and Swinburne at el.

The relatively low frequency of thyroid storm cases caused by thyroiditis is not surprising given the underlying mechanism of the thyrotoxicosis. In severe Graves disease, the massively stimulated thyroid gland is responsible for ongoing production of thyroid hormones. Very high levels of thyroid hormones can be manufactured and the process can be ongoing without treatment due to the continued presence of stimulatory immunoglobulins. With destructive thyroiditis, the degree of thyroid hormone elevation is limited by the content of stored thyroid hormone within the gland and is modulated by the extent and time course of the damage to the thyroid gland. Subacute thyroiditis, for example, could damage the gland over several weeks with ongoing leakage of thyroid hormones and modest thyroid hormone elevation. Alternatively, as might be postulated in this vignette, a massive insult from aggressively progressing leukemia might cause substantial damage at one time and result in much higher thyroid hormone elevation. The precipitous onset of thyroiditis in this patient is supported by the initial report of a normal-appearing thyroid gland on the first CT scan. Thyroiditis is generally self-limited, as once the damaged gland has been emptied of its preformed thyroid hormone stores, circulating thyroid hormone levels should decline—hence, the limited 3- to 6-week duration of most cases of subacute thyroiditis. In addition, the hyperthyroidism associated with thyroiditis is characterized primarily by free T_4 elevation, and less T_3 elevation, reflecting the composition of the stored thyroid hormones within the thyroid gland. Higher T_3 levels, however, are seen in Graves disease and toxic nodular disease. If this patient's condition had stabilized, it would have been predicted that his thyroid hormone levels would have gradually declined, even without treatment. As opposed to a viral insult that is invoked as the cause of subacute thyroiditis, this patient's thyroiditis was postulated to be due to infiltration of the patient's thyroid gland by leukemia cells. Several case reports exist in the literature of patients with lymphoma whose thyroiditis was thought to be due to lymphoma cells infiltrating thyroid tissue.

In this vignette, the patient was started on triple therapy with methimazole, hydrocortisone, and potassium iodide with the assumption that his hyperthyroidism was caused by ongoing production of thyroid hormones. His T_3 levels did decline very slightly, but there was an upward trajectory rather than a downward trajectory in his free T_4. Given the abrupt development of lesions within the patient's thyroid gland (as illustrated by his second CT scan) and the overall clinical picture, the best explanation for the patient's failure to respond to methimazole is that he was suffering from a destructive thyroiditis. Support for this diagnosis is provided by a substantially elevated serum thyroglobulin level of 4880 ng/mL (4880 µg/L), which was reported after the patient died. An elevated thyroglobulin level (Answer A) or absent iodine uptake on a radioiodine uptake and scan are findings that support a diagnosis of destructive thyroiditis. A radioiodine uptake and scan could not be performed in this patient due to his instability, but it most likely would not have been informative because of his exposure to iodinated contrast.

Some of the other answers are not the best choices for elucidating the cause of hyperthyroidism in any clinical scenario. For example, a white blood cell count (Answer D) might provide information about the impact of Graves disease or thionamide therapy on hematologic parameters, but it would not be helpful in determining etiology. A 24-hour urine iodine measurement (Answer B) would probably be elevated in this case given the patient's exposure to iodinated contrast media, but it would be elevated regardless of whether he had hyperthyroidism, and also regardless of whether the iodine load had exacerbated this hyperthyroidism. Iodine exposure can worsen hyperthyroidism due to Graves disease and toxic nodules, but it would not have worsened this patient's thyrotoxicosis, as he would not be expected to have ongoing thyroid hormone synthesis.

Checking levels of thionamide drugs (methimazole or propylthiouracil) (Answer C) has generally been performed as a means of assessing outpatient adherence to therapy, and nonadherence would not be suspected during administration of a medication in a hospital setting. An elevated thyroid-stimulating immunoglobulin titer (Answer E) would point to a diagnosis of Graves disease, but a negative titer can also be seen in some cases of Graves disease and in toxic nodular thyroid disease and thyroiditis. So, this test is not completely discriminatory as far as etiology is concerned. Response to methimazole would certainly be expected if the thyroid-stimulating immunoglobulin were positive, but the value would not really shed light on the failure to respond to thionamides.

Thyroiditis is usually treated with β-adrenergic blockers to ameliorate symptoms of thyrotoxicosis, as well as "tincture of time"—that is, the disease usually has a self-limited course. However, if treatment is indicated by the clinical situation, drugs such as methimazole and propylthiouracil are ineffective, as there is no ongoing thyroid hormone synthesis to block. Therefore, therapy must be directed at removal of circulating thyroid hormones. Cholestyramine has been used in this manner, but it is typically used as one of several therapies due to its modest impact. Surgery could be considered if there is no other option. Other therapies that have been used with varying degrees of success in treating thyroid storm include plasmapheresis, plasma exchange, and charcoal hemoperfusion. These procedures usually lower thyroid hormone levels within 3 days and work because most thyroid hormone is bound to plasma proteins. Although there are case reports of failure to respond to these therapies with lowering of thyroid hormone concentrations, most reports demonstrate success. In plasmapheresis and plasma exchange, the patient's plasma is separated from other blood components and removed. In plasma exchange, the plasma is also replaced by other colloidal solutions. The removal of plasma proteins includes removal of thyroxine-binding globulin and albumin, along with their bound thyroid hormone, thus lowering the thyroid hormone pool. If colloid, including albumin, is infused, this will provide new binding sites for free thyroid hormones, and thus also contribute to lowering circulating thyroid hormones. Concomitant removal of thyroid-stimulating immunoglobulins may possibly contribute to improvement of the hyperthyroid state in Graves disease. However, if there is ongoing production of hormones by the thyroid gland, plasmapheresis or plasma exchange is only transiently effective and will need to be repeated. In the case of charcoal hemoperfusion, blood is passed through charcoal columns or cartridges to remove the circulating thyroid hormones.

Educational Objective
Determine the best options for diagnosing and treating thyrotoxicosis due to thyroiditis.

UpToDate Topic Review(s)
Thyroid storm

Reference(s)

Carhill A, Gutierrez A, Lakhia R, Nalini R. Surviving the storm: two cases of thyroid storm successfully treated with plasmapheresis. *BMJ Case Rep.* 2012;2012. PMID: 23087271

Kreisner E, Lutzky M, Gross JL. Charcoal hemoperfusion in the treatment of levothyroxine intoxication. *Thyroid.* 2010;20(2):209-212. PMID: 20151829

Samuels MH, Launder T. Hyperthyroidism due to lymphoma involving the thyroid gland in a patient with acquired immunodeficiency syndrome: case report and review of the literature. *Thyroid.* 1998;8(8):673-677. PMID: 9737362

Sherman SI, Simonson L, Ladenson PW. Clinical and socioeconomic predispositions to complicated thyrotoxicosis: a predictable and preventable syndrome? *Am J Med.* 1996;101(2):192-198. PMID: 8757360

Swinburne JL, Kreisman SH. A rare case of subacute thyroiditis causing thyroid storm. *Thyroid.* 2007;17(1):73-76. PMID: 17274754

Vyas AA, Vyas P, Fillipon NL, Vijayakrishnan R, Trivedi N. Successful treatment of thyroid storm with plasmapheresis in a patient with methimazole-induced agranulocytosis. *Endocr Pract.* 2010;16(4):673-676. PMID: 20439250

54 ANSWER: A) Pseudohypoparathyroidism type 1a

The woman in this vignette presents with a longstanding history of hypocalcemia and has a high-normal serum phosphate level and a low serum 1,25-dihydroxyvitamin D level despite a significantly elevated serum PTH level, which should raise suspicion for PTH resistance. Pseudohypoparathyroidism (PHP) refers to a group of heterogeneous disorders defined by targeted organ (kidney and bone) unresponsiveness to PTH. Type 1 PHP is caused by pathogenic variants in the *GNAS* gene, which encodes the α subunit of the G-protein coupled to the PTH receptor. *GNAS* is imprinted in humans; therefore, the disease manifestations differ depending on whether the allele is maternally or paternally inherited.

PHP type 1a (Answer A) is an autosomal dominant disease with a loss-of-function pathogenic variant in *GNAS* and it requires maternal transmission of the mutation. Patients with PHP type 1a manifest PTH resistance in addition to Albright hereditary osteodystrophy, which is characterized by round facies, short stature, obesity, short fourth metacarpal bones, subcutaneous calcifications, and developmental delay. This is the most likely diagnosis for the patient in this vignette. Individuals with PHP type 1a may also show resistance to various other G-protein–coupled hormones such as TSH and gonadotropins and manifest reduced insulin sensitivity as compared with healthy control patients who are matched for age, sex, and percentage body fat. Individuals with paternally inherited pathogenic variants in the *GNAS* gene have variable features of Albright hereditary osteodystrophy without hormonal resistance, and such patients are described as having pseudopseudohypoparathyroidism (Answer D). In these patients, the paternal transmission of a *GNAS* mutation results in Albright hereditary osteodystrophy, but the normal maternal allele results in the maintenance of renal responsiveness to PTH. In this vignette, the patient's cousins most likely have pseudopseudohypoparathyroidism.

PHP type 1b (Answer B) is an autosomal dominant disorder caused by pathogenic variants that affect the regulatory elements of *GNAS* (rather than being caused by mutations in *GNAS* itself). These patients manifest resistance to PTH but do not exhibit the phenotypic abnormalities of Albright hereditary osteodystrophy. PHP type 1b is maternally transmitted.

PHP type 1c (Answer C) results from inactivating pathogenic variants that affect the coupling of the G-protein to the PTH receptor. Patients with PHP type 1c are usually phenotypically similar to those with PHP type 1a.

Finally, hereditary resistance to vitamin D (Answer E) is caused by end-organ resistance to 1,25-dihydroxyvitamin D most often because of loss-of-function pathogenic variants in the gene encoding the vitamin D receptor (*VDR*). The typical laboratory abnormalities in this scenario include hypocalcemia, hypophosphatemia, high serum PTH levels, and high serum 1,25-dihydroxyvitamin D levels.

Educational Objective

Identify pseudohypoparathyroidism as a cause of hypocalcemia and describe the effect of genomic imprinting on the inheritance of this disorder.

UpToDate Topic Review(s)

Etiology of hypocalcemia in infants and children

Reference(s)

Levine MA. An update on the clinical and molecular characteristics of pseudohypoparathyroidism. *Curr Opin Endocrinol Diabetes Obes.* 2012;19(6):443-451. PMID: 23076042

Muniyappa R, Warren MA, Zhao X, et al. Reduced insulin sensitivity in adults with pseudohypoparathyroidism type 1a. *J Clin Endocrinol Metab.* 2013;98(11):E1796-E1801. PMID: 24030943

55
ANSWER: C) SHBG measurement

In men, androgen deficiency is a clinical diagnosis confirmed by biochemical testing demonstrating repeatedly reduced circulating testosterone concentrations. Due to circadian rhythmicity and observations that food intake may decrease testosterone, blood draw for testosterone measurement should be done in the morning in the fasted state. The Endocrine Society recommends measurement of total testosterone, by an accurate and reliable assay, as the initial diagnostic test. Total testosterone concentrations are dependent on those of its carrier protein SHBG. Conditions that increase serum SHBG (eg, use of anticonvulsants such as carbamazepine or phenytoin, liver cirrhosis, or hyperthyroidism) can increase total testosterone, sometimes even above the normal range, even though free testosterone may be low. Therefore, reliance on total testosterone can be misleading in situations where circulating SHBG concentrations are abnormal, and measurement of SHBG is indicated. SHBG is necessary for the calculation of free testosterone. Thus, the best test to order now is SHBG measurement (Answer C).

In this patient, because of anticonvulsant treatment, SHBG was markedly increased at 15.5 µg/mL (1.1-6.7 µg/mL) (SI: 138 nmol/L [10-60 nmol/L]), and calculated free testosterone was clearly low at 2.8 ng/dL (9.0-30.0 ng/dL) (SI: 0.098 nmol/L [0.31-1.04 nmol/L]). Moreover, gonadotropin concentrations were increased with an LH value of 21.9 mIU/mL (1.0-9.0 mIU/mL) (SI: 21.9 IU/L [1.0-9.0 IU/L]) and an FSH value of 18.9 mIU/mL (SI: 1.0-13.0 mIU/mL) (SI: 18.9 IU/L [1.0-13.0 IU/L]), consistent with genuine primary hypogonadism.

In many men with conditions that increase SHBG, the subsequent increase in gonadotropins is sufficient to restore normal circulating testosterone concentrations, suggesting that, in this vignette, evaluation for additional central gonadal axis pathology is necessary.

Conversely, in conditions where SHBG is reduced (most commonly obesity and type 2 diabetes), men may not be hypogonadal despite a reduced serum total testosterone concentration because free testosterone may remain in the normal range.

While markedly elevated circulating estradiol (Answer B) can cause secondary hypogonadism due to negative hypothalamic-pituitary feedback, circulating total testosterone would be low. Likewise, although hemochromatosis (Answer D) and hyperprolactinemia (Answer E) can cause hypogonadism, circulating total testosterone would be low.

More than 80% of circulating dihydrotestosterone (Answer A) derives from 5α-reduction of testosterone in peripheral target tissues. Therefore, serum dihydrotestosterone is not a representative measure of testicular function, and its measurement does not contribute to the workup of adult men with suspected hypogonadism. Inability to produce dihydrotestosterone due to genetic 5α-reductase deficiency is very rare and usually presents as a 46,XY disorder of sex development.

Educational Objective
Explain how men can have a low free testosterone concentration due to increased SHBG (eg, caused by anticonvulsant drugs or chronic liver disease).

UpToDate Topic Review(s)
Causes of primary hypogonadism in males

Reference(s)

Bhasin S, Brito JP, Cunningham GR, et al. Testosterone therapy in men with hypogonadism: an Endocrine Society clinical practice guideline. *J Clin Endocrinol Metab.* 2018;103(5):1715-1744. PMID: 29562364

Paragliola RM, Prete A, Kaplan PW, Corsello SM, Salvatori R. Treatment of hypopituitarism in patients receiving antiepileptic drugs. *Lancet Diabetes Endocrinol.* 2015;3(2):132-140. PMID: 24898833

Rastrelli G, O'Neill TW, Ahern T, et al; EMAS study group. Symptomatic androgen deficiency develops only when both total and free testosterone decline in obese men who may have incident biochemical secondary hypogonadism: prospective results from the EMAS. *Clin Endocrinol (Oxf).* 2018;89(4):459-469. PMID: 29855071

56
ANSWER: A) 24-Hour urinary free cortisol and midnight salivary cortisol

In this complicated case, the course of diabetes progression was atypical, and it is important to consider late-onset autoimmune diabetes (LADA) or secondary causes of diabetes. Other important pieces of information include recent deep venous thrombosis, history of fracture, rapid weight gain, and suggestion of proximal muscle weakness. While this constellation points to possible cortisol excess, there are no specific findings of Cushing syndrome such as facial plethora or wide, pigmented striae. How common is subclinical Cushing syndrome in patients with diabetes? Among patients with adrenal incidentalomas, the mean prevalence of subclinical Cushing syndrome is 7.8%. In one study of 90 obese patients with insulin-requiring diabetes who had poor glycemic control and were prospectively screened, 3.3% were subsequently documented to have Cushing syndrome. Similarly, another study identified Cushing syndrome in 3 of 78 women with osteoporosis. These prospective, albeit small, studies suggest that clinicians should be alert to the possibility of Cushing syndrome in patients with diabetes. Thus, measuring 24-hour urinary free cortisol and midnight salivary cortisol (Answer A) is the best option. A 1-mg overnight dexamethasone-suppression test would be a more sensitive test, but it was not provided as a choice. Indeed, this patient was evaluated and found to have ACTH-independent Cushing syndrome.

The Immunology of Diabetes Society has suggested the following criteria for the diagnosis of LADA: age older than 30 years, presence of any islet autoantibody, and at least 6 months of no insulin treatment after diagnosis. While LADA is not an unreasonable consideration, the presence of obesity and other clinical factors make Cushing syndrome more likely. Thus, measuring glutamic acid decarboxylase, IA-2, and ZnT8 antibodies (Answer C) is not the best next step.

Hypothyroidism is a consideration in patients with fatigue and weight gain, but her degree of weight gain is more than expected for hypothyroidism, her heart rate is normal, and there are no other specific features of hypothyroidism. Thus, measuring serum TSH and free T_4 (Answer B) is incorrect.

Although in this case there are features to suggest Cushing syndrome, screening for acromegaly (Answer D) is another consideration, but there is no history of sweating or acral enlargement or evidence of pituitary mass effect to lend support for this diagnosis.

This patient does not have diastolic hypertension or a history of spontaneous or diuretic-induced hypokalemia (and she is on furosemide), so screening for primary aldosteronism (Answer E) is not needed.

Educational Objective
Evaluate for Cushing syndrome in patients with diabetes mellitus and hypertension.

UpToDate Topic Review(s)
Establishing the diagnosis of Cushing syndrome

Reference(s)

Nieman LK, Biller BM, Findling JW, et al. The diagnosis of Cushing's syndrome: an Endocrine Society clinical practice guideline. *J Clin Endocrinol Metab.* 2008;93(5):1526-1540. PMID: 18334580

57   ANSWER: C) Paraganglioma

Although elevated blood pressure in a patient who is in pain is not diagnostic of hypertension, the finding of grade 2 hypertensive retinopathy suggests that he has previously undiagnosed hypertension. In the context of a retroperitoneal mass, secondary causes must be considered.

In the absence of hypokalemia, 11-deoxycorticosterone secretion by an adrenocortical carcinoma (Answer A) is very unlikely even if the radiologic findings are consistent with an adrenocortical carcinoma. 11-Deoxycorticosterone has potent mineralocorticoid activity. In contrast, the absence of hypokalemia does not exclude primary aldosteronism. Due to its high prevalence, primary aldosteronism (Answer B) should be in the differential diagnosis as the cause of hypertension in this patient. However, primary aldosteronism would not be associated with a retroperitoneal mass arising independently of the adrenal gland.

The initial laboratory profile shows a mildly elevated hemoglobin and hematocrit, which, together with the elevated serum urea nitrogen, is suggestive of intravascular volume contraction. This is a recognized manifestation of sustained hypertension in the context of a pheochromocytoma or paraganglioma. Normalization of these indices following α-adrenergic blockade and fluid replacement is a useful indicator of corrected hypovolemia.

Abdominal CT shows a large retroperitoneal mass situated medial and inferior to the left kidney. In the absence of hypertension or other stigmata of endocrine dysfunction, the differential diagnosis for such a mass is broad and includes nonendocrine conditions (eg, sarcoma, lymphoma). However, the discovery of hypertension (especially in a younger patient) mandates consideration of endocrine causes. As indicated above, the left adrenal gland is clearly seen in its normal position and is distinct from the mass. Thus, the mass is not a pheochromocytoma (Answer D).

Although there is a small cyst near the hilum of the right kidney, there are no other features of adult polycystic kidney disease (Answer E). The clinical features and radiologic appearance raise the possibility of an abdominal paraganglioma (Answer C). Further investigation with measurement of plasma free metanephrines and/or 24-hour urinary fractionated metanephrines would help to confirm the diagnosis. Because extraadrenal paraganglioma have increased malignant potential, measurement of the dopamine metabolite 3-methoxytyramine (in plasma) should also be considered where available, although its greatest utility is in the setting of head and neck paragangliomas.

Once acute-phase management has been completed, and with the knowledge of the histologic and immunohistochemical findings of the resected surgical specimen (eg, absent immunohistochemical staining for succinate dehydrogenase B [SDHB]), genetic counseling and screening should be undertaken.

Educational Objective
Recognize that an incidentally discovered retroperitoneal mass may represent a pheochromocytoma or paraganglioma, especially in a patient with hypertension.

UpToDate Topic Review(s)
Paragangliomas: Epidemiology, clinical presentation, diagnosis, and histology

Reference(s)

Fassnacht M, Arlt W, Bancos I, et al. Management of adrenal incidentalomas: European Society of Endocrinology clinical practice guideline in collaboration with the European Network for the Study of Adrenal Tumors. *Eur J Endocrinol.* 2016;175(2):G1-G34. PMID: 27390021

Lenders JW, Duh QY, Eisenhofer G, et al; Endocrine Society. Pheochromocytoma and paraganglioma: an Endocrine Society clinical practice guideline. *J Clin Endocrinol Metab.* 2014;99(6):1915-1942. PMID: 24893135

58 ANSWER: C) Perform rhTSH ^{18}F-fluorodeoxyglucose PET/CT

This patient presents with differentiated thyroid cancer and elevated thyroglobulin levels without thyroglobulin antibodies and a negative radioiodine scan. Therefore, he has persistent thyroid cancer, as his thyroglobulin never became undetectable, and has iodine-refractory differentiated thyroid cancer because his rhTSH radioactive iodine scan was negative. His stimulated thyroglobulin level after thyrotropin injection was 10 ng/mL (10.0 µg/L). In follow-up assessments, his thyroglobulin levels increased from 3.6 to 12.0 ng/mL (3.6-12.0 µg/L) with suppressed TSH. Another radioiodine treatment (Answer A) while the patient is hypothyroid would not be the best option, as his previous rhTSH radioactive iodine scan was negative. However, some studies suggest administering an empiric dose of radioactive iodine in patients with a radioiodine-negative scan and an elevated thyroglobulin level. There are no data to show that this practice affects the prognosis. Repeating the chest CT might reveal more lung nodules, but given that his thyroglobulin levels are rising, the clinician should look for metastases in other locations besides his lungs.

The best next step is to order rhTSH ^{18}F-fluorodeoxyglucose (FDG) PET/CT imaging (Answer C) to look for the non–iodine-avid thyroid cancer metastases, especially given that his thyroglobulin level is rising. FDG PET/CT is primarily considered in patients with high-risk differentiated thyroid cancer and elevated serum thyroglobulin with negative radioiodine imaging. In a meta-analysis of 25 studies that included 789 patients, the sensitivity of FDG PET/CT was 83% (range, 50%-100%) and the specificity was 84% (range, 42%-100%) in non–iodine-avid differentiated thyroid cancer. Tumor dedifferentiation, tumor burden, and TSH stimulation were factors influencing the sensitivity of this imaging. Imaging sensitivity may be slightly increased with TSH stimulation.

This patient's tumor had vascular invasion and extrathyroidal extension and the lymph nodes had extranodal extension, which are features associated with increased recurrence risk. In papillary thyroid carcinoma, several studies have demonstrated that vascular invasion is associated with significantly higher recurrence rates. Additionally, vascular invasion in papillary thyroid carcinoma is also associated with higher rates of distant metastases. Repeated chest CT (Answer B) might reveal more lung nodules, but metastases should be sought in other locations. FDG PET/CT not only assesses for FDG-avid lesions, but also compares those lesions that have FDG avidity with the CT imaging to ensure the presence of a lesion corresponding to those areas. Metastatic lesions with high avidity for glucose in PET imaging are associated with resistance to radioiodine therapy and a worse prognosis. FDG PET/CT can detect lesions as small as 5- to 8 mm depending on the lesion's metabolic activity profile.

Tyrosine kinase inhibitors (Answer D) are well accepted in the treatment of iodine-refractory advanced thyroid cancer. The extent of this patient's metastatic disease has not yet been determined, so initiation of tyrosine kinase inhibitors is not indicated now.

This patient's TSH is already suppressed, and further increasing his thyroid hormone replacement therapy (Answer E) would not add any further beneficial effect to the management of his thyroid cancer. Further TSH suppression can lead to iatrogenic hyperthyroidism, with its own cardiovascular toxicities, as well as osteoporosis.

Educational Objective
Determine when PET imaging is indicated in a patient with well-differentiated thyroid cancer.

UpToDate Topic Review(s)
Differentiated thyroid cancer: Overview of management

Reference(s)

Haugen BR, Alexander EK, Bible KC, et al. 2015 American Thyroid Association management guidelines for adult patients with thyroid nodules and differentiated thyroid cancer: the American Thyroid Association Guidelines Task Force on Thyroid Nodules and Differentiated Thyroid Cancer. *Thyroid.* 2016;26(1):1-133. PMID: 26462967

Wang W, Larson SM, Tuttle EM, et al. Resistance of [18f]-fluorodeoxyglucose-avid metastatic thyroid cancer lesions to treatment with high dose radioactive iodine. *Thyroid.* 2001;11(12):1169-1175. PMID: 12186505

59 ANSWER: C) Rosuvastatin, 5 mg daily

This woman has a longstanding history of dyslipidemia, most likely with a genetic etiology, but no clinical atherosclerotic cardiovascular disease (ASCVD). Moderate- to high-intensity statin therapy has been attempted but was limited by adverse effects.

In general, statins are well tolerated in clinical trials and by most patients in clinical practice. Discontinuation of statin therapy is strongly associated with increased future risk of cardiovascular events. Statin-associated muscle symptoms are the most common adverse effects and are defined as muscle symptoms reported during statin therapy, but they may not necessarily be caused by the drug. Symptoms can include muscle weakness, muscle aches, soreness, stiffness, tenderness, and muscle cramps (but not nocturnal cramping) without significant creatine kinase elevation. Myalgia is more likely to be statin associated if it is bilateral, involves proximal muscles, and has its onset within weeks to months after statin initiation. Although not well defined, predisposing risk factors include older age, female sex, genetic factors, Chinese ancestry, hypothyroidism, preexisting muscle disease, and renal impairment.

When muscle symptoms appear soon after starting treatment with a statin, in the absence of other discernible causes, a 1- to 2-week "statin holiday" can be recommended to determine whether symptoms resolve. If symptoms resolve, a rechallenge with a lower dosage of the same or different statin can be initiated. Up to 60% of individuals tolerate a lower dosage. Sometimes symptoms recur with each rechallenge. Although statin-associated muscle symptoms can usually be explained by patient expectations of harm (the nocebo effect), the symptoms are sometimes real and can be severe.

For patients who experience statin-associated muscle symptoms on daily statin dosing, intermittent dosing with longer-acting statins such as rosuvastatin and atorvastatin may be required; such dosing has been shown to be as effective as daily dosing in reducing LDL cholesterol. However, the effect of intermittent dosing on improving ASCVD outcomes has not been determined. This patient has not tried rosuvastatin, which is metabolized by different cytochrome P pathways (CYP2C19) than those that metabolize simvastatin and atorvastatin (CYP3A4). Hence, a lower statin dosage is indicated. Rosuvastatin, 5 mg daily (Answer C), is equivalent to atorvastatin, 15 mg daily, and simvastatin, 30 mg daily. Metabolism via a different pathway may improve tolerance.

Coenzyme Q10 (Answer A) is a vitamin-like compound widely distributed in the body; there is evidence of significant reductions in plasma coenzyme Q10 levels after statin treatment, but the mechanisms and consequences of this reduction are unknown. However, recent meta-analyses have not demonstrated a beneficial effect of coenzyme Q10 supplementation on statin-associated muscle symptoms. Therefore, addition of coenzyme Q10 is of unclear clinical benefit at this time and is not recommended. Vitamin D deficiency can produce myopathy and could increase statin-associated muscle symptoms, but vitamin D supplementation (cholecalciferol) (Answer B) has shown no demonstrable benefit in randomized clinical trials.

Marine omega-3 fatty acids in high dosages (Answer D) can decrease triglycerides. Recent data from the REDUCE-IT trial (Reduction of Cardiovascular Events with EPA-Intervention Trial) suggest that high dosages of pure eicosapentaenoic acid ethyl ester can provide ASCVD benefit in statin-treated patients with established cardiovascular disease or diabetes and other additional cardiovascular risk factors. In this study, individuals received purified fish oil or placebo in addition to statin therapy. Baseline concentrations of triglycerides and LDL cholesterol were approximately 216 mg/dL (2.44 mmol/L) and 74 mg/dL (1.92 mmol/L), respectively. The benefit in non–statin-treated individuals or in primary prevention of ASCVD is not clear. The VITAL study assessed the use of omega-3 fatty acids with and without vitamin D_3 supplementation in healthy individuals for primary cardiovascular prevention. After 5 years of follow-up, omega-3 fish oil did not show a reduction in the primary composite end points of major cardiovascular events. Hence, addition of omega-3 fatty acids cannot be recommended at this time.

Fenofibrate (Answer E) is a triglyceride-lowering agent. It has modest LDL-cholesterol–lowering effect (up to 20%). Fibrate therapy has not been shown to decrease atherosclerotic cardiovascular disease events and therefore cannot be recommended as the next step until other options have been attempted.

This patient agreed to attempt rosuvastatin, 5 mg daily; she developed myalgias but was able to tolerate every-other-day dosing. Eventually, ezetimibe, 10 mg daily, was added and her LDL-cholesterol level dropped to 121 mg/dL (3.13 mmol/L) on combination therapy. Convincing patients who have adverse effects associated with statin use to continue therapy is among the most challenging tasks of physicians in the outpatient clinic.

Educational Objective
Recommend appropriate treatment of hyperlipidemia in a patient with statin intolerance.

UpToDate Topic Review(s)
Management of elevated low density lipoprotein cholesterol (LDL-C) in primary prevention of cardiovascular disease.

Reference(s)
Grundy SM, Stone NJ, Bailey AL, et al. 2018 AHA/ACC/AACVPR/AAPA/ABC/ACPM/ADA/AGS/APhA/ASPC/NLA/PCNA guideline on the management of blood cholesterol: a report of the American College of Cardiology/American Heart Association Task Force on Clinical Practice Guidelines. *J Am Coll Cardiol.* 2018;pii:S0735-S1097(18)39034-X. PMID: 30423393

Newman CB, Preiss D, Tobert JA, et al; American Heart Association Clinical Lipidology, Metabolism and Thrombosis Committee, a Joint Committee of the Council on Atherosclerosis, Thrombosis and Vascular Biology and Council on Lifestyle and Cardiometabolic Health; Council on Cardiovascular Disease in the Young; Council on Clinical Cardiology; and Stroke Council. Statin safety and associated adverse events: a scientific statement from the American Heart Association. *Arterioscler Thromb Vasc Biol.* 2019;39(2):e38-e81. PMID: 30580575

Rosenson RS, Baker S, Banach M, et al. Optimizing cholesterol treatment in patients with muscle complaints. *J Am Coll Cardiol.* 2017;70(10):1290-1301. PMID: 28859793

Manson JE, Cook NR, Lee IM, et al; VITAL Research Group. Marine n-3 fatty acids and prevention of cardiovascular disease and cancer. *N Engl J Med.* 2019;380(1):23-32. PMID: 30415637

Bhatt DL, Steg G, Miller M, et al; REDUCE-IT Investigators. Cardiovascular risk reduction with icosapent ethyl for hypertriglyceridemia. *N Engl J Med.* 2019;380(1):11-22. PMID: 30415628

60 ANSWER: C) Initiate real-time continuous glucose monitoring

Hypoglycemia is an important limiting step in the treatment of diabetes and it is more common in patients with type 1 than type 2 diabetes. In patients with diabetes, hypoglycemia is defined as a self-monitored or fingerstick blood glucose value of 70 mg/dL or less (≤3.9 mmol/L). Severe hypoglycemia is a hypoglycemic event in which another person must actively treat the hypoglycemia with carbohydrates, glucagon, or other measures to restore plasma glucose to normal. Patients with type 1 diabetes enrolled in the intensive-treatment arm of the Diabetes Control and Complications Trial (DCCT) had a 3-fold higher risk of developing severe hypoglycemia compared with patients in the standard treatment group.

Patients with hypoglycemia unawareness have deficient glucagon and epinephrine response to hypoglycemia, which can lead to blunted symptoms in response to low glucose levels and increase the risk for developing neuroglycopenia. Clinical studies have shown that strict avoidance of hypoglycemia for several weeks after an episode of severe hypoglycemia can prevent further severe hypoglycemic events.

The patient in this vignette has longstanding type 1 diabetes and hypoglycemia unawareness. Tight glucose control under these circumstances is contraindicated. Active measures to reduce the risk of hypoglycemia in this patient are needed. Relaxing the hemoglobin A_{1c} target may be appropriate. However, changing the glucose target to the range of 140 to 190 mg/dL (7.8-10.5 mmol/L) (Answer D) may lead to hyperglycemia.

Real-time continuous glucose monitoring (CGM) (Answer C) has been shown to improve glycemic control and to lower the risk of hypoglycemia in patients with type 1 diabetes treated with insulin pumps or multiple daily insulin injections. The DIAMOND trial was a randomized controlled trial of 158 adults with type 1 diabetes who were treated with multiple daily insulin injections. The study compared conventional fingerstick glucose monitoring with real-time CGM. The trial demonstrated a lower hemoglobin A_{1c} (−1.0%) in the intention-to-treat group compared with a reduction of −0.4% in the aggregate hemoglobin A_{1c} in the conventionally treated group. More importantly, the median daily duration of blood glucose values less than 70 mg/dL (<3.9 mmol/L) was lowered to 43 min/day in the CGM group vs 80 min/day in the conventional glucose monitoring arm (P = .002).

Conventional real-time CGM incorporates low and high glucose alarms and would be an important addition to this patient's treatment regimen to lower the risk of hypoglycemia. Another type of device is the intermittently scanned or "flash" glucose monitor. This glucose monitor does not have alarms or alerts, which is a detriment in some cases. The device reveals a glucose level only when scanned by the patient. In a recent randomized 8-week trial comparing conventional CGM with alarms vs flash monitoring in patients with type 1 diabetes who had hypoglycemia unawareness, conventional CGM was more effective in reducing the amount of hypoglycemia compared with the group using flash glucose monitoring. Initiating intermittently viewed glucose monitoring (Answer B) in this patient could reduce the risk of hypoglycemia, but conventional CGM is a better option.

The high cost of these devices is a real issue for many patients. Some patients will not be able to afford a continuous or flash glucose monitor, in which case conventional fingerstick glucose monitoring will continue to be necessary.

The newer long-acting basal insulins such as insulin degludec (U100 and U200) and U300 insulin glargine (Answer A) have been shown to reduce the risk of nocturnal hypoglycemia in randomized clinical trials of patients with type 1 diabetes. This patient is already treated with insulin degludec and switching to U300 insulin glargine would not reduce nocturnal hypoglycemia events any further.

A patient who has hypoglycemia unawareness is a good candidate for the newer insulin pumps (Answer E) that have glucose suspend technology, as randomized controlled trials have shown that such pumps have led to a lower risk of hypoglycemia compared with conventional insulin pumps. However, the patient in this vignette was treated with an insulin pump in the past and has no interest in restarting this modality.

Educational Objective
Determine the optimal treatment of patients with hypoglycemia unawareness and recurrent severe hypoglycemia.

UpToDate Topic Review(s)
Hypoglycemia in adults with diabetes mellitus

Reference(s)

Cryer PE. The barrier of hypoglycemia in diabetes. *Diabetes.* 2008;57(12):3169-3176. PMID: 19033403

Seaquist ER, Anderson J, Childs B, et al; American Diabetes Association; Endocrine Society. Hypoglycemia and diabetes: a report of a workgroup of the American Diabetes Association and the Endocrine Society. *J Clin Endocrinol Metab.* 2013;98(5):1845-1859. PMID: 2358924

Beck RW, Riddlesworth T, Ruedy K, et al; DIAMOND Study Group. Effect of continuous glucose monitoring on glycemic control in adults with type 1 diabetes using insulin injections: the DIAMOND randomized clinical trial. *JAMA.* 2017;317(4):371-378. PMID: 28118453

Reddy M, Jugnee N, El Laboudi A, Spanudakis E, Anantharaja S, Oliver N. A randomized controlled pilot study of continuous glucose monitoring and flash glucose monitoring in people with type 1 diabetes and impaired awareness of hypoglycaemia. *Diabet Med.* 2018;35(4):483-490. PMID: 29230878

61

ANSWER: C) Reduce the GH dosage by 50%

Treatment of hypopituitarism involves the use of different hormones, which may interact with each other and affect the patient's well-being. The best known interaction is the risk of causing an adrenal crisis when replacing levothyroxine if a patient has undiagnosed adrenal insufficiency (or is undertreated).

Estrogen can also influence the replacement of other hormones. Estrogen therapy can be administered orally or transdermally. When estrogen is given orally, the liver is exposed to a high concentration due to the first-pass effect. Estrogens cause resistance to GH at the level of receptor signaling by inhibiting the Janus kinase/signal transducer, and by inducing expression of suppressor of cytokine signaling-2 (SOCS-2), a protein inhibitor for cytokine signaling. Because serum IGF-1 comes mostly from the liver, women on oral estrogen require a 2- to 3-times higher GH replacement dosage to normalize serum IGF-1 than women on transdermal estrogen or no estrogen. Therefore, in this woman who is switching from oral to transdermal estrogen, the correct change is to reduce the GH dosage to one-half to one-third of the dosage she was taking when on oral estrogen (Answer C). Daily progesterone dosing (Answer A) is not indicated, and it would most likely cause fluid retention and bloating.

Estrogen therapy can also affect the management of central hypothyroidism. Oral estrogens cause an increase in thyroxine-binding globulin. Therefore, it is recommended that when estrogen therapy is started, stopped, or changed, free T_4 levels are monitored and the dosage is adjusted to maintain free T_4 levels within target ranges. In this case, free T_4 measurement will need to be repeated, and it is unlikely that levothyroxine will need to be increased (Answer B). It may possibly need to be reduced.

Although oral estrogen also increases cortisol-binding globulin levels, this patient's peak cortisol level is very robust and rules out adrenal insufficiency. Therefore, repeating the cosyntropin-stimulation test (Answer D) is incorrect.

Prolactin is often mildly elevated after radiation to the hypothalamic/pituitary area, particularly in female patients. As this patient already has central hypogonadism, the mildly increased prolactin has no ill effect, and it does not need to be treated. Therefore, starting cabergoline (Answer E) is unnecessary.

Educational Objective
Explain the effect that the route of estrogen administration has on GH sensitivity and adjust the GH dosage accordingly.

UpToDate Topic Review(s)
Treatment of hypopituitarism

Reference(s)

Fleseriu M, Hashim IA, Karavitaki N, et al. Hormonal replacement in hypopituitarism in adults: an Endocrine Society clinical practice guideline. *J Clin Endocrinol Metab.* 2016;101(11):3888-3921. PMID: 27736313

Mah PM, Webster J, Jönsson P, et al. Estrogen replacement in women of fertile years with hypopituitarism. *J Clin Endocrinol Metab.* 2005;90(11):5964-5969. PMID: 16091478

Constine LS, Woolf PD, Cann D, et al. Hypothalamic-pituitary dysfunction after radiation for brain tumors [published correction appears in *N Engl J Med.* 1993;328(16):1208]. *N Engl J Med.* 1993;328(2):87-94. PMID: 8416438

62

ANSWER: A) Drink enough fluids to ensure at least 2 L of urine output daily

Nephrolithiasis is an extremely common disorder, affecting almost 9% of individuals in the United States during their lifetime. In addition, the economic burden of the disease is estimated to be more than 2 billion dollars annually. Calcium-based stones account for nearly 75% of all cases of nephrolithiasis, with most of those composed primarily of calcium-oxalate. Known mechanisms underlying calcium oxalate–based renal stone disease include hypercalciuria, hyperoxaluria, and hypocitraturia, although other dietary, metabolic, and hereditary factors can also contribute. Many patients do not develop recurrent stones, but 20% experience another stone event within 5 years of the initial episode. Given these observations, it is important to guide patients with an initial calcium stone event on the best approach to reduce their recurrence risk. Although a variety of lifestyle and dietary approaches have been studied, an increase in fluid intake to ensure at least 2 L of urine output daily (Answer A) is recommended to reduce the risk of calcium stone recurrence.

Although clearly effective, thiazide diuretics (Answer B) and other proven agents, such as citrate when indicated based on stone composition and allopurinol, should be reserved for patients with active or recurrent disease despite increased fluid intake and urine volume. High-fiber intake (Answer C) has not been shown to reduce the risk of calcium stones, and restriction of dietary calcium intake (Answer E) is not recommended based on a potential increased risk for recurrent stones. Finally, this patient's calcium (corrected for albumin) is normal (9.9 mg/dL [2.5 mmol/L]), which, combined with normal serum PTH and normal 24-hour urinary calcium excretion, does not support a diagnosis of primary hyperparathyroidism (Answer D), arguing against referral to an endocrine surgeon for neck exploration at this time.

Educational Objective
Determine the best initial therapy in a patient with calcium oxalate–based nephrolithiasis.

UpToDate Topic Review(s)
Options in the management of renal and ureteral stones in adults

Reference(s)

Qaseem A, Dallas P, Forciea MA, Starkey M, Denberg TD; Clinical Guidelines Committee of the American College of Physicians. Dietary and pharmacologic management to prevent recurrent nephrolithiasis in adults: a clinical practice guideline from the American College of Physicians. *Ann Intern Med.* 2014;161(9):659-667. PMID: 25364887

63 **ANSWER: C) Increase the current dosage of phentermine/topiramate to its maximum dosage**

The combination of phentermine/topiramate extended release was approved for long-term weight-loss management in the United States in 2012. Phentermine is a centrally acting sympathomimetic amine that increases the release of norepinephrine, while topiramate modulates γ-aminobutyric acid (GABA) neurotransmitter activity at GABA-A receptors, inhibits carbonic anhydrase, and antagonizes glutamate. By acting on different pathways, the 2 medications have additive effects. Approval of this drug was based on 3 randomized clinical trials. The EQUIP trial was a 56-week study to evaluate the safety and efficacy of phentermine/topiramate in adults with a BMI greater than 35 kg/m². Patients were randomly assigned to phentermine/topiramate 3.75 mg/23 mg daily, phentermine/topiramate 15 mg/92 mg daily, or placebo. Percentage body weight loss was 1.6% for the placebo group, 5.1% for the group taking 3.75 mg/23 mg, and 10.9% for the group taking 15 mg/92 mg. The CONQUER trial was also 56 weeks, but this study enrolled adults with a BMI of 27 to 45 kg/m² who had 2 or more comorbidities. Patients were randomly assigned to phentermine/topiramate 7.5 mg/46 mg daily, phentermine/topiramate 15 mg/92 mg daily, or placebo. Weight loss was greater in the treatment groups than in the placebo group (percentage body weight loss was 1.2% for the placebo group, 6.6% for the group taking 7.5 mg/46 mg, and 8.6% for the group taking 15 mg/92 mg). The SEQUEL study was the extension study of CONQUER. Seventy-eight percent of patients from the CONQUER study agreed to participate in the extension study. Patients were followed up for a total of 108 weeks. As expected, there was greater weight loss in the treatment groups (7.5 mg/46 mg [–7.5%] and 15 mg/92 mg [–8.7%]) than in the placebo group (–1.8%). In these trials, all patients received diet and lifestyle modification counseling based on the Lifestyle, Exercise, Attitudes, Relationship, and Nutrition Program for Weight Management. The most frequent adverse events reported were paresthesia, dry mouth, constipation, upper respiratory tract infection, headaches, dysgeusia, depression, anxiety, and attention disturbance. Phentermine/topiramate is contraindicated in pregnant women, patients with hyperthyroidism or glaucoma, and patients who are taking monoamine oxidase inhibitors or have taken this medication within the preceding 14 days.

Weight-loss medications are a tool to help patients achieve their weight-loss goals. All patients who start a weight-loss medication must follow a lifestyle program, otherwise it is unlikely that they will lose weight. After deciding that a patient is a candidate for a weight-loss medication, the clinician should discuss weight-loss expectations. For most approved long-term weight-loss medications, the goal is for patients to lose 5% of their current weight in 12 weeks. If this weight loss is achieved, then the recommendation is to continue the medication. However, if patients do not lose 5% of their weight during this period, the medication should be stopped and another should be considered. A second weight-loss medication is not added when less than 5% weight loss has been achieved because the first agent was ineffective; when balancing the medication's benefits (losing <5% of weight) and risks (adverse effects, cost, pill burden, etc), it is better to stop the ineffective drug and to try a different one. Although no randomized controlled trials have evaluated combination therapy with weight-loss medications, this is done in clinical practice if patients have achieved the expected weight loss with the initial medication but need further weight loss to achieve their goal.

Phentermine/topiramate has a different titration protocol than other weight-loss medications, as it has a recommended dosage, a maximum dosage, and 2 different titration dosages. Patients on phentermine/topiramate start on 3.75 mg/23 mg daily for 14 days. Then their dosage is increased to the recommended dosage of 7.5 mg/46 mg daily. They continue this dosage for 12 weeks, at which time their weight loss is assessed. Patients who have not lost 3% of their weight (not 5%—the cutoff used for all other weight-loss medications) have 2 options: stop the medication, as it is deemed ineffective, and start a different one or increase the dosage to 11.25 mg/69 mg daily for 14 days and then increase it to the maximum dosage of 15 mg/92 mg daily. After 12 weeks of being on the maximum dosage, the patient should have lost 5% of their initial weight. If this has not occurred, then the medication should be tapered, as there is a risk of seizure if it is stopped abruptly. The recommended taper is to take one 15 mg/92 mg tablet every other day for 1 week.

This patient only lost 2% of her weight while on the regular dosage of phentermine/topiramate, so continuing at this dosage (Answers A, B, and E) is not appropriate. Her options are to stop the medication and start a new one or to increase to the maximum approved dosage. Either option is reasonable. This patient is already taking bupropion extended release, 200 mg daily. If naltrexone/bupropion were added to her regimen (Answer D), she would be taking about 560 mg of bupropion daily, which is higher than the recommended daily dose of this medication. Therefore, the best option of those listed is to increase the current dosage of phentermine/topiramate to its maximum dosage (Answer C).

Educational Objective
Assess adequate weight loss after starting a weight-loss medication and decide whether dosage escalation or drug discontinuation is indicated.

UpToDate Topic Review(s)
Obesity in adults: Drug therapy

Reference(s)

Allison DB, Gadde KM, Garvey WT, et al. Controlled-release phentermine/topiramate in severely obese adults: a randomized controlled trial (EQUIP). *Obesity (Silver Spring)*. 2012;20:330-342. PMID: 22051941

Gadde KM, Allison DB, Ryan DH, et al. Effects of low-dose, controlled-release, phentermine plus topiramate combination on weight and associated comorbidities in overweight and obese adults (CONQUER): a randomised, placebo-controlled, phase 3 trial [published correction appears in *Lancet*. 2011;377(9776):1494]. *Lancet*. 2011;377(9774):1341-1352. PMID: 21481449

Garvey WT, Ryan DH, Look M, et al. Two-year sustained weight loss and metabolic benefits with controlled-release phentermine/topiramate in obese and overweight adults (SEQUEL): a randomized, placebo-controlled, phase 3 extension study. *Am J Clin Nutr*. 2012;95(2):297-308. PMID: 22158731

Saunders KH, Umashanker D, Igel LI, Kumar RB, Aronne LJ. Obesity pharmacotherapy. *Med Clin North Am*. 2018;102(1):135-148. PMID: 29156182

64 ANSWER: D) Abdominal CT

Pheochromocytomas are tumors arising from the adrenal medulla that can secrete catecholamines (such as norepinephrine, epinephrine, and dopamine), which induce adrenergic symptoms and signs, such as palpitations, anxiety, sweating, pallor, and elevations in blood pressure and heart rate. Paragangliomas are tumors that arise from the ganglia of the autonomic nervous system and therefore can occur in any region from the base of the skull to the pelvic floor. Although sympathetic paragangliomas can secrete norepinephrine and dopamine, they are unlikely to synthesize epinephrine as pheochromocytomas do.

Metanephrines are the stable and inactive metabolites of catecholamines that provide the highest sensitivity and specificity for diagnosing pheochromocytoma and paraganglioma. Metanephrine is the metabolite of epinephrine, and normetanephrine is the metabolite of norepinephrine. Typically, pheochromocytomas and paragangliomas that induce clinical symptoms are associated with metanephrine and/or normetanephrine levels that are substantially higher than the upper limit of the reference range—usually 4 times or more (less commonly 2 or 3 times higher). Importantly, mild elevations above the upper limit of the metanephrines reference range (<2 times) are common and are usually attributed to enhanced sympathoadrenergic tone (eg, in a state of anxiety, stress, or illness) and/

or the use of catecholamine reuptake inhibitors (eg, some antidepressants medications and cocaine). In this regard, these milder elevations are a frequent cause of false-positive values.

This patient presents with nausea, fatigue, hypertension, tachycardia, and hyperglycemia. Although this constellation of signs and symptoms could represent many conditions, hyperglycemia in a lean 22-year-old patient should raise concerns for a new diagnosis of type 1 diabetes or secondary diabetes that could be induced by catecholamine excess. The marked elevations in plasma and urinary metanephrines (6- to 10-fold elevations above the upper limit of the reference range) and dopamine, confirm the diagnosis of a catecholamine-secreting tumor, and specifically point to an adrenal pheochromocytoma given the high metanephrine-fraction levels. This degree of elevation in metanephrines is higher than what is typically attributable to medications that inhibit catecholamine reuptake. Thus, a toxicology screen for cocaine or tricyclic antidepressants (Answers A and B) is an incorrect step.

Once the clinical and/or biochemical characteristics confirm a pheochromocytoma, attention should be paid to the radiographic features. Pheochromocytomas are typically 2 cm or larger when a clinical syndrome of adrenergic excess is detected. However, pheochromocytomas can be any size when detected incidentally. Cross-sectional imaging of the abdomen with CT (or MRI) (Answer D) is adequate to visualize symptomatic pheochromocytomas, and the abdomen is also the most likely location to detect paragangliomas. Pheochromocytomas tend to be dense and vascular. Therefore, they often have high attenuation on unenhanced CT imaging (>10 Hounsfield units) or high contrast avidity (often with heterogeneous enhancement) on CT imaging done with intravenous contrast. They have poor delayed contrast washout when CT imaging is performed with an adrenal washout protocol. On MRI, pheochromocytomas tend to display hyperintensity on T2-weighted imaging and have features suggestive of low lipid content (no loss of signal on out-of-phase sequences). Nuclear imaging with meta-iodobenzylguanidine, ^{68}Ga DOTATATE, or FDG-PET (Answers B, C, and E) is not necessary for the initial localization and can be used on a case-by-case basis for assessing functionality of tumors, localizing small tumors or metastases, or before radiation therapy for metastatic disease.

In this patient, abdominal CT revealed a 5-cm left adrenal mass with an unenhanced attenuation value of 45 Hounsfield units. She underwent an uncomplicated left laparoscopic adrenalectomy following hydration with saline and α-adrenergic and β-adrenergic blockade, and pathologic examination revealed a pheochromocytoma. Postoperatively, her blood pressure and pulse normalized, her glycemia normalized, and she no longer needed insulin therapy. Genetic testing for inherited forms of pheochromocytoma-paraganglioma syndromes should be discussed with every patient since they are present in approximately 30% of all affected patients and have implications for the future surveillance of the patient and their family members.

Educational Objective
Devise a diagnostic approach for pheochromocytoma.

UpToDate Topic Review(s)
Clinical presentation and diagnosis of pheochromocytoma

Reference(s)
Lenders JW, Duh QY, Eisenhofer G, et al; Endocrine Society. Pheochromocytoma and paraganglioma: an Endocrine Society clinical practice guideline. *J Clin Endocrinol Metab*. 2014;99(6):1915-1942. PMID: 24893135

65 **ANSWER: D) Perform renal biopsy**

Hyperglycemia, especially in the presence of hypertension, can lead to proteinuria. Incidence of microalbuminuria and diabetic nephropathy increase as hemoglobin A_{1c} rises. However, other causes of proteinuria must be ruled out in patients with diabetes. This patient's urine protein excretion progressed from microalbuminuria to more than 2 g/24 h over the course of a year. A number of elements of this man's history make a secondary cause of proteinuria very likely. He has had a rapid change in proteinuria, he has no evidence of other microvascular complications such as retinopathy, and urinalysis reveals hematuria and proteinuria. In addition, the hypertension has worsened on lisinopril.

In the DCCT (Diabetes Control and Complications Trial), diabetic retinopathy, neuropathy, nephropathy, and microalbuminuria incidence/progression were positively correlated with hemoglobin A_{1c} level. Of the complications, progression of microalbuminuria was the slowest at each hemoglobin A_{1c} level. This patient's data do not fit the pattern demonstrated by the DCCT trial data and should prompt further evaluation. A Cochran review of glycemic targets for preventing diabetic kidney disease showed reduced incidence and decreased progression of microalbuminuria in patients with tightly controlled hemoglobin A_{1c} levels (<7.0% [<53 mmol/mol]). While intensification of glycemic control (Answer A) is important for this patient to prevent microvascular and macrovascular complications, it is not the best next step in this case, as it does not help identify the etiology of the significant proteinuria and hematuria. Similarly, adding an angiotensin-receptor blocker (Answer B) or prescribing a low-protein diet (Answer C) would be incorrect, as each of these steps is a management strategy rather than a diagnostic approach to proteinuria. Also, the addition of an angiotensin-receptor blocker to an ACE inhibitor is not recommended because of the risk of hyperkalemia. Protein restriction can be used to prevent progression of chronic kidney disease in select patients. The restriction should be moderate to prevent malnutrition. Long-term, very low-protein diets have been associated with increased mortality. In patients with a glomerular filtration rate less than 60 mL/min per 1.73 m^2, protein restriction to 0.8 g per kg is recommended. This would also be reasonable to institute for this patient in the future, based on diagnosis and persistence of proteinuria, but it is not the best next step.

Urine sediment evaluation and renal biopsy (Answer D) are the 2 tests that would be most useful in this patient, as they could help identify the specific etiology of nephritic syndrome. In fact, lupus nephritis was diagnosed in this patient on the basis of biopsy findings. Renal ultrasonography (Answer E) would be less useful in narrowing down the differential diagnosis.

Educational Objective
Assess proteinuria in patients with type 1 diabetes mellitus.

UpToDate Topic Review(s)
Moderately increased albuminuria (microalbuminuria) in type 1 diabetes mellitus

Reference(s)
Gilbert S, Weiner D. Hematuria and proteinuria. In: *National Kidney Foundation Primer on Kidney Diseases*. Philadelphia, PA; Elsevier. 2018.

Skyler JS. Diabetic complications. The importance of glucose control. *Endocrinol Metab Clin North Am*. 1996;25(2):243-254. PMID: 8799699

66 ANSWER: C) Central and left neck dissection in the second trimester

The scenario presented in the case is not common, as substantial thought is typically put into a decision as to whether a patient with thyroid cancer should become pregnant and what the optimal timing is. The more commonly encountered situation is a patient who is newly diagnosed with thyroid cancer during pregnancy. On the basis of available data, if there is no evidence of aggressive disease, initial thyroid surgery should probably be postponed until after delivery.

There are many approaches to thyroid surgery that are currently in use, in addition to the standard cervical-approach thyroidectomy. Some robotic or minimally invasive surgeries still involve a cervical approach, and thus a surgical scar. However, due to the use of video-assisted endoscopic approaches with or without carbon dioxide insufflation, the surgery can be performed with smaller surgical scars. Other diverse surgical procedures involve chest, axilla, retroauricular, and transoral approaches, all of which avoid a cervical scar. Most data suggest that outcomes are comparable for these surgeries when compared with conventional surgery, even when the surgery is performed for thyroid cancer. However, some studies suggest that fewer lymph nodes are generally removed and postoperative thyroglobulin levels are higher following robotic surgery. However, as with any surgery, the surgeon's expertise is one of the most important factors. The patient in this vignette had a cervical approach that left her with a very small surgical scar.

Regardless of the initial surgical approach chosen by this patient and her surgeon when she was not pregnant, it is clear from her physical examination, thyroglobulin levels, and imaging studies that her surgery was incomplete and that she requires additional treatment. The selection of the best treatment is made more complicated by the fact that the patient is pregnant. All the therapeutic options offered as answer choices are surgical except external beam radiation with uterine shielding (Answer A). Any approach other than repeated surgery is wrong in this patient who clearly has a substantial volume of residual disease. External beam radiation has considerable morbidity and it is best applied to stabilize rather than remove disease. An example of appropriate use of radiation therapy might be in a patient who has tracheal invasion of her tumor and the tumor has already been resected to the fullest surgical extent possible. A therapeutic option not offered here would be to increase the thyroid hormone dosage to provide a greater degree of thyroid hormone suppression. The risk vs benefit of this would need to be considered on an individual patient basis, but this would not directly address the issue of residual disease that merits surgical resection. However, if it were decided to delay surgical resection until after pregnancy, then suppression of the patient's serum TSH level might be indicated.

Thus, this patient would be best managed by another surgical procedure. Another minimally invasive surgery (not offered as an option) is probably not the best choice, as the success of a second surgery is most likely better with the best field of exposure possible being achieved during surgery. In addition, there is little experience with minimally invasive thyroid surgery performed during pregnancy. This patient appears to have disease that may be invasive into the thyroid cartilage and strap muscles. Because of these features, waiting 8 months before surgically addressing the disease (Answer E) may be unwise and permit disease spread. Low-volume thyroid cancer does not seem to progress during the course of pregnancy, despite the theoretical concern that hCG may stimulate thyroid cancer growth. This often makes surgery after delivery a reasonable option, regardless of whether thyroid cancer is newly diagnosed or residual disease is newly determined to be present.

Once surgery during pregnancy has been decided upon, the remaining answer options involve 3 different timings of a conventional central and left neck dissection. There is a general consensus that if thyroid surgery is deemed necessary during pregnancy, then the best timing is during the second trimester (Answer C). First-trimester surgery (Answer B) appears to carry a greater risk of altered organogenesis and miscarriage. However, third-trimester surgery (Answer D) has an increased risk of premature labor and delivery.

Educational Objective
Determine the optimal management of residual thyroid cancer identified during pregnancy.

UpToDate Topic Review(s)
Overview of thyroid disease in pregnancy

Reference(s)

Alexander EK, Pearce EN, Brent GA, et al. 2017 guidelines of the American Thyroid Association for the diagnosis and management of thyroid disease during pregnancy and the postpartum. *Thyroid.* 2017;27(3):315-389. PMID: 28056690

Mestman JH, Goodwin TM, Montoro MM. Thyroid disorders of pregnancy. *Endocrinol Metab Clin North Am.* 1995;24(1):41-71. PMID: 7781627

Uruno T, Shibuya H, Kitagawa W, Nagahama M, Sugino K, Ito K. Optimal timing of surgery for differentiated thyroid cancer in pregnant women. *World J Surg.* 2014;38(3):704-708. PMID: 24248429

67 ANSWER: D) Hydrocortisone

Nonclassic congenital adrenal hyperplasia (CAH) due to 21-hydroxylase deficiency is the cause of hirsutism in about 4% of cases worldwide and it is commonly misdiagnosed as polycystic ovary syndrome. Screening for nonclassic CAH is appropriate in the evaluation of hirsutism or polycystic ovary syndrome. This is accomplished by measuring 17-hydroxyprogesterone, ideally from a sample drawn in the early morning in the early follicular phase if a woman has regular menses. In this vignette, the early follicular 17-hydroxyprogesterone concentration was greater than 1000 ng/dL (>30.3 nmol/L), which is diagnostic for nonclassic CAH and a cosyntropin-stimulation test is not needed.

Because treatment with corticosteroids in nonclassic CAH often leads to adverse effects of cortisol excess (weight gain and metabolic consequences), they should be reserved for women presenting with infertility and adolescent girls with precocious puberty or rapidly accelerating bone age. Corticosteroid treatment in classic CAH ideally prevents the morning ACTH rise to more effectively decrease 17-hydroxyprogesterone, androgen, and progesterone concentrations that interfere with ovulation and implantation. For this reason, longer-acting corticosteroids such as dexamethasone (Answer C), prednisone, or prednisolone might be prescribed in a "reverse diurnal" pattern with the higher dose at night. However, in nonclassic CAH, studies have shown that shorter-acting and physiologic hydrocortisone therapy (Answer D) improves ovulatory frequency. Compared with hydrocortisone, dexamethasone is typically associated with more adverse effects of cortisol excess and would need to be stopped as soon as pregnancy is diagnosed because it can cross the placenta into the fetal circulation.

Although metformin (Answer B) has been shown to increase ovulation frequency in polycystic ovary syndrome, it has not been studied in nonclassic CAH for this indication.

Spironolactone (Answer A) is an aldosterone antagonist that also acts as a competitive inhibitor of the androgen receptor and it is an effective treatment of hirsutism. Women should be counseled to avoid trying to conceive while on spironolactone. Because this patient's goal is to conceive, spironolactone would not be recommended at this time and would not improve fertility.

Clomiphene (Answer E) is a selective estrogen-receptor modulator that is a competitive inhibitor of estrogen binding to estrogen receptors. By blocking the negative feedback of endogenous estradiol to the hypothalamus, an increase in the GnRH pulse frequency leads to increased FSH and LH, thus improving follicular development and leading to ovulation. In this case, the day 3 progesterone concentration was greater than 3.0 ng/mL (>9.5 nmol/L). Study findings have suggested that pregnancy is more likely in women with CAH when the follicular-phase progesterone is below 3.0 ng/mL (<9.5 nmol/L). Because progesterone might affect or suppress gonadotropin stimulation and folliculogenesis, it would be important to initiate hydrocortisone and optimize progesterone and folliculogenesis before considering ovulation with clomiphene if needed. Therefore, hydrocortisone therapy (Answer D) is the best next step to optimize this patient's chances of conceiving.

Educational Objective
Evaluate and manage nonclassic congenital adrenal hyperplasia in a woman experiencing infertility.

UpToDate Topic Review(s)
Diagnosis and treatment of nonclassic (late-onset) congenital adrenal hyperplasia due to 21-hydroxylase deficiency

Reference(s)

Carmina E, Dewailly D, Escobar-Morreale HF, et al. Non-classic congenital adrenal hyperplasia due to 21-hydroxylase deficiency revisited: an update with a special focus on adolescent and adult women. *Hum Reprod Update.* 2017;23(5):580-599. PMID: 28582566

Bidet M, Bellanne-Chantelot C, Galand-Portier MB, et al. Fertility in women with nonclassical congenital adrenal hyperplasia due to 21-hydroxylase deficiency. *J Clin Endocrinol Metab.* 2010;95(3):1182-1190. PMID: 20080854

68 ANSWER: D) Pioglitazone

Having prediabetes (increased risk for diabetes), obesity, and a sedentary lifestyle increases the risk of developing diabetes. Approximately 5% to 10% of individuals with prediabetes progress to diabetes annually. Patients with a history of impaired fasting glucose and other categories of increased risk for diabetes should be referred to a dietician and counseled on lifestyle modification. This includes modification of diet, weight loss, regular exercise, and smoking cessation.

The table describes the categories used to define prediabetes and diabetes.

Test*	Normal Values	Diagnostic Cutpoints for an Increased Risk for Diabetes (Prediabetes)	Diagnosis of Diabetes Mellitus
8-Hour fasting glucose	<100 mg/dL (SI: <5.6 mmol/L)	100-125 mg/dL (SI: 5.6-6.9 mmol/L)	≥126 mg/dL (SI: ≥7.0 mmol/L)
2-Hour glucose with a 75-g oral glucose tolerance test	<140 mg/dL (SI: <7.8 mmol/L)	140-199 mg/dL (SI: 7.8-11.0 mmol/L)	≥200 mg/dL (SI: ≥11.1 mmol/L)
Elevated hemoglobin A$_{1c}$	<5.7% (<39 mmol/L/mol)	5.7% to 6.4% (39-46 mmol/mol)	≥6.5% (≥48 mmol/mol)

*All tests should be duplicated to confirm the diagnosis of prediabetes or diabetes.

Randomized, placebo-controlled trials, including the Diabetes Prevention Program (DPP) and the Finnish Diabetes Prevention Program, demonstrated that achieving an average weight loss of 5% to 7%, with modification of diet combined with regularly scheduled exercise in patients with prediabetes (impaired glucose tolerance, impaired fasting glucose, or both) led to a 58% reduction in the risk for developing overt diabetes over a 2.8- to 4-year period.

Patients randomly assigned to metformin in the DPP study had a 31% reduced risk of developing diabetes. In a preplanned subset of the DPP cohort, patients with a history of gestational diabetes and impaired glucose tolerance had equivalent risk reduction with metformin and intensive lifestyle modification with regard to developing diabetes.

Given this patient's degree of obesity and her history of gestational diabetes, she is at high risk for progression to diabetes. Metformin would be a good treatment option to prevent onset of diabetes. However, the patient was intolerant to metformin due to gastrointestinal adverse effects in the past, so this is not a treatment option.

Pioglitazone (Answer D) has been shown to be highly effective in preventing progression to diabetes in a high-risk group of Hispanic women who had a history of gestational diabetes. In the Pioglitazone in Prevention of Diabetes (PIPOD) trial, women with a history of gestational diabetes and impaired glucose tolerance were randomly assigned to pioglitazone (30 or 45 mg daily) or placebo and were followed over 3 years. The women treated with pioglitazone had evidence of stabilization of β-cell function and a lower risk of developing diabetes based on intravenous glucose tolerance tests done at baseline, at year 1, and at the study's conclusion. The women treated with pioglitazone gained about 4.4 lb (2 kg) during the trial. Pioglitazone is the best treatment option listed to prevent progression of diabetes in this patient given her history of gestational diabetes.

Liraglutide, 3 mg daily, was shown to reduce the risk of developing diabetes in patients with prediabetes in a randomized, placebo-controlled trial, but it was not listed as a treatment choice in this vignette. No data are available on the efficacy of sitagliptin (Answer A) or dulaglutide (Answer C) in the prevention of diabetes. The current high cost of DPP-4 inhibitors and GLP-1 receptor agonists most likely precludes their use in the prevention of diabetes in routine clinical practice.

Acarbose (Answer B) has been demonstrated to delay progression from impaired glucose tolerance to diabetes in a randomized, placebo-controlled trial. However, the gastrointestinal adverse effects of acarbose are significant and most patients cannot tolerate this medication. Use of acarbose for preventing diabetes would not be the first treatment option in this case.

No data are available on the use of SGLT-2 inhibitors such as canagliflozin (Answer E) to prevent development of diabetes, so this would not be the initial treatment option.

Educational Objective
Recommend the optimal treatment to prevent diabetes in women with a history of gestational diabetes mellitus.

UpToDate Topic Review(s)
Prevention of type 2 diabetes mellitus

Reference(s)

Knowler WC, Barrett-Connor E, Fowler SE, et al; Diabetes Prevention Program Research Group. Reduction in the incidence of type 2 diabetes with lifestyle intervention or metformin. *N Engl J Med.* 2002;346(6):393-403. PMID: 11832527

Toumilehto J, Lindstrom J, Eriksson JG, et al; Finnish Diabetes Prevention Study Group. Prevention of type 2 diabetes mellitus by changes in lifestyle among subjects with impaired glucose tolerance. *N Engl J Med.* 2001;344(18):1343-1350. PMID: 11333990

le Roux CW, Astrup A, Fujioka K, et al; SCALE Obesity and Prediabetes NN8022-1839 Study Group. 3 years of liraglutide versus placebo for type 2 diabetes risk reduction and weight management in individuals with prediabetes: a randomised, double-blind trial. *Lancet.* 2017;389(10077):1399-1409. PMID: 28237263

Xiang AH, Peters RK, Kjos SL, et al. Effect of pioglitazone on pancreatic beta-cell function and diabetes risk in Hispanic women with prior gestational diabetes. *Diabetes.* 2006;55(2):517-522. PMID: 16443789

69 **ANSWER: B) Measure TSH and free T₄**

This patient was diagnosed with esophageal cancer with liver metastases and was started on pembrolizumab. After her third cycle of therapy, she started experiencing fatigue. Three types of immune checkpoint inhibitors have been approved for use in several cancers—antibodies that target cytotoxic T-lymphocyte antigen-4 (CTLA-4), antibodies that target programmed cell death-protein 1 (PD-1), and antibodies that target programmed cell death ligand 1 (PD-L1). This class of medications has several endocrine adverse effects, including thyroid dysfunction, hypophysitis, and diabetes. Pembrolizumab is an immune checkpoint inhibitor that blocks PD-1.

Hypothyroidism was reported in up to 10% of patients receiving pembrolizumab monotherapy, but it could be more frequent (up to 25%) in patients treated with sequential or combined ipilimumab, nivolumab, and pembrolizumab therapy. Hyperthyroidism is less common, and it was reported in up to 5% and 9.9% of patients receiving combined ipilimumab and nivolumab therapy in 2 different studies. In a recent systematic review and meta-analysis including 7551 patients from 38 randomized trials, the overall incidence of significant endocrinopathies was approximately 10% in patients treated with immune checkpoint inhibitors. The incidence of hypothyroidism and hyperthyroidism with pembrolizumab therapy was reported to be 7.0% and 3.2%, respectively. A study reported subclinical hyperthyroidism in 13% of patients receiving anti-PD-1, in 16% of patients receiving ipilimumab, and in 22.2% of patients receiving a combination of nivolumab and ipilimumab. Thyroiditis can be seen with the use of checkpoint inhibitors. Although thyroid dysfunction is for the most part seemingly due to primary thyroid disorders, both TSH and free T_4 levels must be measured in patients taking this class of medication to determine the type of thyroid axis abnormality. In the case of primary hypothyroidism, the patient will need levothyroxine therapy, and for acute thyroiditis a short course of a high-dosage steroid may be helpful.

In secondary hypothyroidism as part of hypophysitis, the common symptoms are fatigue and headaches. The diagnosis is made by documenting low serum TSH and free T_4 levels. The diagnosis of hypophysitis can be supported by a pituitary MRI that shows an enhancement and swelling of the pituitary gland. The incidence of secondary hypothyroidism with pembrolizumab is extremely low (0.4%).

Primary and secondary adrenal insufficiency can also rarely occur, with a very low incidence of adrenal insufficiency in clinical trials (0.7%). When glucocorticoid insufficiency is suspected, cortisol and ACTH levels should be measured in the morning to confirm the etiology of this insufficiency. A cosyntropin-stimulation test may be performed in the event of inconclusive basal measurements, but many factors can influence the interpretation of this test. Thus, before considering glucocorticoid insufficiency as an adverse event of immune checkpoint inhibitors, adrenal and pituitary imaging must be performed to exclude metastasis.

Treatment with immune checkpoint inhibitors has been associated with the onset of type 1 diabetes in a very small number of cases (0.2%). Fasting glucose should be checked; if it is elevated, hemoglobin A_{1c} should be measured. The question has been raised whether these medications should be continued or stopped in the case of endocrine toxicities.

These immune-related adverse events usually develop within the first few weeks to months after treatment initiation. However, immune-related adverse events can present at any point, including after cessation of immune checkpoint blockade therapy, and may wax and wane over time. Some authors have recommended monitoring thyroid function once weekly during the first 2 months of receiving immune checkpoint inhibitor therapy and before each injection from the third month onward. Cortisol and glucose levels should be measured before each injection.

This patient has received 3 cycles of immune checkpoint inhibitor therapy and is now experiencing fatigue. Serum TSH and free T_4 (Answer B) should be measured to assess for thyroid dysfunction. There is no need to measure TPO antibodies (Answer C), as this would not provide more insight. This patient does not have anemia, and a plasma ferritin measurement (Answer A) is not indicated. Because this patient's complete blood cell count is normal, there is no reason to believe she has vitamin B_{12} deficiency, so prescribing supplementation (Answer D) is incorrect. Prednisone (Answer E) can be initiated in patients with confirmed diagnosis of adrenal insufficiency, but this is not the treatment for a patient with hypothyroidism. She does not have any findings consistent with adrenal insufficiency.

Educational Objective
Evaluate for endocrine adverse effects associated with immune checkpoint inhibitor therapy.

UpToDate Topic Review(s)
Patient selection criteria and toxicities with checkpoint inhibitor immunotherapy

Reference(s)
Illouz F, Briet C, Cloix L, et al. Endocrine toxicity of immune checkpoint inhibitors: essential crosstalk between endocrinologists and oncologists. *Cancer Med.* 2017;6(8):1923-1929. PMID: 28719055

Barroso-Sousa R, Barry WT, Garrido-Castro AC, et al. Incidence of endocrine dysfunction following the use of different immune checkpoint inhibitor regimens a systematic review and meta-analysis. *JAMA Oncol.* 2018;4(2):173-182. PMID: 28973656

Postow MA, Sidlow R, Hellmann MD. Immune-related adverse events associated with immune checkpoint blockade. *N Engl J Med.* 2018;378(2):158-168. PMID: 29320654

70

ANSWER: E) 24-Hour urinary calcium

This asymptomatic man has mild hypermagnesemia in the setting of a high-normal serum calcium level and family history of neck surgery in an older sister. Given these findings, one should consider familial hypocalciuric hypercalcemia (FHH) as a cause of mild hypermagnesemia and question whether his sister may have been operated on in error due to a misdiagnosis of primary hyperparathyroidism. FHH is a rare condition inherited in an autosomal dominant pattern, and it results from loss-of-function pathogenic variants in the calcium-sensing receptor gene (*CASR*). The calcium-sensing receptor is expressed in multiple tissues, including the parathyroid glands and the kidneys. In patients with FHH, inactivating *CASR* mutations make the parathyroid glands less sensitive to calcium. In the kidney, this defect leads to an increase in tubular calcium and magnesium reabsorption, resulting in hypercalcemia, hypocalciuria, and high-normal levels of serum magnesium or frank hypermagnesemia. In patients with FHH, serum PTH concentrations are typically inappropriately normal or high in the presence of mild hypercalcemia, and urinary calcium excretion is low, with the calcium-to-creatinine clearance ratio typically less than 0.01. Thus, measuring 24-hour urinary calcium excretion (Answer E), not 24-hour urinary magnesium excretion (Answer D), would be helpful in establishing the diagnosis of FHH and is the best next step in evaluating this patient's hypermagnesemia.

While hypermagnesemia and hypercalcemia can occur in the setting of adrenal insufficiency, perhaps due to volume depletion and hemoconcentration, there is no reason to suspect this condition in an asymptomatic patient with no family history of autoimmune disorders. Therefore, measuring morning serum cortisol (Answer A) would not be the most appropriate next step in evaluating his hypermagnesemia.

Finally, measuring serum PTHrP (Answer B) and serum 1,25-dihydroxyvitamin D (Answer C) would be appropriate in the evaluation of non–PTH-mediated hypercalcemia, but their measurement would not be helpful in this clinical scenario.

Educational Objective

Suspect familial hypocalciuric hypercalcemia in a patient presenting with hypermagnesemia and recommend appropriate evaluation.

UpToDate Topic Review(s)

Disorders of the calcium-sensing receptor: Familial hypocalciuric hypercalcemia and autosomal dominant hypocalcemia
Causes and treatment of hypermagnesemia

Reference(s)

Vargas-Poussou R, Mansour-Hendili L, Baron S, et al. Familial hypocalciuric hypercalcemia types 1 and 3 and primary hyperparathyroidism: similarities and differences. *J Clin Endocrinol Metab.* 2016;101(5):2185-2195. PMID: 26963950

71

ANSWER: B) Hypovolemia due to excessive urine output

This patient has numerous clinical features consistent with acute hypocortisolism, which is confirmed by the finding of a very low serum cortisol level in a patient who is unwell with unprovoked hypoglycemia. However, there is neither accompanying hyponatremia nor hyperkalemia, which should alert the clinician to the possibility that the patient has hypocortisolism (as seen in hypopituitarism) rather than primary adrenal insufficiency with combined glucocorticoid and mineralocorticoid deficiency.

The history of breast cancer, with development of skeletal metastases several years after the primary presentation, is also important to note. Although adrenal metastases are relatively common (eg, in the context of bronchogenic or renal cell carcinoma), they are rarely associated with adrenal insufficiency, even in the presence of bilateral adrenal involvement. In contrast, certain malignancies are known to metastasize to the pituitary gland and may present with anterior, isolated posterior, or panhypopituitarism.

In this patient, the diagnosis of hypocortisolism was made in a timely manner and fluid resuscitation with high-dosage hydrocortisone replacement was instituted. However, several hours later, the patient had a hypotensive periarrest. The dose of hydrocortisone administered should be more than adequate to correct hypocortisolism (intravenous bolus followed by high-dosage maintenance infusion). Thus, inadequate hydrocortisone replacement (Answer C) does not explain this patient's collapse. In addition, even if this patient were mineralocorticoid insufficient, the cover provided with hydrocortisone should be more than adequate because of the mineralocorticoid-like effects of high-dosage hydrocortisone. Thus, failure to commence fludrocortisone replacement (Answer A) is an incorrect explanation.

While it would be important to exclude cardiac decompensation due to overly aggressive fluid resuscitation (Answer D), this would be unusual at this early stage in a patient who was markedly hypovolemic at presentation.

Similarly, pulmonary embolism (Answer E) should be considered, especially in any patient who has been unwell with relative immobility over several weeks. However, no other clinical features are reported that would point to this as the cause of acute collapse following initial resuscitation.

In this case, the patient's hypotensive episode was precipitated by the development of a marked diuresis (a true aquaresis) following institution of hydrocortisone therapy (Answer B). Correction of hypocortisolism allowed the unmasking of diabetes insipidus. Glucocorticoids are key regulators of free water clearance in the kidney, which is therefore impaired in acute adrenal insufficiency. Once cortisol insufficiency has been corrected, the diabetes insipidus becomes apparent and can result in profound hypovolemia if not managed.

Educational Objective
Consider pituitary involvement in a patient with adrenal insufficiency arising in the context of known metastatic malignancy.

UpToDate Topic Review(s)
Causes of hypopituitarism

Reference(s)

Castle-Kirszbaum M, Goldschlager T, Ho B, Wang YY, King J. Twelve cases of pituitary metastasis: a case series and review of the literature. *Pituitary*. 2018;21(5):463-473. PMID: 29974330

Fleseriu M, Hashim IA, Karavitaki N, et al. Hormonal replacement in hypopituitarism in adults: an Endocrine Society clinical practice guideline. *J Clin Endocrinol Metab*. 2016;101(11):3888-3921. PMID: 27736313

72 ANSWER: C) Angiotensin-receptor blocker and calcium-channel blocker

On the basis of the 2017 American Heart Association/American College of Cardiology guideline, this patient would be classified as having stage 2 hypertension. This guideline recommends the use of 2 antihypertensive agents in patients with stage 2 hypertension in whom blood pressure is more than 20/10 mm Hg above target. Similarly, in the 2019 American Diabetes Association Cardiovascular Disease and Risk Management guideline, 2 antihypertensive medications from 2 different classes are recommended if blood pressure assessed in clinic is greater than 160/100 mm Hg. The classes of agents that have been shown to reduce cardiovascular events in patients with diabetes include ACE inhibitors, angiotensin-receptor blockers, thiazide diuretics, and dihydropyridine calcium-channel blockers. β-Adrenergic blockers are recommended in patients with a history of myocardial infarction, active angina, or heart failure. β-Adrenergic blockers are not recommended as first-line therapy because they do not improve mortality in the absence of a history of myocardial infarction, angina, or heart failure. In addition, there is some concern that β-adrenergic blockers would mask symptoms of hypoglycemia in patients with diabetes.

In patients with albuminuria, renin-angiotensin-aldosterone system blockade (with ACE inhibitor or angiotensin-receptor blocker) is considered first-line therapy. In the absence of albuminuria, an agent from any of the 3 classes can be used.

Combination of ACE inhibitors, angiotensin-receptor blockers, or renin blockers (Answers A and E) is not recommended because the risk of hyperkalemia is significant and outweighs any potential cardiovascular advantage. In the absence of known myocardial infarction, angina, or heart failure, a combination that includes a β-adrenergic blocker (Answers B and D) would not be a first choice. In this case, the ACE inhibitor was most likely discontinued because of the patient's cough. Retrial with an ACE inhibitor and calcium-channel blocker or a trial of an angiotensin-receptor blocker and a calcium-channel blocker (Answer C) would be reasonable first choices. Because this patient does not have albuminuria, the use of a calcium-channel blocker with a thiazide diuretic might be a reasonable regimen, although it was not offered as an answer choice. The guidelines suggest initiation of dual therapy; in clinical practice, agents are often started sequentially and the patient's course is followed closely.

Educational Objective
Manage hypertension in patients with type 2 diabetes mellitus.

UpToDate Topic Review(s)
Treatment of hypertension in patients with diabetes mellitus

Reference(s)

American Diabetes Association. 9. Cardiovascular disease and risk management: standards of medical care in diabetes-2018. *Diabetes Care.* 2018;41(Suppl 1):S86-S104. PMID: 29222380

Weber MA, Bakris GL, Jamerson K, et al; ACCOMPLISH Investigators. Cardiovascular events during differing hypertension therapies in patients with diabetes. *J Am Coll Cardiol.* 2010;56(1):77-85. PMID: 20620720

73 **ANSWER: C) Increase topical testosterone and perform regular phlebotomy as needed**
Due to the erythropoietic actions of testosterone, increased hematocrit is one of the most common adverse effects reported in randomized controlled trials of testosterone treatment. Conversely, in hypogonadal men with otherwise unexplained anemia, testosterone treatment can lead to an increase in hematocrit, which may be beneficial.

Current Endocrine Society guidelines recommend checking hematocrit at baseline, 3 to 6 months after starting testosterone treatment, and then annually. Risk factors for development of testosterone treatment-associated erythrocytosis (defined as hematocrit >54% [>0.54]) include older age, higher testosterone dosages, and increased circulating testosterone concentrations during treatment.

If the hematocrit level is greater than 54% (>0.54), testosterone treatment should be withheld, and an individualized workup should be conducted to exclude conditions predisposing to hypoxia (eg, tobacco smoking, untreated obstructive sleep apnea, or pulmonary disease), or primary causes of erythrocytosis (eg, polycythemia rubra vera due to underlying *JAK2* pathogenic variants). Once hematocrit has decreased to a safe level, testosterone can be restarted at a reduced dosage.

In this patient, reducing the testosterone replacement dosage resulted in subtherapeutic testosterone concentrations and insufficient clinical benefit. The best option now is to provide adequate testosterone replacement and perform regular venesection as needed (Answer C) to maintain the hematocrit in a safe range (<52%-54%).

Changing to standard-dose intramuscular testosterone (Answer A) may lead to higher peak serum testosterone concentrations during treatment compared with topical testosterone treatment, and it would not reduce the risk of erythrocytosis.

Given that this patient has organic hypogonadism and a clear beneficial clinical response, stopping testosterone (Answer E) is not appropriate.

While hCG (Answer B) can stimulate testicular testosterone secretion in secondary hypogonadism, long-term treatment of hypogonadal men with hCG is not recommended by current guidelines, and effects on hematocrit relative to testosterone treatment are unknown.

Aromatase inhibitors (Answer D) are likewise not recommended by current guidelines, and effects on hematocrit relative to testosterone replacement are unknown. Moreover, aromatase inhibitors raise serum testosterone by blocking estradiol-mediated negative hypothalamic-pituitary feedback. They require a functioning hypothalamic-pituitary axis and will be ineffective in men with organic pituitary failure. Finally, aromatase inhibitors decrease circulating estradiol and can adversely affect bone health, given evidence that the beneficial effects of testosterone on the skeleton are substantially dependent on its aromatization to estradiol.

Educational Objective
Recommend venesection for hypogonadal men who have elevated hematocrit on testosterone replacement if testosterone is indicated and there is no other underlying cause.

UpToDate Topic Review(s)
Testosterone treatment of male hypogonadism

Reference(s)

Bhasin S, Brito JP, Cunningham GR, et al. Testosterone therapy in men with hypogonadism: an Endocrine Society clinical practice guideline. *J Clin Endocrinol Metab*. 2018;103(5):1715-1744. PMID: 29562364

Roy CN, Snyder PJ, Stephens-Shields AJ, et al. Association of testosterone levels with anemia in older men: a controlled clinical trial. *JAMA Intern Med*. 2017;177(4):480-490. PMID: 28241237

Fernández-Balsells MM, Murad MH, Lane M, et al. Clinical review 1: adverse effects of testosterone therapy in adult men: a systematic review and meta-analysis. *J Clin Endocrinol Metab*. 2010;95(6):2560-2575. PMID: 20525906

74 ANSWER: E) Order 2-dimensional echocardiography

Osteogenesis imperfecta (OI) is a group of molecularly and phenotypically heterogeneous inherited disorders that are characterized by increased skeletal fragility and deformity. Although historically OI has been attributed to pathogenic variants in the type 1 collagen genes that are transmitted in an autosomal dominant fashion, more recent studies have confirmed many additional factors that contribute to normal collagen function and skeletal integrity, including disorders inherited in an autosomal recessive manner. In addition, aberrant production of factors that are critical for osteoblast differentiation also results in disorders of mineralization and bone development that are now considered to be within the spectrum of OI. Nonetheless, most cases of OI are due to pathogenic variants in either the *COL1A1* or *COL1A2* genes, which result in quantitative or qualitative defects in collagen that increase skeletal fragility.

On the basis of this patient's clinical history of multiple childhood fractures, absence of reported skeletal deformities, scleral findings, and dental loss, he has type 1 OI, which is due to an approximately 50% reduction in type 1 collagen production. He has been treated with bisphosphonates in childhood and adulthood, although his skeletal disease is relatively quiescent at present based on stable bone mineral density documented by DXA and no recent low-trauma fractures. Given this, reinitiation of bisphosphonate therapy (either oral or intravenous) (Answers C and D), which does have established effectiveness in patients with type 1 OI, is not indicated now. Additionally, potential adverse effects that occur in patients treated with long-term bisphosphonates (osteonecrosis of the jaw, atypical femoral fractures) are most likely pertinent to patients with OI as well. The measurement of the bone turnover marker C-telopeptide (Answer B), which indirectly reflects osteoclast-mediated bone resorption, has not been established to reliably predict skeletal outcomes (bone density change, fracture-risk reduction) in individual patients with osteoporosis, much less in patients with OI.

Although skeletal and craniofacial manifestations are the hallmark of OI disorders, the effects of abnormal type 1 collagen production can have clinically significant effects in other tissues. Specifically, patients with OI have an apparent increase in risk for valvulopathies, including mitral and aortic regurgitation. On the basis of this patient's significant murmur, referral for echocardiography (Answer E) is appropriate to further characterize his valve disease. Finally, although bluish-gray scleral discoloration is common in OI, other ocular disorders are rare in this disorder. Ectopia lentis, which can be identified through slit-lamp examination (Answer A), occurs in Marfan syndrome, a connective tissue disorder that also can have accompanying valvulopathy but is due to pathogenic variants in the gene encoding fibrillin.

Educational Objective

Recommend appropriate monitoring for patients with osteogenesis imperfecta, bearing in mind the higher risk for valvular heart disease in this population.

UpToDate Topic Review(s)

Osteogenesis imperfecta: Management and prognosis

Reference(s)

Folkestad L, Hald JD, Gram J, et al. Cardiovascular disease in patients with osteogenesis imperfecta - a nationwide, register-based cohort study. *Int J Cardiol*. 2016;225:250-257. PMID: 27741483

Forlino A, Marini JC. Osteogenesis imperfecta. *Lancet*. 2016;16;387(10028):1657-1671. PMID: 26542481

75

ANSWER: C) 75-g oral glucose tolerance test, with fasting and 2-hour glucose values

The prevalence of diabetes in adult patients with cystic fibrosis is approximately 30% to 50%. Therefore, the Cystic Fibrosis Foundation recommends annual screening for diabetes in this patient population. Pursuing no further testing (Answer A) is incorrect. In patients who are clinically stable, the recommended screening method is a 75-g oral glucose tolerance test with measurement of glucose in the fasting state and 2 hours after drinking an oral glucose solution (Answer C). Standard American Diabetes Association criteria apply:

- Fasting glucose ≥126 mg/dL (≥7.0 mmol/L)
- 2-hour glucose value ≥200 mg/dL (≥11.1 mmol/L)

Notably, although hemoglobin A_{1c} (Answer D) is routinely measured, it is not accepted as the screening tool of choice, primarily because of abnormalities in red blood cell turnover in patients with cystic fibrosis.

Fructosamine (Answer E) has not been well studied as a diabetes screening tool in patients with cystic fibrosis. In this vignette, there is no history of ketoacidosis to suggest type 1 diabetes or an autoimmune basis for diabetes. The pathogenesis of diabetes in patients with cystic fibrosis is not lymphocytic destruction of β cells. Therefore, measurement of autoantibodies (Answer B) does not have a routine role in assessing for diabetes in patients with cystic fibrosis.

Dramatic improvement in the care of patients with cystic fibrosis has improved survival rates, with the mean age at death increasing to 40 to 45 years compared with 20 to 25 years about 25 years ago. In patients with cystic fibrosis, the presence of diabetes is a negative predictor of survival and is a risk factor for death in female patients. Prospective studies have established that the degree of insulin deficiency as assessed by oral glucose tolerance testing predicts the rate of pulmonary decline. Finally, retrospective studies suggest that insulin treatment is associated with reversal of lung function decline for a period. A prospective randomized study showed that insulin treatment was associated with improvements in BMI (either stabilization of declining BMI or increased BMI). Both BMI and FEV_1 are positively correlated strongly with survival, so there is good rationale to treat patients with cystic fibrosis–related diabetes. Although the optimal treatment regimen for this patient population has not been established, the most widely accepted treatment is insulin.

Whether the current diagnostic criteria (established to predict microvascular complications) are ideal for patients with cystic fibrosis is unknown. However, these are the recommended guidelines from the Cystic Fibrosis Foundation and the American Diabetes Association.

Educational Objective
Recommend the best diagnostic test for diabetes mellitus in patients with cystic fibrosis.

UpToDate Topic Review(s)
Cystic fibrosis-related diabetes mellitus

Reference(s)

Kelly A, Moran A. Update on cystic fibrosis-related diabetes. *J Cystic Fibros*. 2013;12(4):318-331. PMID: 23562217

Moran A, Brunzell C, Cohen RC, et al; CFRD Guidelines Committee. Clinical care guidelines for cystic fibrosis–related diabetes: a position statement of the American Diabetes Association and a clinical practice guideline of the Cystic Fibrosis Foundation, endorse by the Pediatric Endocrine Society. *Diabetes Care*. 2010;33(12):2697-2708. PMID: 21115772

76 ANSWER: D) Serum very long-chain fatty acids measurement

The symptoms of adrenal insufficiency are often vague, which can lead to a significant delay in diagnosis and increase the risk of a life-threatening adrenal crisis. The pattern of electrolyte abnormalities in this case (hyponatremia, hyperkalemia, elevated serum urea nitrogen), coupled with the markedly elevated plasma ACTH level and abnormal result on cosyntropin-stimulation testing, indicates primary adrenal failure, which is supported by the clinical features (pigmentation and postural hypotension).

The diagnosis of primary adrenal insufficiency in a young man should always mandate consideration of a rare but important cause—adrenoleukodystrophy (ALD)—especially when there are features to suggest associated neurologic dysfunction. ALD is an X-linked disorder caused by pathogenic variants in the *ABCD1* gene (ATP-binding cassette subfamily D member 1), which encodes an ABC transporter. This is critical for the uptake of very long-chain fatty acids into the peroxisome, with subsequent β-oxidation and breakdown. Accumulation of very long-chain fatty acids in the central nervous system, adrenal cortex, and the Leydig cells of the testes leads to the well-recognized clinical features of ALD. Therefore, the best test to identify the cause of his presentation is to measure very long-chain fatty acids (Answer D).

Affected males can present in childhood or adulthood. Childhood onset is typically before age 10 years and the diagnosis may initially be confused with attention-deficit/hyperactivity disorder due to the prominence of behavioral problems and learning difficulties. Neurologic deterioration follows (quadriparesis, vision loss, seizures), and primary adrenal insufficiency is common. A similar form of the disease may manifest in adolescence or adulthood. In contrast, adrenomyeloneuropathy typically has a later age of onset (20-40 years) and presents with progressive stiffness and weakness of the legs (spastic paraparesis), neurogenic bladder, and erectile dysfunction. Again, adrenal insufficiency is a common finding. In the longer term, 20% to 60% eventually develop cerebral involvement. A cerebellar form also exists (with onset in childhood or adolescence). In up to 10% of patients, adrenal insufficiency is the only clinical manifestation. Female carriers may develop symptoms in adulthood (typically after age 30 years) and present with an adrenomyeloneuropathy-like phenotype. However, cerebral involvement and adrenal insufficiency are rare in affected women.

Therefore, once a diagnosis of ALD has been established, it is important to consider genetic counseling and, where appropriate, testing other family members to identify those who merit further assessment and surveillance.

Autoantibodies to the adrenocortical enzyme 21-hydroxylase (Answer A) are characteristic of autoimmune Addison disease, and screening for these would be appropriate in a young patient presenting with primary adrenal insufficiency. However, when boys or young men present with primary adrenal failure and have neuromuscular findings on physical examination, the clinician should be most concerned about a possible diagnosis of adrenoleukodystrophy.

Adrenal CT (Answer B) may be helpful (and indeed some clinicians advocate performing this in all patients presenting with primary adrenal failure) if there is suspected invasion/infiltration (eg, due to underlying malignancy with a known propensity to metastasize to the adrenal glands [such as melanoma] or infectious causes [such as tuberculosis, histoplasmosis]). However, there are no other features to suggest systemic upset in this patient, and the adrenal CT would most likely be reported as normal. Reliably diagnosing adrenal atrophy is difficult, even in the hands of an experienced radiologist.

Primary adrenal failure is a recognized complication of opportunistic infection (eg, cytomegalovirus adrenalitis) in individuals with AIDS due to HIV infection (Answer C). However, this patient was previously fit and well until 4 months ago, and there are no other clinical features to suggest HIV infection. In the era of highly active antiretroviral therapy, far fewer cases of opportunistic infections and malignancies are seen now than in the early days of the AIDS epidemic.

The *AIRE* gene (Answer E) encodes the autoimmune regulator protein, which is involved in thymic elimination of self-reactive T cells. More than 90 pathogenic variants in *AIRE* have been identified in persons with autoimmune polyendocrinopathy-candidiasis-ectodermal dystrophy (APECED, also referred to as autoimmune polyendocrine syndrome type 1 [APS-1]). Chronic mucocutaneous candidiasis is a major feature of the condition. Endocrine manifestations include hypoparathyroidism and primary adrenal insufficiency, but other autoimmune endocrinopathies may also occur (eg, premature ovarian failure, Hashimoto hypothyroidism, type 1 diabetes mellitus). Given the lack of other endocrine manifestations in this patient, sequencing the *AIRE* gene is not indicated.

Educational Objective
Suspect adrenoleukodystrophy in a young man with adrenal insufficiency, especially when associated with neurologic features.

UpToDate Topic Review(s)
Adrenoleukodystrophy

Reference(s)

Berger J, Forss-Petter S, Eichler FS. Pathophysiology of X-linked adrenoleukodystrophy. *Biochimie*. 2015;98:135-142. PMID: 24316281

Burtman E & Regelmann MO. Endocrine dysfunction in X-linked Adrenoleukodystrophy. *Endocrinol Metab Clin North Am*. 2016;45(2):295-309. PMID: 27241966

77 ANSWER: E) Change her basal insulin dose to 40 units NPH in the morning

This vignette highlights the value of using the blood glucose graph in the electronic medical record to identify a glucose excursion pattern over several days. The graph shows a cyclic pattern of point-of-care glucose values, with the nadir blood glucose occurring at 7 AM, a rise in glucose during the day peaking at 11 PM, then dropping overnight. The history provides clues to the cause of this pattern—the patient is receiving prednisone, 40 mg orally each morning. Prednisone, given in the morning, increases postprandial glucose during the day by impairing insulin action and increasing hepatic glucose production. This effect can last for up to 12 hours and is nicely depicted in the graph: a staircase pattern with each daytime glucose value higher than the preceding one, peaking at bedtime. By midnight each day, the period of fasting coincides with the waning effect of the steroids, causing glucose to drop to near hypoglycemia by morning. The clinician is asked to select an insulin regimen that will best optimize her blood glucose levels.

Of the listed choices, changing her basal insulin dose to 40 units NPH in the morning (Answer E) is the best fit, as the action of morning NPH will peak in 9 to 10 hours and wane over the next few hours to zero. The extra basal insulin during the day provided by NPH, in addition to the prandial insulin lispro, may be sufficient to flatten out the daytime glucose curve.

Initiating an intravenous insulin infusion (Answer A) would be effective, but it requires additional nursing resources and hourly blood glucose testing. Increasing the dose of the rapid-acting insulin for meals (Answer B) or increasing the correction scale to more aggressive coverage (Answer C) would correct the postprandial hyperglycemia, but these actions would not prevent the morning hypoglycemia. Switching the timing of the basal insulin glargine from bedtime to morning (Answer D) may have modest benefit, but morning hypoglycemia could still occur.

Educational Objective
Identify glucose patterns in hospitalized patients and make appropriate adjustments to reduce hyperglycemic and hypoglycemic excursions.

UpToDate Topic Review(s)
Management of diabetes mellitus in hospitalized patients

Reference(s)

American Diabetes Association. 15. Diabetes care in the hospital: standards of medical care in diabetes-2019. *Diabetes Care*. 2019;42(Suppl 1):S173-S181. PMID: 30559241

Brady V, Thosani S, Zhou S, Bassett R, Busaidy NL, Lavis V. Safe and effective dosing of basal-bolus insulin in patients receiving high-dose steroids for hyper-cyclophosphamide, doxorubicin, vincristine, and dexamethasone chemotherapy. *Diabetes Technol Ther*. 2014;16(12):874-879. PMID: 25321387

Clement S, Braithwaite SS, Magee MF, et al; American Diabetes Association Diabetes in Hospitals Writing Committee. Management of diabetes and hyperglycemia in hospitals. *Diabetes Care*. 2004;27(2):553-591. PMID: 14747243

78 ANSWER: B) Another inferior petrosal sinus sampling

The differential diagnosis of hypercortisolism is often challenging and must proceed in steps. The initial step is to determine whether the patient has pathologic hypercortisolism. This can be done with a combination of tests, including measuring 24-hour urinary free cortisol and bedtime salivary cortisol and performing a low-dose dexamethasone suppression test. Only after this requirement is met should the physician start determining the etiology of the hypercortisolism. To this end, the first step is to measure plasma ACTH, which is low or unmeasurable in adrenal Cushing syndrome, while it is normal or elevated in ACTH-dependent Cushing syndrome. After ACTH-dependent Cushing syndrome is diagnosed, the source of abnormal ACTH secretion should be sought.

This patient has an established diagnosis of ACTH-dependent Cushing syndrome. The most common cause of ACTH-dependent Cushing syndrome is a pituitary adenoma (Cushing disease). In a patient with ACTH-dependent Cushing syndrome and an obvious pituitary adenoma (≥6 mm), it is reasonable to refer the patient to an experienced pituitary surgeon. When an adenoma is smaller or not obviously visible, inferior petrosal sinus sampling can be performed. The presence of a central-to-peripheral ACTH gradient (>2 at baseline and >3 after corticotropin-releasing hormone or desmopressin injection) indicates that the abnormal ACTH secretion is pituitary-dependent (Cushing disease). The lack of such a gradient suggests an ectopic source of ACTH, which should trigger the search for an extrapituitary neuroendocrine tumor (most frequently a lung carcinoid).

Inferior petrosal sinus sampling has a significant percentage (5%-9%) of false negativity in diagnosing Cushing disease. This may be due to inappropriate catheter placement or cyclical activity of the adenoma (for this reason, some centers measure urine or serum cortisol immediately before the procedure to help interpret the data). Furthermore, statistically, Cushing disease is more frequent than ectopic ACTH secretion. Therefore, at this point, the best option is to repeat inferior petrosal sinus sampling (Answer B) in the hope that a gradient might be observed to help diagnose Cushing disease. Other possible alternatives (proceed directly for exploratory pituitary surgery or bilateral adrenalectomy) could also be considered at this point, but they were not offered as options.

This patient has already undergone chest and abdomen CT, as well as a gallium (^{68}Ga) DOTATATE scan, which is a radioconjugate consisting of the somatostatin analogue tyrosine-3-octreotate (Tyr3-octreotate or TATE) labeled with the PET tracer ^{68}Ga via the chelating agent dodecane tetraacetic acid (DOTA). This agent binds to somatostatin receptors present on the cell membranes of many types of neuroendocrine tumors and is now used as a somatostatin receptor imaging agent in conjunction with PET. In this patient, the ^{68}Ga DOTATATE scan failed to show a suspicious lesion. This imaging has a higher sensitivity than MRI (Answer E) and ^{111}In octreotide scan (Answer A) in detecting ectopic sources of ACTH. Another pituitary MRI (Answer C) would not help; even if a small adenoma were observed, there would be no obvious proof that it is the source of ACTH. Adrenal CT (Answer D) is not useful, as this patient's Cushing syndrome is ACTH-dependent, and the discovery of a small adrenal mass that had escaped the abdominal CT would not be clinically relevant.

Educational Objective
Identify the limitations of inferior petrosal sinus sampling in the diagnosis of ACTH-dependent Cushing syndrome.

UpToDate Topic Review(s)
Establishing the cause of Cushing's syndrome

Reference(s)

Guaraldi F, Salvatori R. Cushing syndrome: maybe not so uncommon of an endocrine disease. *J Am Board Fam Med.* 2012;25(2):199-208. PMID: 22403201

Carroll TB, Findling JW. The diagnosis of Cushing's syndrome. *Rev Endocr Metab Disord.* 2010;11(2):147-153. PMID: 20821267

Isidori AM, Sbardella E, Zatelli MC, et al; ABC Study Group. Conventional and nuclear medicine imaging in ectopic Cushing's syndrome: a systematic review. *J Clin Endocrinol Metab.* 2015;100(9):3231-3244. PMID: 26158607

Swearingen B, Katznelson L, Miller K, et al. Diagnostic errors after inferior petrosal sinus sampling. *J Clin Endocrinol Metab.* 2004;89(8):3752-3763. PMID: 15292301

Sheth SA, Mian MK, Neal J, et al. Transsphenoidal surgery for cushing disease after nondiagnostic inferior petrosal sinus sampling. *Neurosurgery.* 2012;71(1):14-22. PMID: 22353796

79

ANSWER: B) Perform liver ultrasonography

This patient presents with very low cholesterol levels, a condition called hypobetalipoproteinemia in which plasma LDL-cholesterol and apolipoprotein B levels are below the fifth percentile. Hypobetalipoproteinemia can occur secondary to eating a strict vegetarian or vegan diet, intestinal fat malabsorption (chronic pancreatitis), severe liver disease, and hyperthyroidism. Primary causes occur due to genetic defects along the chylomicron/VLDL production and secretion pathway. Most patients with familial hypobetalipoproteinemia are asymptomatic but may present with nonalcoholic fatty liver and mild elevations in liver enzymes.

There is no indication that the patient in this vignette is a vegetarian, and she takes no lipid-lowering medications. She does not have symptoms or signs of conditions that cause secondary hypobetalipoproteinemia. Therefore, phenotypically, she most likely has primary hypobetalipoproteinemia. Abetalipoproteinemia and homozygous familial hypobetalipoproteinemia have a severe phenotype with clinical presentation in childhood and neurologic signs due to deficiency of fat-soluble vitamins. This patient's mild phenotype suggests heterozygous familial hypobetalipoproteinemia.

Familial hypobetalipoproteinemia can be caused by pathogenic variants in the gene encoding apolipoprotein B (*APOB*), which result in the formation of a truncated apolipoprotein B protein that has a reduced capacity to export triglycerides from hepatocytes. Thus, hepatic steatosis can occur, the course of which is not always benign. Steatohepatitis, cirrhosis, and hepatocellular carcinoma have all been described in individuals with pathogenic variants in the *APOB* gene; therefore, triglyceride accumulation can lead to progression of liver disease. Ultrasonography of the liver (Answer B) is indicated, as well as eventual referral to a hepatologist for ongoing surveillance. Given that the patient's family history included an aunt with cryptogenic cirrhosis and growing evidence that patients with heterozygous familial hypobetalipoproteinemia might be at risk of developing more severe liver disease in the presence of other factors that can cause liver injury, molecular diagnosis was confirmed by identifying a pathogenic variant in the *APOB* gene.

Genetic defects in the gene encoding microsomal triglyceride transfer protein, a protein that facilitates assembly of lipids with apolipoprotein B during lipoprotein synthesis, result in extremely low plasma cholesterol and LDL-cholesterol levels and an almost complete absence of apolipoprotein B. This condition is extremely rare and is called abetalipoproteinemia. Abetalipoproteinemia is usually diagnosed early in life (first and second decades), and it presents with steatorrhea, oral fat intolerance, retinitis pigmentosa, and debilitating neurologic abnormalities due to deficiency of fat-soluble vitamins A, D, and E (Answer A). LDL-cholesterol levels are unmeasurable. Acanthocytosis of red blood cells on the peripheral blood smear (Answer C) is a feature that distinguishes this condition from heterozygous hypobetalipoproteinemia. This patient does not have clinical evidence of abetalipoproteinemia.

Serum protein electrophoresis (Answer D) is a test used to separate proteins based on their electrical charge, and it is commonly used to diagnosed multiple myeloma and other paraproteinemias. There is no clinical indication for serum protein electrophoresis in this vignette.

Loss-of-function pathogenic variants in the *PCSK9* gene are another cause of familial hypobetalipoproteinemia. Mutations decrease the degradation of the LDL receptor and thus make more LDL receptors available on the surface of the liver, thereby lowering LDL-cholesterol levels. In contrast to pathogenic variants in *APOB*, *PCSK9* mutations are rare, not associated with any clinical symptoms, and have been associated with a decreased risk of cardiovascular disease. Therefore, genetic testing for pathogenic variants in the *PCSK9* gene (Answer E) is not likely to add clinical benefit at this time.

Patients with heterozygous hypobetalipoproteinemia do not appear to have increased cardiovascular risk; risk is in fact quite low. This patient should be reassured that her low lipid levels are secondary to an underlying genetic disorder; no lipid-lowering therapy is indicated.

Educational Objective
Appropriately manage the care of an individual with very low lipid levels (hypobetalipoproteinemia).

UpToDate Topic Review(s)
Low LDL-cholesterol

Reference(s)

Welty FK. Hypobetalipoproteinemia and abetalipoproteinemia. *Curr Opin Lipidol.* 2014;25(3):161-168. PMID: 24751931

Hooper AJ, Burnett JR. Update on primary hypobetalipoproteinemia. *Curr Atheroscler Rep.* 2014;16(7):423. PMID: 24781598

80

ANSWER: B) Left adrenalectomy

This patient has a pheochromocytoma (left adrenal mass) and a lipid-rich adrenocortical adenoma (right adrenal mass). The treatment of choice for pheochromocytoma is surgical adrenalectomy (Answer B), preferably without delay following preoperative adrenergic blockade. Thus, repeated imaging in 3 months (Answer D) is incorrect.

Pheochromocytomas are tumors arising from the adrenal medulla that can secrete catecholamines (such as norepinephrine, epinephrine, and dopamine), which induce adrenergic symptoms and signs, such as palpitations, anxiety, sweating, pallor, and elevations in blood pressure and heart rate. Paragangliomas are tumors that arise from the ganglia of the autonomic nervous system and therefore can occur in any region from the base of the skull to the pelvic floor. Although sympathetic paragangliomas can secrete norepinephrine and dopamine, they are unlikely to synthesize epinephrine as pheochromocytomas do.

Metanephrines are the stable and inactive metabolites of catecholamines that provide the highest sensitivity and specificity for diagnosing pheochromocytoma and paraganglioma. Typically, pheochromocytomas and paragangliomas that induce clinical symptoms are associated with metanephrine and/or normetanephrine levels that are substantially higher than the upper limit of the reference range—usually 4 times or more (less commonly 2 or 3 times higher). However, some pheochromocytomas do not secrete high concentrations of catecholamines, and in some instances, even when high catecholamine concentrations are detected, some patients do not exhibit the classic hyperadrenergic symptoms (such as this patient). Importantly, mild elevations above the upper limit of the metanephrines reference range (<2 times) are common and are usually attributed to enhanced sympathoadrenergic tone (eg, in a state of anxiety, stress, or critical illness) and/or the use of catecholamine reuptake inhibitors (eg, some antidepressant medications and cocaine). In this regard, these milder elevations are a frequent cause of false-positive values. The absence of classic adrenergic symptoms in this patient does not exclude a pheochromocytoma; however, the marked elevation in normetanephrine levels (approximately 15 times the upper limit of the reference range) strongly suggests that one or both of the adrenal tumors is a pheochromocytoma.

Determining which adrenal mass represents a pheochromocytoma requires understanding the radiographic features of adrenal masses. Cross-sectional imaging of the abdomen with CT or MRI is adequate to visualize symptomatic pheochromocytomas. Pheochromocytomas tend to be dense and vascular. Therefore, they almost always have high attenuation on unenhanced CT imaging (>10 Hounsfield units) or high contrast avidity (often with heterogeneous enhancement) on CT imaging done with intravenous contrast, or they have poor delayed contrast washout when CT imaging is performed with an adrenal washout protocol. Adrenal masses with unenhanced attenuation well below 10 HU are almost never pheochromocytomas. On MRI, pheochromocytomas tend to display hyperintensity on T2-weighted imaging and have features suggestive of low lipid content (no loss of signal on out-of-phase sequences). In contrast, lipid-rich adrenal adenomas display low attenuation on unenhanced CT (<10 Hounsfield units) and greater than 40% relative and 60% absolute washout on delayed protocols. Therefore, the right adrenal mass is not consistent with a pheochromocytoma and does not need to be removed (Answers A and C).

The role of adrenal biopsy (Answer E) is generally limited to 2 scenarios: (1) confirmation of an extraadrenal metastasis to determine staging and consequent management and (2) confirmation of an invasive infectious infiltration of the adrenal glands. Both scenarios can be either unilateral or bilateral processes. There is no role for adrenal biopsy when the biochemical confirmation of a pheochromocytoma has been made. Biopsy of a pheochromocytoma is generally contraindicated due to the concern that the procedure or needle trauma may precipitate a catecholamine crisis.

This patient underwent an uncomplicated left adrenalectomy following α-adrenergic and β-adrenergic blockade, and pathologic examination revealed a pheochromocytoma. Postoperatively, his blood pressure was lower and he needed fewer antihypertensive medications.

Educational Objective
Distinguish the radiographic characteristics of a pheochromocytoma from those of a benign adrenocortical adenoma.

UpToDate Topic Review(s)
Clinical presentation and diagnosis of pheochromocytoma
Treatment of pheochromocytoma in adults

Reference(s)

Vaidya A, Hamrahian A, Bancos I, Fleseriu M, Ghayee HK. The evaluation of incidentally discovered adrenal masses. *Endocr Pract.* 2019;25(2):178-192. PMID: 30817193

Lenders JW, Duh QY, Eisenhofer G, et al; Endocrine Society. Pheochromocytoma and paraganglioma: an Endocrine Society clinical practice guideline. *J Clin Endocrinol Metab.* 2014;99(6):1915-1942. PMID: 24893135

Fassnacht M, Arlt W, Bancos I, et al. Management of adrenal incidentalomas: European Society of Endocrinology clinical practice guideline in collaboration with the European Network for the Study of Adrenal Tumors. *Eur J Endocrinol.* 2016;175(2):G1-G34. PMID: 27390021

81 ANSWER: E) Measure tissue transglutaminases IgA and IgG

This patient has a history of vitamin D deficiency and hypothyroidism. She takes levothyroxine every day on an empty stomach and her levothyroxine dosage was adjusted 6 months earlier due to an elevated TSH level despite taking levothyroxine daily. Her thyroid function test results are still abnormal and her levothyroxine dosage requires further adjustment. In addition, her vitamin D level is low despite taking vitamin D, 50,000 IU weekly. Interestingly, her levothyroxine dosage is much higher than her weight-based calculated levothyroxine dosage (weight in kg × 1.6 mcg per day = ~88 mcg daily). These findings should raise concern for malabsorption. The patient is not taking any calcium or iron supplements that might interfere with levothyroxine absorption. Her personal diagnosis of hypothyroidism and vitamin D deficiency raise concern that she may have another autoimmune condition such as celiac disease.

Patients with celiac disease can present with symptoms related to malabsorption, including diarrhea, weight loss, and nutrient and vitamin deficiencies. However, most patients with celiac disease exhibit minor gastrointestinal symptoms or nongastrointestinal manifestations or they are completely asymptomatic. Serum tissue transglutaminases IgA and IgG (Answer E) should be measured to check for celiac disease. An IgA level should also be ordered at the same time to ensure there is no IgA deficiency, which can cause a falsely normal tissue transglutaminase IgA result. If this patient's levels of serum tissue transglutaminases IgA and IgG are elevated, she should be referred to a gastroenterologist for an esophagogastroduodenoscopy with several biopsies of the duodenum to confirm celiac disease. Once celiac disease is confirmed, she should follow a gluten-free-diet to improve absorption of vitamin D and levothyroxine.

Patients with one autoimmune disorder can exhibit other autoimmune diseases. This patient has hypothyroidism due to Hashimoto thyroiditis, confirmed by her elevated TPO antibodies (also, Hashimoto thyroiditis is the most common cause of hypothyroidism in the United States). In prospective studies, the prevalence of celiac disease is noted to be 1% to 19% in patients with type 1 diabetes mellitus, 2% to 5% in patients with autoimmune thyroid disorders, and 3% to 7% in patients with primary biliary cirrhosis. Following a gluten-free diet improves glycemic control in patients with type 1 diabetes mellitus and enhances the absorption of medications for associated hypothyroidism and osteoporosis. It probably does not change the natural history of associated autoimmune disorders.

Increasing the levothyroxine dosage to 150 mcg daily (Answer A) could be considered once celiac disease has been excluded. Likewise, celiac disease should be ruled out before increasing the dosage of vitamin D (Answer C).

This patient's laboratory test results show subclinical hypothyroidism (mildly elevated TSH with normal free T_4 and free T_3), probably related to malabsorption of levothyroxine due to untreated celiac disease. At this time, there is no reason to add liothyronine (Answer B) and her free T_3 is within normal range. A levothyroxine absorption test (Answer D) could be recommended once celiac disease has been ruled out and other reasons for abnormal TSH have been evaluated.

Educational Objective
Explain the effect of untreated celiac disease on the management of hypothyroidism.

UpToDate Topic Review(s)
Pathogenesis, epidemiology, and clinical manifestations of celiac disease in adults
Diagnosis of celiac disease in adults

Reference(s)

Ch'ng CL, Jones MK, Kingham JG. Celiac disease and autoimmune thyroid disease. *Clin Med Res.* 2007;5(3):184-192. PMID: 18056028

Gujral N, Freeman HJ, Thomson AB. Celiac disease: prevalence, diagnosis, pathogenesis and treatment. *World J Gastroenterol.* 2012;18(42):6036-6059. PMID: 23155333

82 ANSWER: E) Insulin 70/30 twice daily

Glucocorticoid-induced hyperglycemia refers to the rise in blood glucose caused by initiation of steroids. The pathophysiology of glucocorticoid-induced hyperglycemia is not well understood, but it is thought to be due to multiple mechanisms, including increased hepatic gluconeogenesis and decreased glucose uptake in adipocytes. There are limited data on optimal blood glucose management in these patients. The only guideline available on inpatient management of glucocorticoid-induced hyperglycemia is from the Joint British Diabetes Societies. This guideline provides management strategies based on presteroid use status (type 1 diabetes, type 2 diabetes, no previous diabetes history, hyperglycemia in pregnancy, etc). In those with type 2 diabetes, the recommendation is titration of oral agents if the patient is not on insulin therapy. In patients treated with insulin, the guidance is to intensify insulin administration in a stepwise fashion. Administration of basal insulin in the morning should be considered if it is currently given in the evening (presumably to avoid nocturnal hypoglycemia). If needed, the basal insulin dosage can be increased (10% every 24-48 hours), and finally mealtime short-acting insulin can be added as needed.

In this patient with preexisting type 2 diabetes that is fairly well controlled, the addition of an SGLT-2 inhibitor (Answer D) or liraglutide (Answer B) would not be the best choice since there are no data on use of these agents for glucocorticoid-induced hyperglycemia, especially in the short term. In addition, the liraglutide dosage is typically titrated over 2 or more weeks, which would be longer than the duration of oral steroid use. In patients with hematologic malignancies being treated with dexamethasone, a comparison study showed that a basal-bolus insulin regimen was superior to basal and supplemental insulin on a scale. Therefore, mixed insulin (Answer E) would most likely be superior to adding only insulin glargine (Answer C) or only supplemental insulin (Answer A) to his regimen. Glucocorticoids are most likely to cause postprandial hyperglycemia with meals close to the time of administration. If this patient takes prednisone at 8 AM, blood glucose after breakfast and lunch would most likely be higher than glucose concentrations after dinner. Since steroids are typically given in the morning, the use of 70/30 insulin would also allow for a larger dose in the morning when the steroid-induced rise in blood glucose would be most pronounced. Insulin glargine is often avoided due to its long duration of action and associated risk of nocturnal hypoglycemia. Other choices to treat hyperglycemia during the day and avoid nocturnal hypoglycemia might be the use of just NPH insulin in the morning or insulin 70/30 in the morning. Use of a short-acting sulfonylurea in the morning could be considered in some cases, but it is not usually potent enough to control glucose levels during treatment with glucocorticoids.

Educational Objective

In a patient with diabetes mellitus, adjust the insulin regimen to treat glucocorticoid-induced hyperglycemia.

UpToDate Topic Review(s)
Major side effects of systemic glucocorticoids

Reference(s)

Gosmanov AR, Goorha S, Stelts S, Peng L, Umpierrez GE. Management of hyperglycemia in diabetic patients with hematologic malignancies during dexamethasone therapy. *Endocr Pract.* 2013;19(2):231-235. PMID: 23337144

Roberts A, James J, Dhatariya K; Joint British Diabetes Societies (JBDS) for Inpatient Care. Management of hyperglycaemia and steroid (glucocorticoid) therapy: a guideline from the Joint British Diabetes Societies (JBDS) for Inpatient Care group. *Diabet Med.* 2018;35(8):1011-1017. PMID: 30152586

83 ANSWER: E) Initiate potassium iodide

This patient with poorly controlled Graves disease has elected to undergo thyroidectomy as definitive treatment. Although thyroidectomy was only selected by 0.9% of US endocrinologists and 1% of European endocrinologists in a 2011 survey of treatment approaches for Graves disease, it is an excellent treatment, as not only does it remove the source of the excessive production of thyroid hormone, but it may also render the autoimmune process responsible for Graves orbitopathy and Graves dermopathy more quiescent. Usually total thyroidectomy is performed, as subtotal thyroidectomy is associated with an unacceptable risk of recurrent hyperthyroidism. However, one caveat for this patient is that she will still have to adhere to taking a daily medication, and adherence to her methimazole regimen appears to be difficult for her.

The complications of thyroidectomy for Graves disease are similar to the complications of thyroidectomy performed for other reasons. These complications including bleeding, hypoparathyroidism, and recurrent laryngeal nerve damage. Some studies suggest that bleeding may be more common in association with surgery for Graves disease than other benign diseases or thyroid cancer. In addition, for Graves disease specifically, there is the risk of worsening hyperthyroidism, particularly if the patient is not euthyroid at the time of surgery.

In this vignette, the goal is to minimize the potential for blood loss during surgery such that the need for blood transfusion will not arise. Only potassium iodide (Answer E) has efficacy in this capacity. Decreased blood loss with potassium iodide use has been clearly demonstrated in several randomized controlled studies (*see table*).

Author, Year	Potassium Iodide Use Described in Study	Blood Loss Without Potassium Iodide (mL)	Blood Loss With Potassium Iodide (mL)	P value
Erbil et al 2007	Lugol solution (10 drops per day orally, 3 times a day for 10 days)	108	54	<.001
Yilmaz et al 2017	Lugol iodine (0.8 mg/kg for 10 days)	172	76	.0001
Whalen et al 2017	SSKI (8 drops in a glass of water daily for a week before operation)	161	61	.05

Some experts have questioned the recommendation to use a potassium iodide preparation before surgery for Graves disease presented in the 2017 American Thyroid Association Guidelines for the Treatment of Hyperthyroidism. They cite failure to show differences in surgical outcomes. However, a recent trial published in 2018 showed less transient hypoparathyroidism and less transient hoarseness when potassium iodide was used.

With respect to preventing worsening hyperthyroidism during thyroid surgery, the best strategy is to render the patient euthyroid before surgery. However, even in cases of patients who undergo surgery while hyperthyroid, there are surprisingly few adverse events. Three of the choices offered in this vignette are agents that act to control hyperthyroidism. High-dosage steroids (Answer A) are often used to help control severe hyperthyroidism when it is necessary, based on the overall medical situation, for the patient to undergo surgery without optimal control of hyperthyroidism. Steroids act by decreasing the conversion to T_4 to T_3, thereby decreasing the levels of the active hormone. However, steroids are not known to decrease the vascularity of the thyroid gland and decrease perioperative bleeding.

Increasing this patient's methimazole dosage before surgery (Answer B) in an attempt to achieve euthyroidism is clearly indicated. However, methimazole will only reduce thyroid hormone synthesis and will not directly affect the risk of perioperative blood loss.

Lithium (Answer D) prevents release of thyroid hormones from the thyroid gland and is mostly used when first-line therapies to treat hyperthyroidism have failed or have resulted in toxicity. It has a track record in assisting in the control of hyperthyroidism, but no similar record with respect to controlling blood loss during surgery.

Rituximab (Answer C) has been successfully used to treat Graves orbitopathy, but it has not been shown to decrease thyroid gland vascularity or perioperative blood loss.

Educational Objective
List the effects of potassium iodide used as preoperative preparation for thyroidectomy for Graves disease.

UpToDate Topic Review(s)
Surgical management of hyperthyroidism

Reference(s)
Erbil Y, Barbaros U, Salmaslioglu A, et al. Determination of remnant thyroid volume: comparison of ultrasonography, radioactive iodine uptake and serum thyroid-stimulating hormone level. *J Laryngol Otol.* 2008;122(6):615-622. PMID: 17605833

Hope N, Kelly A. Pre-operative Lugol's iodine treatment in the management of patients undergoing thyroidectomy for Graves' disease: a review of the literature. *Eur Thyroid J.* 2017;6(1):20-25. PMID: 28611944

Randle RW, Bates MF, Long KL, Pitt SC, Schneider DF, Sippel RS. Impact of potassium iodide on thyroidectomy for Graves' disease: Implications for safety and operative difficulty. *Surgery.* 2018;163(1):68-72. PMID: 29108701

Whalen G, Sullivan M, Maranda L, Quinlan R, Larkin A. Randomized trial of a short course of preoperative potassium iodide in patients undergoing thyroidectomy for Graves' disease. *Am J Surg.* 2017;213(4):805-809. PMID: 27769543

Yilmaz Y, Kamer KE, Ureyen O, Sari E, Acar T, Karahalli O. The effect of preoperative Lugol's iodine on intraoperative bleeding in patients with hyperthyroidism. *Ann Med Surg (Lond).* 2016;9:53-57. PMID: 27408715

84 ANSWER: A) Fasting glucose and/or hemoglobin A₁c measurements

Turner syndrome is a condition of primary or hypergonadotrophic hypogonadism due to a chromosomal disorder affecting phenotypic females with one intact X chromosome and complete or partial absence of the second X chromosome in association with one or more clinical features. In this patient with coarctation of the aorta, Turner syndrome was diagnosed on the basis of karyotype analysis during the evaluation of growth failure and delayed puberty. Because of her known history of coarctation of the aorta, she requires annual follow-up with cardiology, ideally with cardiologists who have expertise in congenital heart disease. Women diagnosed with Turner syndrome without cardiac disease should have baseline echocardiography or cardiac MRI to screen for valvular disease, aortic root dilatation, or other cardiac abnormalities. The frequency of imaging and cardiology referral depends on any baseline abnormalities and aortic size index. Regardless of known cardiac anomalies, women with Turner syndrome should have screening with cardiac imaging before trying to conceive or if hypertension is newly diagnosed.

When patients with Turner syndrome transition to adulthood, it is important to recognize the need to screen for other associated conditions on a regular basis. For example, patients with Turner syndrome have a higher prevalence of hypothyroidism, so annual thyroid function testing is recommended. This patient was already diagnosed with hypothyroidism in childhood. Because of the higher prevalence of type 2 diabetes in women with Turner syndrome, adult patients should undergo annual assessment of fasting glucose and/or hemoglobin A₁c (Answer A).

While the risk for celiac disease is modestly increased in Turner syndrome, it tends to present in childhood. In this patient who has not presented with celiac disease by age 20, the risk is relatively low. Screening for celiac disease using tissue transglutaminase IgA antibody assessment (Answer C) could be considered, but it is not necessary in the absence of gastrointestinal symptoms, unexplained weight loss, or vitamin D deficiency at this age. However, it is important to note that a negative tissue transglutaminase IgA antibody assessment does not rule out the diagnosis and referral to gastroenterology for endoscopy should be considered if suspicion for celiac disease exists.

Although primary ovarian insufficiency is associated with primary adrenal insufficiency, Turner syndrome is not, so annual measurement of ACTH and cortisol (Answer B) is not indicated.

Women with Turner syndrome do have an increased risk for osteoporosis and fractures. Although screening recommendations include monitoring serum 25-hydroxyvitamin D every 3 to 5 years in adulthood, PTH and calcium (Answer D) do not need to be assessed annually because there is no association of Turner syndrome with primary hyperparathyroidism.

Women with Turner syndrome are not at increased risk for IGF-1 excess or other pituitary tumors. Therefore, measuring IGF-1 (Answer E) on an annual basis is not recommended. A history of GH deficiency in childhood might warrant testing in adulthood if symptoms of adult GH deficiency are present. Annual screening is not recommended in asymptomatic patients with Turner syndrome or asymptomatic adults with a history of childhood GH deficiency or treatment.

Educational Objective
Recommend appropriate screening in a woman with Turner syndrome.

UpToDate Topic Review(s)
Management of Turner syndrome in adults

Reference(s)

Gravholt CH, Anderson NH, Conway GS, et al; International Turner Syndrome Consensus Group. Clinical practice guidelines for the care of girls and women with Turner syndrome: proceedings from the 2016 Cincinnati International Turner Syndrome Meeting. *Eur J Endocrinol*. 2017;177(3):G1-G70. PMID: 28705803

85 ANSWER: C) Increase the basal insulin rate at midnight, 4 AM, and 4 PM

Self-monitoring of blood glucose is critical for patients with diabetes treated with insulin or antiglycemic medications that can cause hypoglycemia. For patients with type 1 diabetes, more frequent monitoring of glucose is needed to attain good glycemic control and to lower the risk of hypoglycemia.

Continuous glucose monitoring (CGM) has been available as an adjunct to fingerstick glucose testing for several years. CGM measures glucose in the interstitial fluid as opposed to the blood. Real-time CGM has been shown to improve glycemic control and quality of life, and it decreases the amount of time spent in hypoglycemia and hyperglycemia (ie, improves the time in the target range [usually 70-180 mg/dL (3.9-10.0 mmol/L)]) and lowers the risk of moderate to severe hypoglycemia in children and adults with type 1 diabetes treated with either insulin pump therapy or multiple daily insulin injections. Most of the real-time CGM devices available require daily calibration with fingerstick glucose testing. Patients who are well educated and comfortable with technology (eg, use smart phones and computers) are able to use CGM to gain insight into glucose trends before and after meals and during and after exercise. Finally, patients who are motivated and use CGM consistently most of the time (wearing the sensor for 6 or more days per week) have better glycemic control and less hypoglycemia than patients who use CGM intermittently.

Real-time CGM is especially useful for patients with hypoglycemia unawareness. An appropriate hemoglobin A_{1c} range for this patient is 7.5% to 8.0% (58-64 mmol/mol). Improvement in glucose control is warranted, but any changes in basal insulin rates and the insulin-to-carbohydrate ratio must be made judiciously.

Pattern recognition of glucose data from self-monitoring of blood glucose and CGM by both the provider and the patient can lead to improved glycemic control and a lowered risk of hypoglycemia. Reviewing the 2-week CGM tracing in this case demonstrates elevated and rising mean glucose levels from midnight to 6:30 AM. The glucose levels trend downward from 7:30 AM to 8 AM, then reach a reasonable level by midday. The glucose levels start to rise gradually at 2 PM and reach a peak at about 6 PM, then trend downward and are stable until midnight.

Changing the insulin-to-carbohydrate ratio from 1:10 to 1:8 for all meals (Answers A, B, and E) is inappropriate, as the glucose levels trend downward or are stable after breakfast and lunch. Providing a stronger insulin-to-carbohydrate ratio at dinner may be an acceptable treatment change, but the glucose levels start to rise at 4 PM and continue through 6:30 PM, so raising the basal insulin rate at 4 PM is more appropriate. Increasing the basal rate at midnight, 4 AM, and 7:30 AM (Answer D) is not appropriate, as the patient does not need a higher basal insulin rate at 7:30 AM because the glucose values trend downward. The most appropriate action in this case is to increase the basal insulin rates at midnight, 4 AM, and 4 PM (Answer C).

Educational Objective

Use glucose patterns from continuous glucose sensors to make appropriate changes in basal insulin and the insulin-to-carbohydrate ratio to optimize glucose control.

UpToDate Topic Review(s)

Self-monitoring of blood glucoses in management of adults with diabetes mellitus

Reference(s)

Juvenile Diabetes Research Foundation Continuous Glucose Monitoring Study Group. Effectiveness of continuous glucose monitoring in a clinical care environment: evidence from the Juvenile Diabetes Research Foundation continuous glucose monitoring (JDRF-CGM) trial. *Diabetes Care*. 2010;33(1):17-22. PMID: 19837791

Battelino T, Conget I, Olsen B, et al; SWITCH Study Group. The use and efficacy of continuous glucose monitoring in type 1 diabetes treated with insulin pump therapy: a randomized controlled trial, *Diabetologia*. 2012;55(12):3155-3162. PMID: 22965294

Danne T, Nimri R, Battelino T, et al. International consensus on use of continuous glucose monitoring. *Diabetes Care*. 2017;40(12):1631-1640. PMID: 29162583

Heinemann L, Freckmann G, Ehrmann D, et al. Real-time continuous glucose monitoring in adults with type 1 diabetes and impaired hypoglycaemia awareness or severe hypoglycaemia treated with multiple daily insulin injections (HypoDE): a multicentre, randomized controlled trial. *Lancet*. 2018;391(10128):1367-1377. PMID: 29459019

86

ANSWER: B) Low-calorie diet (1200 calories per day)

A diet plan is a key component of any weight-loss program. When discussing which meal plan is the most appropriate, one must consider the patient's food preferences, medical history, goals, and budget. It is important to explain that in order for weight loss to occur, the patient must have a negative energy balance. This reduction in intake can be achieved by following different dietary approaches (low-fat, high-protein, low-carbohydrate, etc). In most cases, weight loss is achieved when there is good adherence to the program regardless of the diet's macronutrient composition.

A patient following a very low-calorie diet (Answer A) eats a maximum of 800 calories/day and obtains all calories from meal replacements. This caloric restriction results in an average weight loss of 31 to 46.2 lb (14.2-21.0 kg) over 11 to 14 weeks. A very low-calorie diet is usually recommended when rapid weight loss is desired—for example, when patients must undergo surgery in the next 2 to 4 months and their weight is a contraindication to having the procedure. One of the problems with this diet is that it is usually only followed for a short period (about 12 weeks), and when the plan is stopped, weight regain occurs. This patient wants a long-term plan, so following a very low-calorie diet does not meet her needs.

The hallmark of a ketogenic diet (Answer C) is dietary restriction of carbohydrates (usually less than 20 to 50 g of carbohydrates per day) with unlimited intake of protein and fat. On average, patients following a ketogenic diet obtain 60% to 70% of their calories from fat. One study that included 64 participants with diabetes who followed a ketogenic diet for 56 weeks achieved weight loss of 56.8 ± 14.1 lb (25.8 ± 6.4 kg). There are no studies comparing a ketogenic diet with other types of diets. There is concern that ketogenic diets can raise LDL cholesterol, but data in this regard are mixed. It would be reasonable not to recommend this type of diet to someone with hypercholesterolemia (as this patient has) until there are more definitive data on the effect of a ketogenic diet on LDL cholesterol and non-HDL cholesterol.

When following a low-fat diet (Answer D), less than 20% of calories come from fat. In a meta-analysis, when a low-fat diet was compared with a typical diet, the group following the low-fat diet lost 11.9 lb (95% confidence interval [CI], 7.7-16.7 lb) (5.4 kg [95% CI, 3.5-7.6 kg]) more than the control group at 1 year; however, when the low-fat diet was compared with a higher-fat dietary plan at 1 year, there was no weight-loss difference between groups (−0.8 lb [95% CI, −1.5 to −3.0 lb]; −0.36 kg [95% CI, −0.66 to −1.37 kg]). This type of diet leads to lower LDL cholesterol without significant change in triglycerides or HDL cholesterol. Long-term adherence is poor when meal plans restrict fat intake. The low-fat diet offers no additional weight loss compared with other plans and it has the limitation of low long-term adherence. This patient followed a macronutrient-restricted meal plan in the past and she struggled with adherence, so a low-fat diet would not be the best plan to recommend.

When following a high-protein diet (Answer E), 25% to 30% of the daily energy requirement comes from protein. A meta-analysis comparing long-term weight loss between high- and low-protein diets found no significant difference in weight change between groups (−0.39 kg [95% CI, −1.43 to 0.65, P = 0.46]). Adherence to a high-protein diet is easier because protein increases satiety more than carbohydrates or fat, which can be helpful when trying to adhere to a plan with lower energy content. This meal plan could be a good choice for this patient, as it provides the same weight loss as lower-protein meal plans and has overall good adherence. However, the amount of protein recommended in this answer option (1 g/kg) is too much for someone with chronic kidney disease stage 3. If this patient wanted to follow a high-protein diet, her protein allowance would be 0.8 g/kg. When recommending a high-protein meal plan, patients must be reminded that they should adhere to lean proteins (chicken, fish, turkey) and avoid proteins high in fat, as the latter can increase their total calories and blunt weight loss. Patients following a high-protein diet must also restrict their number of daily calories to achieve weight loss.

General recommendations for a low-calorie diet (Answer B) are 1200 to 1500 kcal/d for women and 1500 to 1800 kcal/d for men. This can be further personalized by calculating the individual's caloric requirement using standardized formulas (for example the Mifflin-St. Jeor formula). An advantage of this plan is that there are no restrictions regarding macronutrients, so patients have more food choices and adherence is usually better. The only restriction patients have is the lower daily caloric allowance. Patients must have a daily calorie deficit of 500 calories to achieve, after 1 week, a weight loss of about 1 lb (0.5 kg). Given this patient's desire to follow a plan with less restrictions and good long-term adherence, this is the best recommendation.

There are no data regarding benefits on cardiovascular outcomes for any of the diet plans listed above.

Educational Objective
Recommend a dietary plan based on a patient's preferences and comorbidities.

Reference(s)

Bray GA, Heisel WE, Afshin A, et al. The science of obesity management: an Endocrine Society scientific statement. *Endocr Rev.* 2018;39(2):79-132. PMID: 29518206

Tobias DK, Chen M, Manson JE, Ludwig DS, Willett W, Hu FB. Effect of low-fat diet interventions versus other diet interventions on long-term weight change in adults: a systematic review and meta-analysis. *Lancet Diabetes Endocrinol.* 2015;3(120):968-979. PMID: 26527511

Schwingshackl L, Hoffmann G. Long-term effects of low-fat diets either low or high in protein on cardiovascular and metabolic risk factors: a systematic review and meta-analysis. *Nutr J.* 2013;12:48. PMID: 23587198

Clinical practice guidelines for nutrition in chronic renal failure. K/DOQI, National Kidney Foundation. *Am J Kidney Dis.* 2000;35(6 Suppl 2):S1-S140. PMID: 10895784

Paoli A. Ketogenic diet for obesity: friend or foe? *Int J Environ Res Public Health.* 2014;11(2):2092-2107. PMID: 24557522

Dashti HM, Mathew TC, Khadada M, et al. Beneficial effects of ketogenic diet in obese diabetic subjects. *Mol Cell Biochem.* 2007;302(1-2):249-256. PMID: 17447017

87 ANSWER: A) Start cinacalcet

This patient presents with a clinical constellation of longstanding hypercalcemia, bony pain, and elevated PTH, which could be consistent with a diagnosis of primary hyperparathyroidism. Additionally, because parathyroid imaging with technetium sestamibi is only approximately 80% sensitive for detecting parathyroid adenomas, a negative study, as in this woman's case, is inadequate to exclude a diagnosis of primary hyperparathyroidism. Nonetheless, this patient clearly has evidence of hypocalciuria (fractional excretion of calcium [FeCa] = 0.004; FeCa = urine calcium × serum creatinine / serum calcium × urine creatinine), which is more consistent with familial hypocalciuric hypercalcemia (FHH). Her biochemical profile of slightly elevated PTH (elevated in 15%-20% of patients with FHH) and magnesium (elevated due to enhanced renal reclamation) is also consistent with FHH. Confirmation of serum calcium elevation in first-degree relatives, which was not possible for this patient, would also support a diagnosis of FHH. Finally, genetic analysis could be pursued to search for pathogenic variants in the calcium-sensing receptor gene (*CASR*) and other genes that, when mutated, are mechanistically responsible for FHH (as detailed below). However, such testing may not be diagnostic, particularly in patients presenting with de novo disease.

FHH is an inherited disorder due to abnormal calcium sensing. Although most patients with FHH have inactivating pathogenic variants in the *CASR* gene, which encodes a classic G-protein–coupled receptor that tightly regulates PTH production and secretion by chief cells within the parathyroid gland and causes type 1 FHH, affected patients may also have pathogenic variants in the CASR-associated G protein alpha 11 gene (*GNA11*) (type 2 FHH) and in the adaptor-related protein complex 2 sigma 1 subunit gene (*AP2S1*) (type 3 FHH). In contrast to historical teaching, patients with FHH may have significant symptoms, including bone pain, muscle cramps, memory loss, or pancreatitis. Additionally, in vitro assessment to date has revealed that most patients with *CASR* pathogenic variants are sensitive to cinacalcet. Symptomatic patients with FHH appear to benefit from the use of cinacalcet at a dosage of 30 to 90 mg daily for up to 3 years. Therefore, a therapeutic trial of cinacalcet (Answer A) seems reasonable for this patient.

Given the apparent diagnosis of FHH and the absence of evidence for primary hyperparathyroidism, referral to an endocrine surgeon (Answer D) is inappropriate. Use of an intravenous bisphosphonate such as pamidronate (Answer C), which has some utility in neonatal severe hyperparathyroidism (due to homozygous mutations in *CASR*), has no role in the management of patients with FHH. Pregabalin (Answer B) is indicated for a diagnosis of fibromyalgia, which is not associated with hypercalcemia and is a diagnosis of exclusion. Finally, no further testing or treatment (Answer E) is not the best course of action given the patient's clinical presentation of symptomatic hypercalcemia.

Educational Objective

Explain the benefit of cinacalcet for patients with symptomatic hypercalcemia due to familial hypocalciuric hypercalcemia.

Disorders of the calcium-sensing receptor: Familial hypocalciuric hypercalcemia and autosomal dominant hypocalcemia

Reference(s)

Mayr B, Schnabel D, Dörr HG, Schöfl C. Genetics in endocrinology: gain and loss of function mutations of the calcium-sensing receptor and associated proteins: current treatment concepts. *Eur J Endocrinol.* 2016;174(5):R189-R208. PMID: 26646938

Rasmussen AQ, Jørgensen NR, Schwarz P. Clinical and biochemical outcomes of cinacalcet treatment of familial hypocalciuric hypercalcemia: a case series. *J Med Case Rep.* 2011;5:564. PMID: 22142470

88 ANSWER: A) TSH

This patient has papillary thyroid cancer with progressive distant metastases. His radioiodine scan was negative with no iodine-avid foci. Therefore, another radioiodine treatment is not recommended. Besides suppressive thyroid hormone therapy in patients with radioiodine-refractory differentiated thyroid cancer with distant metastases, tyrosine kinase inhibitor (TKI) therapy is now available. TKIs such as sunitinib, lenvatinib, sorafenib, motesanib, cabozantinib, and vandetanib have been studied in solid tumor and radioiodine-refractory thyroid cancer. TKIs are associated with numerous adverse effects, including diarrhea, fatigue, induced hypertension, liver toxicity, skin changes, nausea, increased levothyroxine dosage requirement, changes in taste, and weight loss. These adverse effects can have an impact on quality of life and require dosage reductions and even treatment discontinuation in some cases. Furthermore, these agents are also associated with more serious adverse effects such as thrombosis, bleeding, heart failure, hepatotoxicity, gastrointestinal tract fistula formation, and intestinal perforation. Currently, the incidence of TKI-induced hypothyroidism is estimated to be present in more than 50% of treated patients. Among cases of TKI-induced thyroid dysfunction, sunitinib has been the most studied medication. Desai et al reported on thyroid function in 42 euthyroid patients treated with sunitinib for imatinib-resistant gastrointestinal stromal tumors in a phase I/II trial. An abnormal TSH level was documented in 62% of patients: TSH was greater than 20 mIU/L in 21%, greater than 7.0 mIU/L in 14%, between 5.0 and 7.0 mIU/L in 17%, and less than 0.5 mIU/L in 10%.

Lenvatinib is a TKI that targets VEGFR1-3, FGFR1-4, PDGFR-α, RET, and c-KIT. Since 2015, lenvatinib has been FDA-approved in the United States for the treatment of radioiodine-refractory differentiated thyroid cancer with locally recurrent or metastatic progressive disease. In an international randomized, double-blind, phase III trial, this medication was associated with severe toxicities in 75% of patients and therapy-attributed mortality in 2.3%. Sorafenib is another TKI that has been FDA-approved for radioiodine-refractory differentiated thyroid cancer since 2013.

Several mechanisms have been proposed regarding how TKIs affect the hypothalamic-pituitary-thyroid axis, including thyroid gland integrity and thyroid hormone biosynthesis (capillary dysfunction caused by TKI leading to direct destruction of the thyroid gland); thyroid hormone transport (monocarboxylate transporter 8 [MCT8] inhibited by TKI); thyroid hormone metabolism (enhanced type 3 deiodinase activity); and TSH metabolism. Hypothyroidism may occur in patients with previously normal thyroid function tests and may be preceded by a destructive thyroiditis and transient suppression of TSH. In patients with preexisting hypothyroidism, thyroid hormone requirements may increase. TKIs can have effects on thyroid hormone metabolism. Accelerated conversion of T_4 to reverse T_3 due to activation of the D3 deiodinase enzyme has been suggested to be one of the mechanisms by which TKIs increase the levothyroxine requirement in hypothyroid patients. This is the case in this vignette. Additionally, TKIs can affect the activities of other deiodinases. The development of hypothyroidism during TKI therapy has been identified as an independent predictor of effectiveness in patients with other metastatic cancers such as renal cell carcinoma. The onset of TKI-induced thyroid dysfunction ranges from 4 to 94 weeks after treatment. Therefore, close monitoring of serum TSH (Answer A) is recommended in patients receiving TKI therapy.

Although TKIs can also cause adrenal insufficiency (more subclinical glucocorticoid deficiency than overt adrenal insufficiency), a recent publication showed that primary adrenal insufficiency can occur with lenvatinib treatment. Low or elevated glucose levels have been observed during TKI treatment.

This patient has normal blood pressure and heart rate and there are no electrolyte abnormalities. He probably does not have adrenal insufficiency, so cortisol measurement (Answer B) is not indicated. Lenvatinib does not cause vitamin D deficiency, so vitamin D measurement (Answer C) is not needed. As he has normal libido, he most likely has a normal testosterone level and does not require testosterone measurement (Answer D). He does not have symptoms of hypoglycemia or hyperglycemia, and his glucose level is normal. Therefore, measurement of hemoglobin A_{1c} (Answer E) is not indicated.

Educational Objective
Explain the effect of tyrosine kinase inhibitors on thyroid hormone levels.

UpToDate Topic Review(s)
Drug interactions with thyroid hormones

Reference(s)

Haugen BR, Alexander EK, Bible KC, et al. 2015 American Thyroid Association management guidelines for adult patients with thyroid nodules and differentiated thyroid cancer: the American Thyroid Association Guidelines Task Force on Thyroid Nodules and Differentiated Thyroid Cancer. *Thyroid*. 2016;26(1):1-133. PMID: 26462967

Illouz F, Braun D, Briet C, Schweizer U, Rodien P. Endocrine side-effects of anti-cancer drugs: thyroid effects of tyrosine kinase inhibitors. *Eur J Endocrinol*. 2014;171(3):R91-R99. PMID: 24833135

Desai J, Yassa L, Marqusee E, et al. Hypothyroidism after sunitinib treatment for patients with gastrointestinal stromal tumors. *Ann Intern Med*. 2006;145(9):660-664. PMID: 17088579

Rizzo LFL, Mana DL, Serra HA. Drug-induced hypothyroidism. *Medicina (B Aires)*. 2017;77(5):394-404. PMID: 29044016

Colombo C, De Leo S, Di Stefano M, Vannuchhi G, Persani L, Fugazzola L. Primary adrenal insufficiency during lenvatinib or vandetanib and improvement of fatigue after cortisone acetate therapy. *J Clin Endocrinol Metab*. 2019;104(3):779-784. PMID: 30383218

89   ANSWER: D) Improved bone density

The recently published Testosterone Trials (T-Trials) have provided substantial new data on organ-specific outcomes for testosterone treatment in older men. The T-Trials were a coordinated set of trials (a main trial and several substudies) conducted in the United States that included 790 men aged 65 years or older who were randomly assigned to receive transdermal testosterone (dosed to maintain serum testosterone within the normal range for healthy young men) or placebo for 12 months. Eligible participants had a baseline testosterone concentration less than 275 ng/dL (<9.5 nmol/L), averaged from at least 2 measurements, and at least 1 symptom or sign consistent with hypogonadism (eg, decreased libido, difficulty walking, or low vitality). Men with pathologic hypogonadism were excluded. Most men enrolled in the T-Trials had cardiovascular risk factors such as obesity (63%) and hypertension (72%), and men participating in the bone trial had normal bone mineral density as quantified by DXA, with T-scores ranging from –0.3 to 1.3 at baseline. The clinical characteristics of the patient in this vignette are similar to those of eligible T-trial participants.

In the bone trial, testosterone treatment substantially improved volumetric bone mineral density in the spine, increasing 6.8% more in testosterone-treated patients than in placebo-treated patients) (thus, Answer D is correct). Testosterone also improved estimated bone strength. The study was not powered for fracture outcomes.

In the main trial, testosterone treatment improved all aspects of sexual function (libido and sexual activity more so than erectile function) and improved mood and depressive symptoms to a small degree. Although men with marked symptoms of prostatic hypertrophy, defined as an International Prostate Symptom Score (a questionnaire assessing parameters such as urinary flow and nocturia) of more than 19 out of 35 were excluded, the change in the score did not differ significantly between the 2 groups (thus, Answer B is incorrect).

The mobility trial reported that testosterone therapy consistently improved self-reported walking ability and modestly improved walking distance. However, testosterone did not affect falls; fall frequency was identical between testosterone- and placebo-treated men (27% of patients in both groups had at least 1 fall) (thus, Answer A is incorrect).

The cardiovascular trial reported a greater increase in coronary plaque volume in testosterone-treated men than in placebo-treated men, raising a possible concern over adverse cardiovascular effects of testosterone (thus, Answer C is incorrect). While there was no difference in cardiovascular events between groups, the trial was not large enough or long enough to assess cardiovascular outcomes. Considering the literature as a whole, the evidence regarding cardiovascular effects of testosterone in older men remains inconclusive.

In the cognitive function trial, testosterone treatment did not improve aspects of cognition such as memory, spatial ability, recall, or global cognitive function (thus, Answer E is incorrect).

In the anemia trial, testosterone increased hemoglobin and corrected mild to moderate anemia.

While in men with organic hypogonadism, testosterone replacement is usually indicated irrespective of age, more research is needed to clarify the role for testosterone therapy in older men without organic hypogonadism. Of note, testosterone treatment is FDA-approved as replacement therapy only for men who have low testosterone levels due to disorders of the testicles, pituitary gland, or brain—conditions that cause organic hypogonadism. In most older men, low testosterone is a marker of poor health and should prompt a holistic approach with focus on lifestyle measures and optimization of comorbidities.

Educational Objective
Counsel older men regarding the expected effects of testosterone therapy.

UpToDate Topic Review(s)
Approach to older men with low testosterone

Reference(s)

Snyder PJ, Bhasin S, Cunningham GR, et al; Testosterone Trials Investigators. Effects of testosterone treatment in older men. *N Engl J Med.* 2016;374(7):611-624. PMID: 26886521

Snyder PJ, Bhasin S, Cunningham GR, et al. Lessons from the testosterone trials. *Endocr Rev.* 2018;39(3):369-386. PMID: 29522088

Grossmann M, Matsumoto AM. A perspective on middle-aged and older men with functional hypogonadism: focus on holistic management. *J Clin Endocrinol Metab.* 2017;102(3):1067-1075. PMID: 28359097

90 ANSWER: E) Overactive secretion of GLP-1

Bariatric surgery is increasing in popularity as a treatment for obesity. Although postoperative problems in the short-term are typically handled by the surgical team, postprandial hypoglycemia is commonly addressed by the primary care physician or the endocrinologist. In many situations, postprandial symptoms are mild and consist of nausea, bloating, or epigastric fullness. Less commonly, affected patients have adrenergic symptoms of tremors and shakiness. More severe manifestations are neuroglycopenic symptoms of hypoglycemia (ie, blurry vision, difficulty with memory, or delayed reaction time while driving). When evaluating patients with possible postprandial hypoglycemia, it is important to investigate whether the symptoms fulfill the Whipple triad (hypoglycemic symptoms, confirmed hypoglycemia by laboratory testing at the time of symptoms, and relief of symptoms after glucose ingestion). This vignette describes a patient who fulfills the Whipple triad.

Research into the mechanism of postprandial hypoglycemia after bariatric surgery is new. The typical pattern is hypoglycemia that occurs 1 to 3 hours after eating and occasionally after exercise. It rarely occurs during fasting. Although much research is still needed to understand the mechanism of this disorder, GLP-1 levels are up to 10-fold higher in patients after gastric bypass surgery, causing the β cells to have increased sensitivity to glucose. In the fasting state, the glucose level is low, resulting in minimal insulin release. In the context of high GLP-1 levels, the increase in postprandial glucose appears to trigger the pancreas to release excess insulin, causing hypoglycemia. Therefore, overactive secretion of GLP-1 (Answer E) is correct. Treatment of the condition includes avoiding high glycemic-index foods and possibly medications such as acarbose or octreotide in patients with debilitating symptoms. Use of continuous glucose monitoring may be helpful.

Although carbohydrates appear to be involved in triggering the insulin response (Answer A), it seems that postprandial hypoglycemia can be treated by modifying the type of carbohydrate (ie, consuming carbohydrates that have a low glycemic index). Malabsorption of carbohydrates or fat (Answers B and C) is not part of this syndrome. Insulinoma (Answer D) is associated with hypoglycemia during fasting.

Educational Objective
Discern the etiology of postprandial hypoglycemia after bariatric surgery.

UpToDate Topic Review(s)
Hypoglycemia in adults without diabetes mellitus: Clinical manifestations, diagnosis, and causes

Reference(s)

Busetto L, Dicker D, Azran C, et al. Practical recommendations of the Obesity Management Task Force of the European Association for the Study of Obesity for the post-bariatric surgery medical management. *Obes Facts*. 2017;10(6):597-632. PMID: 29207379

Lembo E, Lupoli R, Ciciola P, et al. Implementation of low glycemic index diet together with cornstarch in post-gastric bypass hypoglycemia: two case reports. *Nutrients*. 2018;10(6). pii:E670. PMID: 29799438

Patti M, Goldfine AB. Hypoglycemia after gastric bypass: The dark side of GLP-1. *Gastroenterology*. 2014;146(3):605-608. PMID: 24468184

Goldfine AB, Patti ME. How common is hypoglycemia after gastric bypass? *Obesity (Silver Spring)*. 2016;24(6):1210-1211. PMID: 27225595

Laguna Sanz AJ, Mulla CM, Fowler KM, et al. Design and clinical evaluation of a novel low-glucose prediction algorithm with mini-dose stable glucagon delivery in post-bariatric hypoglycemia. *Diabetes Technol Ther*. 2018;20(2):127-139. PMID: 29355439

91 ANSWER: A) Maintain current regimen

This patient has a macroprolactinoma causing central hypogonadism and central hypothyroidism. Dopaminergic therapy is the universally accepted treatment for macroprolactinomas. Two drugs are approved for this purpose in the United States: bromocriptine and cabergoline. Cabergoline is generally better tolerated and more effective than bromocriptine. Therefore, it is the drug of choice in this patient, particularly because the possible right-sided cavernous sinus invasion would make full surgical cure unlikely.

A 24-month prospective study of cabergoline outcomes in men with prolactinoma showed that the prolactin level normalized in 76.5% of patients without any difference between those with macroprolactinomas vs microprolactinomas, and that most patients achieved tumor shrinkage. Additionally, about two-thirds of the patients recovered from testosterone, GH, and ACTH deficiencies during treatment. Finally, sperm volume and number and serum testosterone normalized in all patients during the first 12 months, whereas motility normalized in more than 80% of patients after 24 months of dopaminergic therapy. Therefore (particularly because his thyroid axis has already normalized), the odds are good that this patient's testosterone level will recover in the next few months. Indeed, a delay in the timing of testosterone normalization after prolactin normalization has been reported in several studies. Therefore, particularly in view of his desired fertility (which would be reduced by testosterone replacement therapy [Answer C]), the best approach is to continue cabergoline therapy (Answer A) and reassess his testosterone level in the following months.

While hCG (Answer B) would most likely normalize his testosterone and increase his sperm count, this therapy is expensive and not yet justified. Similarly, clomiphene (Answer D) has been reported to increase testosterone in some patients with prolactinoma, but its use in men is off-label and not yet justified in this scenario. The use of aromatase inhibitors (Answer E) has been reported to be useful in patients with macroprolactinomas in whom testosterone therapy (by aromatization to estradiol) has caused tumor growth. This is not the case in this patient.

Educational Objective
Explain the timing of testosterone normalization in men with prolactinoma.

UpToDate Topic Review(s)
Management of hyperprolactinemia

Reference(s)

Melmed S, Casanueva FF, Hoffman AR, et al; Endocrine Society. Diagnosis and treatment of hyperprolactinemia: an Endocrine Society clinical practice guideline. *J Clin Endocrinol Metab*. 2011;96(2):273-288. PMID: 21296991

Walia R, Bhansali S, Dutta P, Khandelwal N, Sialy R, Bhadada S. Recovery pattern of hypothalamo-pituitary-testicular axis in patients with macroprolactinomas after treatment with cabergoline. *Indian J Med Res*. 2011;134(3):314-319. PMID: 21985814

De Rosa M, Zarrilli S, Vitale G, et al. Six months of treatment with cabergoline restores sexual potency in hyperprolactinemic males: an open longitudinal study monitoring nocturnal penile tumescence. *J Clin Endocrinol Metab*. 2004;89(2):621-625. PMID: 14764772

Colao A, Vitale G, Cappabianca P, et al. Outcome of cabergoline treatment in men with prolactinoma: effects of a 24-month treatment on prolactin levels, tumor mass, recovery of pituitary function, and semen analysis. *J Clin Endocrinol Metab*. 2004;89(4):1704-1711. PMID: 15070934

92 **ANSWER: C) Perform pelvic ultrasonography**

This woman developed androgenetic alopecia after menopause. Androgenetic alopecia is a common type of hair loss in men involving the anterior, mid, or temporal scalp and/or the vertex of the scalp. Menopause can be associated with symptoms of mild hirsutism because of relative excess ovarian androgen production from high postmenopausal gonadotropin levels, which is in contrast to the more abrupt fall in estrogens in menopause. In a premenopausal or postmenopausal woman, factors that increase concern for an androgen-producing tumor include new or significantly worsening hirsutism with a rapid pace or other signs of virilization such as voice deepening and clitoromegaly. In this case, the patient did not have any signs of virilization. However, it was reasonable to measure androgen concentrations in this patient because of the new symptoms and her level of concern. The normal range for total testosterone is not clearly defined for postmenopausal women, but it should be on the lower end of the reference range given the known decline in ovarian androgens produced during menopause. Therefore, this patient's mild elevation of total testosterone is more notable than it would be in a premenopausal woman. The DHEA-S level was mildly elevated, but this could represent conversion of androstenedione or testosterone to DHEA, which is then sulfated from the circulation by the adrenal gland, rather than suggesting an adrenal source. If the adrenal nodule were autonomously producing cortisol, one would observe lower-than-normal DHEA-S (usually <50 µg/dL [<1.4 µmol/L]) due to ACTH suppression.

Her total testosterone did not decrease after a 48-hour low-dose (2 mg) dexamethasone suppression test, so further evaluation for an ovarian tumor or increased volume (ovarian volume of 6 cc or greater indicating possible ovarian hyperthecosis) is the best next step. Pelvic ultrasonography (Answer C), not MRI (Answer E), is recommended at this point to evaluate the ovaries. However, MRI might be considered if a mass cannot be clearly seen on ultrasonography.

Even if a tumor is not specifically identified on ovarian ultrasound, ovarian pathology could still be the source of androgen excess. Leydig-cell tumors can present with symptoms of androgen excess even when not visible on imaging. Ovarian hyperthecosis is a non-neoplastic condition of androgen excess classically described by the presentation of significant and progressive hirsutism or virilization due to differentiation of ovarian interstitial cells into active luteinized theca cells capable of producing androstenedione and testosterone. It is more common in postmenopausal women and is associated with severe, progressive hirsutism or even virilization. Premenopausal women with ovarian hyperthecosis tend to have even more severe hirsutism or virilization with higher total testosterone concentrations. In some cases, ultrasonography might demonstrate homogeneous, hyperechogenic ovarian stroma. Especially in a postmenopausal woman, this might be more difficult to appreciate, and the diagnosis is often made by pathologic examination. Although the gold standard is a histologic diagnosis with nests of steroidogenically active luteinized stromal cells throughout the ovarian stroma, cases have also been described with normal ovarian histology. Other clinical features suggestive of ovarian hyperthecosis include postmenopausal status with symptoms of hyperandrogenism, ovarian volume of 6 cc or greater, or total testosterone concentration of 150 ng/dL or greater (≥5.2 nmol/L). Yet, as many as 50% of androgen-secreting ovarian tumors are associated with total testosterone levels less than 150 ng/dL (<5.2 nmol/L) and can be associated with normal ovarian volume.

Ovarian and adrenal venous sampling (Answer D) can be particularly helpful in distinguishing between an ovarian or adrenal source when an adrenal nodule/adenoma is present, or to confirm an ovarian source if imaging does not reveal a tumor or characteristics of ovarian hyperthecosis. This is a technically difficult test that should only be performed in a tertiary care center by an experienced interventional radiologist. However, adrenal tumors are a very rare cause of hirsutism in women. If pelvic ultrasonography reveals an ovarian mass, the next step would be to consult gynecology given the rare occurrence of adrenal tumors causing hirsutism or virilization.

If this patient's total testosterone had suppressed below 40% after a dexamethasone suppression test, initiation of therapy, such as spironolactone (Answer B), GnRH agonists (Answer A), oral contraceptives, or hormone replacement therapy, might have been considered to address symptoms.

Educational Objective
Diagnose and treat hirsutism in a postmenopausal woman presenting with an adrenal nodule.

UpToDate Topic Review(s)
Ovarian hyperthecosis
Female pattern hair loss (androgenetic alopecia in women): Treatment and prognosis

Reference(s)

Alpañés M, González-Casbas JM, Sánchez J, Pián H, Escobar-Morreale HF. Management of postmenopausal virilization. *J Clin Endocrinol Metab.* 2012;97(8):2584-2588. PMID: 22669303

Markopoulos MC, Kassi E, Alexandraki KI, Mastorakos G, Kaltsas G. Hyperandrogenism after menopause. *Eur J Endocrinol.* 2015;172(2):R79-R91. PMID: 25225480

Kaltsas GA, Isidori AM, Kola BP, et al. The value of the low-dose dexamethasone suppression test in the differential diagnosis of hyperandrogenism in women. *J Clin Endocrinol Metab.* 2003;88(6):2634-2643. PMID: 12788867

93 ANSWER: B) Add fenofibrate

Diabetic retinopathy is the most common cause for new-onset blindness and it affects a large proportion of patients with diabetes. While mild nonproliferative diabetic retinopathy is not associated with vision loss, more advanced forms of this disease are associated with loss of central vision due to macular edema, retinal detachment, and preretinal or vitreous hemorrhage. Therefore, there is a strong rationale to make efforts to reduce progression of eye disease. Factors associated with disease progression include duration of diabetes, glycemic control, blood pressure, and dyslipidemia. Further, higher levels of baseline retinopathy are associated with greater likelihood of progression.

This patient has characteristic dyslipidemia associated with retinal hard exudates and vision loss. Findings from 2 trials in patients with type 2 diabetes (FIELD [Fenofibrate Intervention and Event Lowering in diabetes] and ACCORD [Action to Control Cardiovascular Risk in Diabetes]) suggest that use of fenofibrate (Answer B) reduces the need for laser photocoagulation (hazard ratio, 0.69) and is associated with less macular edema (hazard ratio, 0.66) and less progression of diabetic retinopathy. This effect was lost after fenofibrate was stopped and was more pronounced in those with existing diabetic retinopathy. Taken together, there is evidence that fenofibrate at either a dosage of 160 mg daily or 200 mg daily may be helpful in reducing diabetic retinopathy progression. Fenofibrate is fibric acid derivative that is typically used to treat hypertriglyceridemia. The mechanism of action is thought to be related to agonism of PPAR-α, which reduces free fatty acid levels, inhibits formation of triglycerides and VLDLs, and also has antiinflammatory and antiangiogenic effects.

Blood pressure lowering is associated with 34% reduced progression of diabetic retinopathy as documented in the UKPDS (United Kingdom Prospective Diabetes Study), when mean systolic blood pressure is lowered from 154 to 144 mm Hg. However, more recent data from the ACCORD Eye Study suggest neither benefit nor harm from further lowering of systolic blood pressure from 140 to 120 mm Hg. Therefore, adding verapamil (Answer C) is unlikely to be helpful.

Epidemiologic investigations have determined that statin use may be associated with less diabetic retinopathy or reduced need for diabetic retinopathy treatments. Many large randomized controlled trials of statins have been conducted in patients with type 2 diabetes mellitus. A beneficial effect of statins on eye disease has not been shown, although these studies were not designed to address this question specifically. Therefore, increasing this patient's atorvastatin dosage (Answer A) is incorrect.

Given that platelet dysfunction exists in patients with diabetes and patients with diabetic retinopathy are at risk for retinal bleeding, numerous studies investigating the use of aspirin (Answer E) or dipyridamoles have been conducted in patients with diabetic retinopathy. A systematic review suggests that aspirin is neither beneficial nor harmful with regard to progression of diabetic retinopathy.

Finally, improved glycemic control has long been associated with reduced microvascular complications in both the DCCT (Diabetes Control and Complications Trial) and UKPDS studies. However, this patient already has good glycemic control and additional benefit from glycemic lowering is likely to be very modest and must be balanced against the risk of hypoglycemia. Therefore, adding a rapid-acting insulin analogue with meals (Answer D) is not the best choice for reducing progression of diabetic retinopathy.

Educational Objective
Recommend strategies to reduce the progression of diabetic retinopathy.

UpToDate Topic Review(s)
Diabetic retinopathy: Prevention and treatment

Reference(s)

Solomon SD, Chew E, Duh EJ, et al. Diabetic retinopathy: a position statement by the American Diabetes Association. *Diabetes Care*. 2017;40(3):412-418. PMID: 28223445

Bergerhoff K, Clar C, Richter B. Aspirin in diabetic retinopathy. A systematic review. *Endocrinol Metab North Am*. 2002;31(3):779-793. PMID: 12227131

94 ANSWER: A) TPO antibody titer

Multiple studies have attempted to determine the risk factors for developing hypothyroidism after lobectomy. The data available about the incidence of developing hypothyroidism and the need for thyroid hormone replacement after lobectomy are variable. This is in part due to different follow-up durations, different frequency of TSH assessments, different TSH cut-offs used to initiate levothyroxine therapy, and different rates of normalization of elevated TSH values when levothyroxine treatment was not initiated. However, 2 helpful meta-analyses are available and some consistent predictive factors have been identified. A 2012 meta-analysis by Verloop et al combined the results of 32 studies (comprising 4899 patients) and suggested that 22% of patients developed hypothyroidism. This analysis showed both TPO antibodies and lymphocytic infiltration to be significant predictors of the risk of developing hypothyroidism. The 2013 meta-analysis by Kandil et al also included 32 studies, most of which were also used in the Verloop analysis. These studies included 15,412 patients. The authors found predictors of hypothyroidism following lobectomy to be preoperative TSH values greater than 2.5 mIU/L, preoperative thyroid antibodies, and evidence of thyroiditis identified on pathology. A summary of the findings from this analysis is shown (*see box*).

Prediction Based on TPO Antibody Status
• Meta-analysis of 15,412 patients undergoing hemithyroidectomy, incidence of hypothyroidism in the included studies was 11% to 49%
• Preoperative thyroid antibodies pooled relative risk of hypothyroidism was 3.52 (95% confidence interval, 2.55-4.86)
• Thyroiditis on histopathology pooled relative risk of hypothyroidism was 3.30 (95% confidence interval, 2.49-4.36)

On the basis of these large analyses, TPO antibody titer (Answer A) is correct.

Some individual studies have examined additional risk factors for developing hypothyroidism after lobectomy. One study of 117 patients found that lymphocytic infiltration and germinal center formation within the resected thyroid lobe predicted the development of hypothyroidism. Hypothyroidism was defined as a TSH value greater than 7.0 mIU/L or a TSH value greater than 5.5 mIU/L with accompanying symptoms. Another study of 136 patients found that higher preoperative TSH values, presence of TPO antibodies, and lymphocytic infiltration of the thyroid lobe were all associated with the development of hypothyroidism. Hypothyroidism was defined either as overt hypothyroidism (TSH >4.0 mIU/L and free T_4 <0.7 ng/dL) or subclinical hypothyroidism (TSH >4.0 mIU/L, free T_4 >0.7 ng/dL) and symptoms. Preoperative free T_4 values (Answer B) and patient age were not identified as risk factors for developing hypothyroidism. Hypothyroidism generally developed 1 to 6 months after lobectomy. A study of 98 patients also found that a preoperative TSH value greater than 2.5 mIU/L and lymphocytic thyroiditis predicted ultimate development of hypothyroidism. Every unit increase in preoperative TSH increased the likelihood of needing postoperative thyroid hormone by 55%. The median time to postoperative thyroid hormone initiation was 16 months. An algorithm for monitoring for postlobectomy hypothyroidism has been proposed by Johner et al.

Regarding the other answer choices, preoperative total T_3 (Answer C) or free T_3 measurements were documented in some studies, but were not found to have predictive value. A repeated TSH measurement (Answer D) would allow this patient's TSH value to be confirmed, but the TSH value already provided was obtained recently, so a repeated measurement is likely to be similar. However, a more valuable piece of information could be obtained by measuring TPO antibodies. Thyroglobulin levels (Answer E) were only assessed in one study and were not found to be useful.

Educational Objective
List the risk factors for developing hypothyroidism following thyroid lobectomy.

UpToDate Topic Review(s)

Differentiated thyroid cancer: Overview of management

Reference(s)

Johner A, Griffith OL, Walker B, et al. Detection and management of hypothyroidism following thyroid lobectomy: evaluation of a clinical algorithm. *Ann Surg Oncol.* 2011;18(9):2548-2554. PMID: 21547704

Kandil E, Krishnan B, Noureldine SI, Yao L, Tufano RP. Hemithyroidectomy: a meta-analysis of postoperative need for hormone replacement and complications. *ORL J Otorhinolaryngol Relat Spec.* 2013;75(1):6-17. PMID: 23486083

Koh YW, Lee SW, Choi EC, et al. Prediction of hypothyroidism after hemithyroidectomy: a biochemical and pathological analysis. *Eur Arch Otorhinolaryngol.* 2008;265(4):453-457. PMID: 17978827

Morris LF, Iupe IM, Edeiken-Monroe BS, et al. Pre-operative ultrasound identification of thyroiditis helps predict the need for thyroid hormone replacement after thyroid lobectomy. *Endocr Pract.* 2013;19(6):1015-1020. PMID: 24013973

Verloop H, Louwerens M, Schoones JW, Kievit J, Smit JW, Dekkers OM. Risk of hypothyroidism following hemithyroidectomy: systematic review and meta-analysis of prognostic studies. *J Clin Endocrinol Metab.* 2012;97(7):2243-2255. PMID: 22511795

95   ANSWER: A) Vitamin D

In this clinical scenario, the 25-hydroxyvitamin D level is extremely low, in single digits, resulting in secondary hyperparathyroidism and an elevated alkaline phosphatase level. This suggests that the most likely diagnosis is nutritional osteomalacia rather than primary osteoporosis. Therefore, treatment with vitamin D replacement (Answer A) is the most appropriate initial therapy at this time.

Osteomalacia is characterized by decreased mineralization of newly formed osteoid at sites of bone turnover. Individuals with osteomalacia may present with bone pain, muscle weakness, and difficulty walking. In nutritional osteomalacia, laboratory abnormalities include a very low serum 25-hydroxyvitamin D level (<10 ng/mL [<25 nmol/L]), low to low-normal serum calcium and phosphate levels, high PTH and alkaline phosphatase levels, and low urinary calcium excretion. The serum concentration of 1,25-dihydroxyvitamin D may be normal, low, or high, depending on the severity and duration of vitamin D deficiency, and its measurement is therefore not helpful in making the diagnosis. Radiologic abnormalities may include markedly reduced bone density, Looser zones (or pseudofractures), and occasionally findings characteristic of secondary hyperparathyroidism, including subperiosteal resorption of the phalanges, bone cysts, and resorption of the distal ends of long bones.

Populations at risk for vitamin D deficiency include dark-skinned individuals, obese individuals, patients with malabsorption syndromes (such as gastric bypass or celiac disease), patients on anticonvulsant drug therapy, homebound older adults or institutionalized individuals who have little sun exposure, those with limited sun exposure due to clothing that covers most of the body or restrictions related to skin conditions, individuals with liver or kidney disease, and patients with cystic fibrosis.

Vitamin D supplementation in patients who are deficient leads to significant improvement in muscle strength and bone tenderness within weeks, with the effects being most dramatic when adequate calcium intake occurs simultaneously. In most cases, serum calcium and phosphate are normal after a few weeks of treatment, but alkaline phosphatase may remain elevated for several months. Bone mineral density improves within 3 to 6 months. Healing of osteomalacia is considered to have occurred when there are increases in urinary calcium excretion and bone mineral density and this can take many months to a year or more, varying with the degree and duration of the deficiency. Patients with osteomalacia associated with osteoporosis should undergo treatment for osteomalacia first; 6 to 12 months later, osteoporosis should be reevaluated and treated appropriately. Therefore, all the other listed options, including starting alendronate (Answer B), zoledronic acid (Answer C), denosumab (Answer D), or teriparatide (Answer E) in 3 months, all of which are approved therapies for osteoporosis, would not be appropriate. Furthermore, it is important to emphasize that antiresorptive osteoporosis therapy in the context of osteomalacia is contraindicated as it may aggravate the hypocalcemia.

Educational Objective

Identify nutritional osteomalacia as a cause of low bone density and fractures and recommend appropriate treatment.

Reference(s)

Lips P. Vitamin D deficiency and secondary hyperparathyroidism in the elderly: consequences for bone loss and fractures and therapeutic implications. *Endocr Rev.* 2001;22(4):477-501. PMID: 14493580

Holick MF, Siris ES, Binkley N, et al. Prevalence of vitamin D inadequacy among postmenopausal North American women receiving osteoporosis therapy. *J Clin Endocrinol Metab.* 2005;90(6):3215-3224. PMID: 15797954

Holick MF, Binkley NC, Bischoff-Ferrari HA, et al; Endocrine Society. Evaluation, treatment, and prevention of vitamin D deficiency: an Endocrine Society clinical practice guideline [published correction appears in *J Clin Endocrinol Metab.* 2011;96(12):3908]. *J Clin Endocrinol Metab.* 2011;96(7):1911-1930. PMID: 21646368

Lips P. Relative value of 25(OH)D and 1,25(OH)2D measurements. *J Bone Miner Res.* 2007;22(11):1668-1671. PMID: 17645404

96 ANSWER: A) Lorcaserin

Weight-loss medications are a tool to consider for patients who are participating in a weight-loss program for whom lifestyle changes are not providing the desired results. Candidates for weight-loss medications include individuals with a BMI of 27 kg/m² or greater and an obesity-related comorbidity or those with a BMI of 30 kg/m² or greater. The patient described in this vignette is struggling with hunger, so to help her weight-loss efforts it was appropriate to start a medication that targets this symptom. When deciding which medication to choose, it is important to consider adverse effects, adverse reactions, contraindications, drug interaction, route of administration, cost, and patient preference. Given the patient's symptoms (tremors, diaphoresis, and diarrhea) and her regular use of paroxetine, this patient was most likely started on lorcaserin (Answer A). She experienced a mild form of serotonin syndrome.

Lorcaserin is a selective serotonin-2C receptor agonist that binds to serotonin-2C receptors on proopiomelanocortin/cocaine- and amphetamine-responsive transcript neurons in the arcuate nucleus of the hypothalamus. This binding triggers the release of α-melanocyte–stimulating hormone, which leads to appetite suppression. This medication is approved for long-term weight management and there are 2 formulations available: an immediate-release (10-mg tablet twice daily) and an extended release (20-mg tablet once daily).

The most common adverse effects associated with lorcaserin are headaches, upper respiratory tract infections, nasopharyngitis, dizziness, and dry mouth. Other than pregnancy, there are no contraindications to taking this medication. However, prescribers should use the medication with caution in patients who are also taking selective serotonin reuptake inhibitors, serotonin and norepinephrine reuptake inhibitors, monoamine oxidase inhibitors, bupropion, and St. John's wort, as taking these medications together may increase the risk of developing serotonin syndrome.

Serotonin syndrome is a drug reaction due to excess of serotonergic agonism of central and peripheral serotonergic receptors. Affected patients present with a range of symptoms that have an acute onset after a change in medication. Milder forms include tremors, diaphoresis, and diarrhea. Moderate cases include tachycardia, hypertension, and hyperthermia. In severe cases, patients have agitated delirium, hypertonicity, muscular rigidity, and life-threatening hyperthermia (core body temperature >106°F). Most cases of mild serotonin syndrome are missed because of variable and unspecific symptoms. Therefore, clinicians must have a high degree of suspicion when patients are using 2 serotoninergic agents and present with the symptoms described above. Management of serotonin syndrome includes removal of the precipitating agents, supportive care, and, in severe cases, control of agitation, hyperthermia, and autonomic instability and administration of serotonin antagonists. Once the patient's condition is stable, it is important to contact the physician who was prescribing the serotoninergic agent to assess whether a different medication should be started.

Lorcaserin's product insert states that the safety of its use with other serotonergic agents has not been evaluated. Caution and observation are recommended when using lorcaserin in combination with another serotoninergic agent.

Liraglutide (a GLP-1 analogue) (Answer B), phentermine (a sympathomimetic amine) (Answer C), orlistat (an inhibitor of gastric and pancreatic lipase) (Answer D), and topiramate (a GABA agonist) (Answer E) are not serotonergic agents, so they cannot cause serotonin syndrome when administered in conjunction with a selective serotonin reuptake inhibitor.

To help this patient with her weight-loss efforts, she could be offered a different weight-loss medication. Given that she is struggling with hunger, orlistat would not be the best choice. This medication works by decreasing fat absorption, not by decreasing hunger. Topiramate by itself is not FDA approved for weight loss; however, it is used off label for patients who struggle with cravings. Because the patient has other FDA-approved treatment options, topiramate would not be the first choice. Medications she could try next include liraglutide or phentermine. Both are FDA approved for weight loss. Cost, adverse effects, and route of administration are factors that will help determine which medication to try next.

Educational Objective
Identify symptoms of serotonin syndrome in a patient who is taking 2 serotoninergic agents.

UpToDate Topic Review(s)
Serotonin syndrome (serotonin toxicity)

Reference(s)

Greenway FL, Shanahan W, Fain R, Ma T, Rubino D. Safety and tolerability review of lorcaserin in clinical trials. *Clin Obes.* 2016;6(5):285-295. PMID: 27627785

Boyer EW, Shannon M. The serotonin syndrome [published corrections appear in *N Engl J Med.* 2007;356(23):2437 and *N Engl J Med.* 2009;361(17):1714]. *N Engl J Med.* 2005;352(11):1112-1120. PMID: 15784664

Nguyen CT, Zhou S, Shanahan W, Fain R. Lorcaserin in obese and overweight patients taking prohibited serotonergic agents: a retrospective analysis. *Clin Ther.* 2016;38(6):1498-1509. PMID: 27206567

97 ANSWER: D) Stop insulin glargine and start mixed insulin (70/30) twice daily

Hereditary hemochromatosis (HH) is an autosomal recessive disorder that can lead to abnormal absorption of iron from the gut with subsequent development of iron overload. Most patients with HH are homozygous for a single nucleotide substitution (C282Y) in the hemochromatosis gene (*HFE*), which encodes a major histocompatibility complex class-I molecule. Iron deposition in the liver, pancreas, heart, skin, joints, and pituitary gland results in end-organ damage. Iron overload in the pancreas can lead to apoptosis and impaired insulin release by β cells. Animal and human studies have shown that HH also increases insulin resistance. The iron overload can be manifested by hepatomegaly, elevated transaminases, and an increased risk for fibrosis and cirrhosis. Patients who present with "bronze diabetes" accumulate iron in the skin and have the triad of cirrhosis, diabetes mellitus, and hyperpigmentation of the skin (bronze coloration). This is a late manifestation of the disease and it has become less prevalent over time.

HH should be suspected in patients with chronic liver disease, cardiac enlargement, diabetes mellitus, hypogonadism, and other manifestations and in families that have an iron overload syndrome. Liver biopsy is the gold standard in diagnosing cirrhosis in patients with iron overload.

The frequency of diabetes in patients with clinical hemochromatosis ranges from 20% to 50%. With earlier screening for HH, the prevalence of diabetes has decreased over time. The patient in this vignette has HH and was diagnosed with diabetes 7 years ago. He is being treated with insulin glargine and metformin. Metformin is safe in the treatment of diabetes in patients with compensated cirrhosis, but it would need to be stopped if the cirrhosis worsens or if he is hospitalized.

Due to the cirrhosis, red blood cell survival time is reduced in this case. Therefore, hemoglobin A_{1c} is not reliable as a measure of glycemic control. Recommending no changes to his management on the basis of his hemoglobin A_{1c} value (Answer E) is incorrect. Review of fingerstick glucose data is a more appropriate method to manage this patient's diabetes. In this vignette, his fasting glucose values are well controlled, but his glucose levels increase throughout the course of each day. Increasing the insulin glargine dose (Answer C) would most likely lead to only minor improvement in his nonfasting glucose levels and could increase the risk of nocturnal hypoglycemia. Switching from basal insulin to a premixed insulin given twice daily (Answer D) would allow for better control of fasting and daytime glucose levels and is the correct answer.

Adding an SGLT-2 inhibitor such as empagliflozin (Answer A) to the treatment regimen would most likely improve this patient's glycemic control without resorting to intensified insulin therapy. However, SGLT-2 inhibitors increase the risk of developing urinary tract infections and candidiasis and would not be a good choice given that he has had recurrent urinary tract infections. There are no randomized controlled clinical trials using GLP-1 analogues such as dulaglutide (Answer B) or SGLT-2 inhibitors in the treatment of patients with cirrhosis and diabetes.

Educational Objective
Identify secondary form of diabetes, including hemochromatosis, and determine when it is appropriate to intensify insulin therapy.

UpToDate Topic Review(s)
Clinical manifestations and diagnosis of hereditary hemochromatosis.

Reference(s)

Utzschneider KM, Kowdley KV. Hereditary hemochromatosis and diabetes mellitus: implications for clinical practice. *Nature Rev Endocrinol.* 2010;6(1):26-33. PMID: 20010968

McClain DA, Abraham D, Rogers J, et al. High prevalence of abnormal glucose homeostasis secondary to decreased insulin secretion in individuals with hereditary haemochromatosis. *Diabetologia.* 2006;49(7):1661-1669. PMID: 16538487

Clar C, Gill JA, Court R, Waugh N. Systematic review of SGLT2 receptor inhibitors in dual or triple therapy in type 2 diabetes. *BMJ Open.* 2012;2(5):pii:e001007. PMID: 23087012

98 ANSWER: E) Start levothyroxine

Patients with pituitary adenomas can develop partial or total pituitary failure. This means that they can lack the function of one or more axes, but also that the individual axis failure may be partial. This patient has had longstanding central hypogonadism, but had documented otherwise normal pituitary function. After surgery, MRI shows a resection cavity and midline pituitary stalk, but the volume of the normal pituitary is rather small. He therefore may have failure of another axis. The GH axis is most likely to be affected, but others should be considered. A random serum cortisol value greater than 15 μg/dL (>413.8 nmol/L) correlates with a normal result on cosyntropin-stimulation testing. His morning cortisol value rules out adrenal insufficiency. Therefore, repeating a cosyntropin-stimulation test (Answer A) is not necessary.

When interpreting thyroid function tests in patients who are known or suspected to have a malfunctioning pituitary gland, one cannot rely on TSH levels, but must rather consider symptoms and free T_4 levels. "Normal" free T_4 levels are a population range, but the free T_4 level is relatively stable in each person. Therefore, in the absence of established predisease historical values for an individual patient, the general recommendation in patients with central hypothyroidism is to maintain free T_4 levels in the mid to upper reference range. Because this patient's free T_4 is at the low end of normal (and the presurgery free T_4 level is not available), the most logical and inexpensive approach is to start levothyroxine therapy (Answer E) and monitor symptoms and free T_4 levels. Because levothyroxine replacement causes a peak concentration about 2 to 4 hours after ingestion, blood should be drawn for laboratory tests before the ingestion of levothyroxine tablets to avoid measuring at peak levels.

This patient's testosterone level is normal and age appropriate. To date, there is no evidence that bringing the testosterone level into the upper normal range or changing its delivery method helps with fatigue. Therefore, increasing the testosterone dosage (Answer C) or switching to injectable testosterone (Answer E) is incorrect.

While this patient has a high likelihood of being GH deficient, optimization of thyroid status should be done before considering a GH-stimulation test (Answer B). This could be considered in the future, but it would not be the best next step now.

Educational Objective
Interpret tests of pituitary function and explain how central hypothyroidism can occur even when free T_4 is within normal limits.

UpToDate Topic Review(s)
Treatment of hypopituitarism

Reference(s)

Fleseriu M, Hashim IA, Karavitaki N, et al. Hormonal replacement in hypopituitarism in adults: an Endocrine Society clinical practice guideline. *J Clin Endocrinol Metab.* 2016;101(11):3888-3921. PMID: 27736313

Beck-Peccoz P, Rodari G, Giavoli C, Lania A. Central hypothyroidism - a neglected thyroid disorder. *Nat Rev Endocrinol.* 2017;13(10):588-598. PMID: 28549061

de Carvalho GA, Paz-Filho G, Mesa Junior C, Graf H. Management of endocrine disease: pitfalls on the replacement therapy for primary and central hypothyroidism in adults. *Eur J Endocrinol.* 2018;178(6):R231-R244. PMID: 29490937

99 ANSWER: D) Long-duration taper (weeks-to-months) of supplemental glucocorticoid therapy

This patient has Cushing syndrome, biochemically confirmed hypercortisolism, and an undetectable ACTH level in this context. Collectively, these findings indicate ACTH-independent hypercortisolism and implicate an adrenal cause. The abdominal CT indicates a unilateral right-sided adenoma and the treatment of choice is right-sided adrenalectomy to cure the hypercortisolism.

Although this patient is hypercortisolemic now, postoperatively she is expected to manifest secondary adrenal insufficiency and will need supplemental glucocorticoids. Excess cortisol secretion from the adrenal adenoma will result in suppression of corticotropin-releasing hormone and ACTH, and consequently this ACTH deficiency will result in decreased stimulation of the contralateral adrenal cortex. With prolonged ACTH deficiency, as has likely been the case for this patient, the contralateral zona fasciculata will gradually atrophy since ACTH is not only a secretagogue of cortisol, but also a trophic factor. Importantly, aldosterone production is regulated by angiotensin II and potassium in addition to ACTH, and therefore should remain normal despite ACTH deficiency. Thus, this patient will need glucocorticoid, but not mineralocorticoid (Answers C and E), supplementation.

The chronic suppression of the hypothalamic-pituitary-adrenal (HPA) axis by endogenous or exogenous glucocorticoids can result in a deep inhibition in the ability to secrete corticotropin-releasing hormone and ACTH that can take weeks to months to recover, even when glucocorticoid levels have fallen to subphysiologic levels. In parallel, chronic deficiency of ACTH can result in a deep inhibition of the zona fasciculata that can similarly take weeks to months to fully recover since it relies on normalization of, and exposure to, physiologic and/or supraphysiologic ACTH levels.

The time required for the HPA axis to recover depends on several factors. The severity and duration of hypercortisolism are possibly the most important determinants; patients with severe hypercortisolism and multiple metabolic abnormalities consistent with Cushing syndrome have the most profound suppression of the HPA axis that may take many months to recover fully. It is anticipated that this patient may need many months, possibly even 1 year or more, to withdraw fully from supplemental glucocorticoids and have a normally functioning HPA axis (Answer D). Another concomitant factor is the amount of supplemental glucocorticoids prescribed postoperatively and the patient's tolerance to tapering the dosage. Often, patients with Cushing syndrome have acclimatized to supraphysiologic glucocorticoid exposure and need higher dosages of glucocorticoids immediately postoperatively. The ability to taper these dosages is often limited by the symptoms of relative adrenal insufficiency experienced by the patient (such as fatigue, nausea, difficulty thinking, etc) and can prolong the time to full HPA axis recovery.

Options to assess HPA axis recovery include measurement of morning cortisol and ACTH 24 hours following the last dose of a glucocorticoid such as hydrocortisone or prednisone. After adrenalectomy, this patient had a morning cortisol value of 2.0 µg/dL (55.2 nmol/L) with an ACTH value less than 5 pg/mL (<1.1 pmol/L) 3 days following adrenalectomy, indicating a fully suppressed HPA axis. She was treated with hydrocortisone and, 3 months later, after holding her hydrocortisone dose of 15 mg daily for 24 hours, her morning ACTH concentration was 77 pg/mL (10-60 pg/mL) (SI: 16.9 pmol/L [2.2-13.2 pmol/L]) with a morning cortisol concentration of 4.0 µg/dL (110.4 nmol/L), indicating a supraphysiologic surge in ACTH in response to decreasing hydrocortisone doses, but insufficient cortisol production from the zona fasciculata (ie, an endogenous cosyntropin-stimulation test). Six months postoperatively, she stopped taking all exogenous glucocorticoids, and her morning cortisol concentration was 15.0 µg/dL (413.8 µg/dL) with an ACTH concentration of 33 pg/mL (7.3 pmol/L), indicating a relatively normal HPA axis. Alternatively, the HPA axis and adrenal responses can be monitored with serial cosyntropin-stimulation tests.

Educational Objective

Guide the postoperative management of adrenal Cushing syndrome.

Reference(s)

Hurtado MD, Cortes T, Natt N, Young WF Jr, Bancos I. Extensive clinical experience: hypothalamic-pituitary-adrenal axis recovery after adrenalectomy for corticotropin-independent cortisol excess. *Clin Endocrinol (Oxf)*. 2018;89(6):721-733. PMID: 29968420

100 ANSWER: B) Methimazole and prednisone

This patient with a history of coronary artery disease and mitral valve insufficiency developed atrial fibrillation following mitral valve replacement and maze surgery and requires amiodarone treatment. Despite amiodarone, his atrial fibrillation persists and his heart rate remains uncontrolled. Thyroid function tests are ordered and the results are consistent with hyperthyroidism. This patient has amiodarone-induced thyrotoxicosis (AIT).

Amiodarone is a common drug used in the treatment of refractory atrial or ventricular arrhythmias. Amiodarone has a high iodine content, which is 37% of its molecular weight. The half-life of this medication is 100 days. AIT occurs in up to 6% of patients taking amiodarone in iodine-sufficient areas and in up to 10% in iodine-deficient areas. There are 2 proposed mechanisms for the development of AIT: type 1 AIT, which is defined as iodine-induced hyperthyroidism due to the high iodine content of amiodarone and type 2 AIT, which is a destructive thyroiditis due to direct toxicity of amiodarone in follicular cells. Type 1 AIT usually occurs in patients with underlying thyroid autonomy such as Graves disease or nodular goiter, whereas type 2 AIT occurs as a result of direct damage of follicular cells by amiodarone. In many cases, mixed forms of AIT exist, making both diagnosis and treatment challenging. A color-flow Doppler study can distinguish between type 1 AIT (increased vascularity) and type 2 AIT (absent vascularity). However, interpretation of color-flow Doppler requires an experienced sonographer. It has been reported that the onset of thyrotoxicosis was significantly earlier in type 1 AIT (median of 3.5 months) compared with that of type 2 AIT (median 30 months). If thyrotoxicosis occurs after amiodarone has been stopped, the diagnosis is usually type 2 AIT.

Antithyroid drugs are used to treat type 1 AIT, whereas corticosteroids are used to treat type 2 AIT. Combined antithyroid drugs and corticosteroid therapy should be initiated in patients with AIT who are clinically unstable, in patients who did not respond to single treatment, or when the etiology of thyrotoxicosis cannot be determined.

In this case, the patient's thyroid gland is palpable and irregular and his TSH concentration was 0.5 mIU/L 1 year ago. He has nodular goiter, possibly with some degree of autonomy. The high iodine content of amiodarone could have caused him to become hyperthyroid (ie, type 1 AIT). However, his 24-hour thyroid uptake is low, which is commonly observed in type 2 AIT, but it can be seen in type 1 AIT due to the large amount of iodine in amiodarone. He has shortness of breath at rest and a rapid heart rate despite medical therapy. Therefore, the best option is to initiate combination therapy with methimazole and prednisone (Answer B) because the etiology of thyrotoxicosis cannot be determined with certainty and he is symptomatic clinically. Prescribing only methimazole (Answer A) or only prednisone (Answer C) is incorrect. In general, if patients respond quickly to combination therapy, this would favor type 2 AIT and methimazole can be stopped. However, steroids should be continued for several months with slow taper. If patients do not respond quickly to combination therapy, methimazole should be continued along with steroids and when thyroid hormone levels start decreasing, steroids can be stopped.

Patients with AIT who fail to respond to medical therapy should be offered thyroidectomy. While thyroidectomy in this setting has a high mortality rate (9%), delay or deferral of thyroid surgery has a higher risk of death. If amiodarone is discontinued in patients with AIT, definitive therapy with radioiodine treatment or thyroid surgery should be recommended to facilitate reinitiation of amiodarone.

Radioiodine treatment (Answer E) can be recommended for patients with type 1 AIT who have a high 24-hour thyroid uptake. This patient's 24-hour thyroid uptake is low. Therefore, radioiodine treatment would not be appropriate now. Amiodarone has a long half-life, so radioiodine treatment can only be prescribed several months after discontinuation of amiodarone.

Educational Objective

Manage amiodarone-induced thyrotoxicosis.

UpToDate Topic Review(s)
Amiodarone and thyroid dysfunction

Reference(s)

Ross DS, Burch HB, Cooper DS, et al. 2016 American Thyroid Association guidelines for diagnosis and management of hyperthyroidism and other causes of thyrotoxicosis. *Thyroid.* 2016;26(10):1343-1421. PMID: 27521067

Tomisti L, Rossi G, Bartalena L, Martino E, Bogazzi F. The onset time of amiodarone-induced thyrotoxicosis (AIT) depends on AIT type. *Eur J Endocrinol.* 2014;171(3):363-368. PMID: 24935933

101 ANSWER: D) Administer a correction bolus via insulin syringe

Insulin pumps are now in widespread use for both type 1 and type 2 diabetes. Pumps deliver insulin continuously, thereby providing both basal insulin and nutritional and correction dosing based on user input. Some pumps are integrated with continuous glucose monitors. For others, such as the one used by the patient in this vignette, the user enters blood glucose values obtained via fingerstick monitoring. Many users prefer insulin pumps to multiple daily injections.

Insulin pumps deliver insulin stored in a reservoir through an infusion set and a cannula inserted subcutaneously. Mechanical problems with a pump can lead to interruption of insulin delivery and metabolic effects. Blockages in the infusion set or cannula or heat exposure of the insulin in the reservoir can affect insulin delivery. Temperature extremes (both high and low) can lead to denaturing of the insulin. Insulin in the reservoir and infusion sets should be replaced every 3 days to limit risk of heat inactivation and/or infusion blockages. However, this patient reports changing her infusion set yesterday. While many pumps alert or alarm if an insulin blockage is detected, this is not always completely reliable. Lack of insulin for as few as 60 minutes in a patient with type 1 diabetes can lead to hyperglycemia and development of diabetic ketoacidosis. The patient in this vignette has rising blood glucose and positive urine ketones despite a lack of alerts/alarms on the pump and reported use of insulin boluses and may be evolving into mild ketoacidosis. The rates of adverse pump events vary by population studied and provider experience, with some studies finding increased and some decreased rates of ketoacidosis among individuals using insulin pumps compared with individuals using multiple daily injections. Thus, all pump users should receive comprehensive instruction in troubleshooting insulin delivery problems.

The answer options provided are all potential actions for this patient to take. However, the most important thing to do now is to deliver a dose of fast-acting insulin via an insulin syringe (Answer D) to prevent worsening of ketosis. Using an insulin syringe guarantees insulin delivery, whereas administering increased insulin via the pump (Answer B), even if the insulin, reservoir, and infusion set are all changed (Answer C) would not guarantee delivery. Moreover, the delay in changing out her insulin sets would extend her period of insulin deficiency and increase her risk for progressing to overt ketoacidosis. Administering long-acting insulin (Answer E) may be needed, but this is not the best next step due to its extended action; this patient needs fast-acting insulin now. While she has positive urinary ketones, she does not necessarily need to seek emergency medical care at this point (Answer A). As long as she can tolerate oral fluids and receive insulin via injection, she may be able to reverse her present course and avoid worsened ketoacidosis. She should be advised to drink water and to monitor her blood glucose hourly until she is normoglycemic. She can then either restart the insulin pump (changing the insulin, infusion set, and infusion site is recommended) and closely monitor her glucose readings to ensure insulin delivery or revert to insulin syringes for administration of basal and bolus insulin until the pump can be checked by the manufacturer. She should also monitor urine ketones to make sure they resolve.

All patients using insulin pumps should ensure they have a few insulin syringes or insulin pen/needle devices available as back-up in case of pump failure, and they should be trained to switch to insulin injections if there is the potential for pump delivery failure. Reminding patients of their basal and bolus doses and the importance of carrying back-up supplies when traveling is important.

Educational Objective

Manage unexplained hyperglycemia in patients with type 1 diabetes who are on insulin pump therapy.

UpToDate Topic Review(s)
Management of blood glucose in adults with type 1 diabetes mellitus

Reference(s)

Pickup JC. Insulin-pump therapy for type 1 diabetes mellitus. *N Engl J Med*. 2012;366(17):1616-1624. PMID: 22533577

Pala L, Dicembrini I, Mannucci E. Continuous subcutaneous insulin infusion vs modern multiple injection regimens in type 1 diabetes: an updated meta-analysis of randomized clinical trials. *Acta Diabetol*. 2019;56(9):973-980. PMID: 30945047

102 ANSWER: E) Add evolocumab

Familial hypercholesterolemia is an autosomal dominant disorder characterized by very high blood LDL-cholesterol levels. The condition is due to pathogenic variants in the genes involved in LDL-receptor–mediated cholesterol uptake pathways, including *LDLR*, *APOB*, and *PCSK9*. The severity of the phenotype depends on residual LDL-receptor activity. Pathogenic variants in the *LDLR* gene are the most common cause of elevated LDL-cholesterol levels in patients with familial hypercholesterolemia. Most individuals with familial hypercholesterolemia are heterozygous for mutations in one of the genes and therefore, have heterozygous familial hypercholesterolemia.

The lifetime exposure to high cholesterol levels is independently associated with a high risk of cardiovascular disease in patients with heterozygous familial hypercholesterolemia. Treatment involves starting lipid-lowering therapy as early as possible. In addition to lifestyle modification, LDL-cholesterol lowering using statins is first-line therapy, with a goal of at least 50% reduction in LDL-cholesterol levels. When LDL-cholesterol–lowering targets cannot be reached by statins alone, other drug therapies are added.

Evolocumab (Answer E) is a proprotein convertase subtilisin/kexin type 9 (PCSK9) inhibitor antibody that lowers LDL cholesterol. PCSK9 is a serine protease that is secreted by the liver and targets the LDL receptor for degradation. Monoclonal antibodies such as evolocumab and alirocumab bind to PCSK9 and prevent LDL-receptor degradation, leading to more available LDL receptors and therefore lower LDL-cholesterol levels in the blood. When a PCSK9 inhibitor is added to high-intensity statin therapy, up to 100% of PCSK9 is bound by the antibody, resulting in a 50% reduction in LDL cholesterol. A recent randomized controlled trial of evolocumab vs placebo added to regimens of individuals with known atherosclerotic cardiovascular disease (ASCVD) already receiving statin therapy showed a 15% reduction in cardiovascular events. Similarly, alirocumab added to statin therapy 1 to 10 months postacute coronary syndrome showed a 15% relative risk reduction of cardiovascular events. Currently, PCSK9 inhibitors are approved for use in patients with heterozygous familial hypercholesterolemia, as well as in patients with known cardiovascular disease who are on a maximum tolerated statin dosage and need further LDL-cholesterol lowering due to the presence of additional cardiovascular risk factors. PCSK9 inhibitor therapy does not appear to affect glycemic control. Before the availability of PCSK9 inhibitors, multiple drug combination therapy was used for LDL-cholesterol lowering in individuals with familial hypercholesterolemia. Despite the higher cost of PCSK9 therapy and burdensome prior authorization process, this patient should be offered treatment with evolocumab in combination with statin therapy due to his high-risk status (diabetes, ASCVD). Niacin and ezetimibe can be discontinued after starting injectable therapy.

Two large cardiovascular disease outcome trials (AIM-HIGH [Atherothrombosis Intervention in Metabolic Syndrome with Low HDL/High Triglycerides: Impact on Global Health Outcomes] and HPS2-THRIVE [Heart Protection Study 2-Treatment of HDL to Reduce the Incidence of Vascular Events]), studied the use of extended-release niacin formulations added to statins, and both failed to show clinical ASCVD benefit. These studies were conducted in individuals with known ASCVD who were on statin therapy with the goal of raising HDL cholesterol, and they highlighted several safety effects of niacin. Worsening insulin resistance can develop with high niacin dosages. Therefore, ongoing niacin therapy cannot be recommended for this patient who has impaired fasting glucose.

Marine omega-3 fatty acids (Answer B) (eicosapentaenoic acid, C20:5n-3 [EPA] and docosahexaenoic acid, C22:6n-3 [DHA]) lower fasting and postprandial triglyceride levels in a dosage-dependent fashion by decreasing VLDL synthesis and increasing catabolism. A recent clinical trial (REDUCE-IT [Reduction of Cardiovascular Events with EPA-Intervention Trial]) showed significant reduction in major adverse cardiovascular events with the addition of pure EPA to statin therapy in individuals with known ASCVD or diabetes with additional risk factors. In this study, individuals had relatively well-controlled LDL-cholesterol levels and moderate triglyceride elevations (baseline triglycerides ~216 mg/dL [2.44 mmol/L]). Although the patient in this vignette has known ASCVD, he does not have elevated triglycerides and therefore there is no indication to add omega-3 fatty acids now.

Metformin (Answer C) is the first-line therapy for type 2 diabetes and it can beneficially influence body weight, lipid profile, and liver fat. The United Kingdom Prospective Diabetes Study reported that use of metformin monotherapy in obese patients with type 2 diabetes decreased cardiovascular disease–related endpoints such as myocardial infarction and stroke. Nevertheless, evidence that metformin is beneficial for overall cardiovascular primary risk reduction is very limited. Metformin also has modest beneficial lipid-lowering effects, including lowering triglycerides and LDL cholesterol and raising HDL cholesterol.

Semaglutide (Answer D) is a GLP-1 receptor agonist that is approved for once-weekly treatment of type 2 diabetes. GLP-1 receptor agonists enable glucose lowering and weight loss by decreasing energy intake and inducing appetite suppression. There is some evidence that liraglutide, 3 mg, decreases progression to type 2 diabetes in individuals with obesity and prediabetes (SCALE Obesity and Prediabetes study). Similar data with semaglutide in prediabetes are lacking, although semaglutide has significant hemoglobin A_{1c}–reducing and weight-loss effects. Semaglutide can decrease triglycerides and LDL cholesterol and has demonstrated cardiovascular benefit in individuals with type 2 diabetes and known ASCVD. This patient does not have type 2 diabetes (yet), so semaglutide is not the best choice now.

Educational Objective
Determine when to appropriately prescribe PCSK9 inhibitor therapy for a patient with increased cardiovascular risk.

UpToDate Topic Review(s)
Familial hypercholesterolemia in adults: Treatment

Reference(s)

Defesche JC, Gidding SS, Harada-Shiba M, Hegele RA, Santos RD, Wierzbicki AS. Familial hypercholesterolaemia. *Nat Rev Dis Primers*. 2017;3:17093. PMID: 29219151

Sabatine MS. PCSK9 inhibitors: clinical evidence and implementation. *Nat Rev Cardiol*. 2019;16(3): 155-165. PMID: 30420622

103 ANSWER: A) Elemental phosphorus

Although not as common as osteoporosis, osteomalacia is a metabolic bone disorder that is periodically encountered by endocrine specialists. Classically, osteomalacia presents with bone pain, a wide-based waddling gait, muscular weakness that is often proximal in location, and lower-extremity insufficiency or stress fractures, although affected patients often have subtle or nonspecific symptoms. Once osteomalacia is diagnosed, as in this patient who presents with symptomatic (localized bone pain), biochemical (high alkaline phosphatase), and radiographic (femoral stress fracture) evidence of disease, the clinician must determine whether the condition is hereditary or acquired. This patient presented in childhood, which is consistent with an inherited disorder, although this is not a definitive finding. Additionally, he has biochemical derangements (low phosphate, high 1,25-dihydroxyvitamin D, high 24-hour urinary calcium excretion) that are inconsistent with the most common acquired form of osteomalacia (ie, rickets) in childhood—vitamin D deficiency. On the basis of this reasoning, the clinician must next determine the specific genetic abnormality to most accurately and safely guide management.

Hereditary hypophosphatemic osteomalacia refers to a group disorders that have in common abnormal renal and/or intestinal phosphorus handling. However, the diseases can be further stratified into whether they are FGF-23 dependent or independent. FGF-23 is phosphate-regulating hormone that is primarily produced by osteocytes and actively lowers serum phosphorus through down-regulation of both renal reabsorption and intestinal absorption of phosphorus. Pathogenic variants in the gene encoding FGF-23 that render the protein resistant to catabolism (autosomal dominant hypophosphatemic rickets) or increase the systemic levels and availability of FGF-23 (X-linked hypophosphatemic rickets due to pathogenic variants in *PHEX*; autosomal recessive hypophosphatemic rickets types 1, 2, and 3 due to pathogenic variants in *DMP1*, *ENPP1*, and *FAM20C*, respectively) result in hypophosphatemia, inappropriately low or normal 1,25-dihydroxyvitamin D, and inappropriately normal or elevated plasma FGF-23 levels. In contrast, patients with FGF-23–independent hypophosphatemic osteomalacia exhibit disease that is due primarily to reduced renal phosphorus reabsorption.

On the basis of clinical data, this patient most likely has hereditary hypophosphatemic rickets with hypercalciuria due to a pathogenic variant in the *SLC34A3* gene, which encodes the renal proximal tubule transport protein NPT2c. Patients with homozygous or compound heterozygous mutations in *SLC34A3* have renal phosphate wasting and hypophosphatemia due to defective renal phosphorus reabsorption. In addition, hypophosphatemia results in a secondary increase in 1,25-dihydroxyvitamin D production, which in turn results in enhanced intestinal calcium absorption and attendant hypercalciuria that increases the risk for nephrolithiasis. Furthermore, patients who are heterozygous for pathogenic variants in the *SLC34A3* gene are themselves at a higher risk for renal calcifications.

Given this patient's hypophosphatemia and femoral stress fracture, treatment with elemental phosphorus (Answer A) is indicated. In contrast, calcitriol treatment (Answer B), which is typically central to the management of FGF-23–dependent hypophosphatemic osteomalacia, is contraindicated for patients with hereditary hypophosphatemic rickets with hypercalciuria, as it will increase urinary calcium excretion and increase the risk for renal stones. Although this patient's hypercalciuria may benefit from hydrochlorothiazide (Answer D), it will not address his hypophosphatemia and stress fracture. Teriparatide (Answer E) is not FDA-approved for this purpose, but it is sometimes used off-label in patients with delayed fracture healing. It does not address the underlying primary disorder and also increases urinary calcium excretion. Finally, although hypophosphatasia is an inherited osteomalacic disorder that can be treated with the FDA-approved therapy asfotase alfa (Answer C), it is due to pathogenic variants in the gene encoding tissue nonspecific alkaline phosphatase that result in low alkaline phosphatase with no alterations in systemic phosphorus metabolism.

Educational Objective
Determine appropriate therapy in a patient with an insufficiency fracture due to hereditary hypophosphatemia with hypercalciuria.

UpToDate Topic Review(s)
Evaluation and treatment of hypophosphatemia

Reference(s)

Dasgupta D, Wee MJ, Reyes M, et al. Mutations in SLC34A3/NPT2c are associated with kidney stones and nephrocalcinosis. *J Am Soc Nephrol*. 2014;25(10):2366-2375. PMID: 24700880

Goldsweig BK, Carpenter TO. Hypophosphatemic rickets: lessons from disrupted FGF23 control of phosphorus homeostasis. *Curr Osteoporos Rep*. 2015;13(2):88-97. PMID: 25620749

104 ANSWER: D) Discontinue metformin and continue glipizide

This vignette highlights the new guideline issued by the US FDA regarding the use of metformin in patients with impaired renal function. The guideline was issued in 2016 and is part of the prescribing information for all metformin-containing compounds. According to the guideline, serum creatinine alone is no longer recommended as the best method to measure kidney function. The recommended method is to calculate the estimated glomerular filtration rate using an equation. The estimated glomerular filtration rate equation accounts for the patient's age, sex, and race. The most commonly used equation is the MDRD equation (Modification of Diet in Renal Disease), which is available on most apps for medical equations:

$$\text{glomerular filtration rate (mL/min per 1.73 m}^2\text{)} = 175 \times (\text{serum creatinine})^{-1.154} \times (\text{age})^{-0.203} \times (0.742 \text{ if female}) \times$$
$$(1.212 \text{ if African American}) \text{ (conventional units)}$$

The equation does not require weight because the results are reported normalized to 1.73 m^2 body surface area, which is an accepted average adult surface area. (The MDRD equation is available at: https://www.niddk.nih.gov/health-information/communication-programs/nkdep/laboratory-evaluation/glomerular-filtration-rate-calculators/mdrd-adults-conventional-units)

The guideline states:

- Before starting metformin, obtain the patient's estimated glomerular filtration rate.

- Metformin is contraindicated in patients with an estimated glomerular filtration rate below 30 mL/min per 1.73 m^2.

- Starting metformin in patients with an estimated glomerular filtration rate between 30 and 45 mL/min per 1.73 m² is not recommended.

- Obtain an estimated glomerular filtration rate at least annually in all patients taking metformin. In patients at increased risk for the development of renal impairment such as elderly individuals, renal function should be assessed more frequently.

- In patients taking metformin whose estimated glomerular filtration rate later falls below 45 mL/min per 1.73 m², assess the benefits and risks of continuing treatment. Discontinue metformin if the patient's estimated glomerular filtration rate later falls below 30 mL/min per 1.73 m².

- Discontinue metformin at the time of or before an iodinated contrast imaging procedure in patients with an estimated glomerular filtration rate between 30 and 60 mL/min per 1.73 m²; in patients with a history of liver disease, alcoholism, or heart failure; or in patients who will be administered intra-arterial iodinated contrast. Reevaluate the estimated glomerular filtration rate 48 hours after the imaging procedure; restart metformin if renal function is stable.

The guideline was issued to reduce the potential risk for lactic acidosis, which may occur in patients with diabetes. Because metformin is cleared by the kidney, a low estimated glomerular filtration rate results in higher blood levels of metformin, thus placing the patient at higher risk for lactic acidosis.

Based on the MDRD formula, the patient's estimated glomerular filtration rate is 28.92 mL/min per 1.73 m², which is the below the guideline cutoff of 30 mL/min per 1.73 m².

Of the possible answers, discontinuing metformin and continuing glipizide (Answer D) is the best next step, as the patient is elderly and her hemoglobin A_{1c} may not increase to such a degree that insulin (Answer A) is needed. Starting a GLP-1 receptor agonist (Answer B) is incorrect, as there are limited data regarding their use in the setting of renal failure, and some of these agents are renally excreted and need dosage adjustment when a patient has renal insufficiency. Simply reducing the metformin dosage (Answer C) is not recommended in the FDA guideline. Discontinuing metformin and starting an SGLT-2 inhibitor (Answer E) is incorrect, as SGLT-2 inhibitors are contraindicated when the estimated glomerular filtration rate is less than 30 mL/min per 1.73 m².

Educational Objective
Apply the US FDA warning regarding the use of metformin in patients with reduced kidney function.

UpToDate Topic Review(s)
Metformin in the treatment of adults with type 2 diabetes mellitus

Reference(s)
US Food and Drug Administration. FDA Drug Safety Communication: FDA revises warnings regarding use of the diabetes medicine metformin in certain patients with reduced kidney function. Available at: https://www.fda.gov/Drugs/DrugSafety/ucm493244.htm. Accessed for verification July 2019.

105 ANSWER: A) Adrenocortical adenoma
This patient has reassuring radiographic findings that suggest the adrenal mass is a lipid-poor adrenocortical adenoma (Answer A). The radiographic characteristics of an adrenal mass are critical in evaluating whether the mass is benign or potentially malignant. Reassuring features that are suggestive of a benign adrenal mass include small size (generally <4 cm), round and uniform shape, homogenous appearance, and high lipid content (such as low attenuation on unenhanced CT [<10 Hounsfield units] or loss of signal on out-of-phase sequencing on MRI), and high contrast washout on delayed contrast CT imaging (>60% absolute washout and >40% relative washout).

Importantly, this patient's original CT was done with an intravenous contrast bolus, as is often the case when evaluating the cause of abdominal pain. Therefore, the adrenal mass CT attenuation value of 41 Hounsfield units is not interpretable, since it is the unenhanced attenuation that best characterizes lipid content. However, on a subsequent CT dedicated to assessing the adrenal mass, the unenhanced attenuation was 24 Hounsfield units, suggesting a lipid-poor entity, but the absolute washout was greater than 60% and the relative washout was greater than 40%, suggesting that the mass is most likely a lipid-poor adenoma.

Adrenocortical carcinoma (Answer B), metastasis (Answer C), and pheochromocytoma (Answer E) would most likely have much lower washout values. A myelolipoma (Answer D) is enriched for lipid content and typically has very low unenhanced attenuation values, usually less than zero Hounsfield units (ranging from −10 to −50). Myelolipomas can be large and heterogeneous, despite having lipid content.

Features that raise concern for a malignant process include larger size (generally >4 to 6 cm), irregular shape or contours, heterogeneous content, calcifications, low lipid content on CT or MRI, and poor washout on delayed contrast CT imaging. A pheochromocytoma can have poor lipid content and poor washout on delayed contrast CT imaging, but it generally presents with a round contour and shape and with substantial elevations in metanephrines. Pheochromocytomas almost never exhibit an unenhanced CT attenuation less than 10 Hounsfield units.

Educational Objective
Interpret the radiographic characteristics of an adrenal mass.

UpToDate Topic Review(s)
Clinical presentation and evaluation of adrenocortical tumors

Reference(s)

Vaidya A, Hamrahian A, Bancos I, Fleseriu M, Ghayee HK. The evaluation of incidentally discovered adrenal masses. *Endocr Pract.* 2019;25(2):178-192. PMID: 30817193

Fassnacht M, Arlt W, Bancos I, et al. Management of adrenal incidentalomas: European Society of Endocrinology Clinical Practice Guideline in collaboration with the European Network for the Study of Adrenal Tumors. *Eur J Endocrinol.* 2016;175(2):G1-G34. PMID: 27390021

106 ANSWER: C) 17α-hydroxyprogesterone

While insufficient suppression of circulating testosterone ("testosterone escape") may occur in some men with prostate cancer receiving pharmacologic androgen deprivation therapy, testosterone escape after surgical orchidectomy is distinctly uncommon. In postpubertal men, more than 95% of circulating testosterone is produced by the testes, and the remainder is produced by the adrenal glands. In congenital adrenal hyperplasia (CAH), most commonly due to 21-hydroxylase deficiency, the contribution of adrenal androgens to the circulating pool of testosterone is more substantial, and circulating adrenal androgens, such as DHEA-S and androstenedione, are typically increased. The phenotype of CAH is variable and depends on the residual activity of 21-hydroxylase deficiency. While classic CAH can present with salt-wasting and adrenal crises in infancy, less severe forms of CAH can escape detection because residual 21-hydroxylase activity prevents symptomatic mineralocorticoid deficiency, and latent glucocorticoid deficiency is compensated by pituitary ACTH hypersecretion. Clues to the diagnosis include a history of precocious puberty, short stature due to premature closure of the epiphyses, pigmentation, and bilateral adrenal gland enlargement on imaging due to tonic ACTH hypersecretion.

In this vignette, the patient's relatively short stature, evidence of pigmentation, and increased DHEA-S level are consistent with a diagnosis of CAH, and the best initial diagnostic test is measurement of the 17α-hydroxyprogesterone concentration (Answer C), which is increased in CAH, especially after ACTH stimulation. In this man, treatment with glucocorticoids reduced ACTH-stimulated production of excess adrenal androgen precursors and consequently reduced circulating testosterone concentrations to the castrate range. Abiraterone, a potent CYP17A1 inhibitor, blocks both testicular and extratesticular testosterone synthesis (eg, by adrenal glands, prostate cancer cells) and prolongs survival in men with castrate-resistant prostate cancer. Due to its ability to reduce adrenal androgens, abiraterone can lower circulating androgens in classic 21-hydroxylase deficiency. Abiraterone, which is usually administered together with glucocorticoids, may have been successful in achieving castrate testosterone concentrations before orchidectomy in this patient.

While hCG-producing tumors can increase serum testosterone, hCG does so via stimulation of testicular LH receptors. Following orchidectomy, testosterone concentrations should be in the castrate range. Thus, measuring hCG (Answer A) is incorrect.

Eighty percent of dihydrotestosterone is produced by 5α-reduction in target tissues, and dihydrotestosterone (Answer E) is not a representative measure of testicular function. Dihydrotestosterone measurement does not contribute to assessment of androgen status in men.

In men, 25% to 50% of estradiol is produced from aromatization of androgens in peripheral tissues. While some of the biologic effects of androgens in men (eg, on the skeleton) are dependent on aromatization to estradiol, there is no established clinical usefulness for routine estradiol measurement (Answer D) in male patients. Estradiol measurement would not help elucidate the cause for the insufficient suppression of circulating testosterone in this case.

Likewise, measuring SHBG (Answer B) would not be helpful in this clinical scenario. While a man with an inactivating pathogenic variant in the *SHBG* gene who presented with undetectable circulating SHBG, low testosterone, and relatively normal androgenization has been reported, abnormalities in circulating SHBG do not cause persistently detectable testosterone after surgical castration.

Educational Objective
Suspect nonclassic congenital adrenal hyperplasia as a cause of nonsuppressible testosterone concentrations after castration.

UpToDate Topic Review(s)
Genetics and clinical presentation of nonclassic (late-onset) congenital adrenal hyperplasia due to 21-hydroxylase deficiency

Reference(s)
Speiser PW, Arlt W, Auchus RJ, et al. Congenital adrenal hyperplasia due to steroid 21-hydroxylase deficiency: an Endocrine Society clinical practice guideline. *J Clin Endocrinol Metab.* 2018;103(11):4043-4088. PMID: 30272171

Ragnarsson O, Johannsson G, Geterud K, Lodding P, Dahlqvist P. Inadequate testosterone suppression after medical and subsequent surgical castration in a patient with prostate cancer. *BMJ Case Rep.* 2013;2013. PMID: 23943809

Feng X, Kline G. Massive adrenal incidentalomas and late diagnosis of congenital adrenal hyperplasia in prostate cancer. *Endocrinol Diabetes Metab Case Rep.* 2017;2017. pii: 17-0108. PMID: 29118987

Auchus RJ, Buschur EO, Chang AY, et al. Abiraterone acetate to lower androgens in women with classic 21-hydroxylase deficiency. *J Clin Endocrinol Metab.* 2014;99(8):2763-2770. PMID: 24780050

107 ANSWER: A) Metformin

In this woman with a personal history of a pulmonary embolism provoked by combined oral contraceptives (COCs), use of COCs without anticoagulation represents an unacceptable health risk. The Centers for Disease Control have published resources to guide prescribers of contraception for women with specific risk factors and medical conditions. Before prescribing a COC, care providers should screen for factors that might increase the risk of adverse events, including stroke and venous thrombosis. In addition to older age, cigarette smoking, hypertension, and migraine headaches with aura, other factors that further increase stroke risk in women taking a COC include obesity, dyslipidemia, and genetic variants predisposing to thrombosis. Although a COC taken with anticoagulation (Answer C) might lower the risk for a woman with a higher risk of complications during pregnancy, there are other treatment options to consider.

Guidelines recommend metformin (Answer A) to improve ovulatory frequency and menstrual regularity in women with polycystic ovary syndrome who cannot take or tolerate oral contraceptives or in women trying to conceive. Metformin has been shown to improve ovulatory frequency and menstrual regularity even in lean women and those who have no evidence of prediabetes or diabetes. Metformin would be reasonable and is the lowest-risk option in this case to improve cycle regularity without the use of hormones. Because metformin can improve ovulatory frequency, she should be counseled about the use of nonhormonal forms of contraception when sexually active if pregnancy is not desired.

Spironolactone (Answer B) is an aldosterone antagonist that also acts as a competitive inhibitor of the androgen receptor. It is considered second-line therapy for the treatment of hirsutism or first-line therapy in a patient who cannot be prescribed COCs. Spironolactone is also an appropriate addition to a COC when symptoms are not controlled by the COC alone. However, spironolactone alone would be more likely to cause irregular or more frequent vaginal bleeding. Therefore, it would not be the best next step to effectively treat this patient's irregular menses. It is recommended to use spironolactone in combination with COCs or an intrauterine device that releases levonorgestrel to prevent conception while on an antiandrogen and to prevent irregular uterine spotting or bleeding that might occur with spironolactone.

In women with infrequent menses, progesterone taken for 10 days can help induce a withdrawal bleed to avoid endometrial hyperplasia. It is typically recommended every 3 months if no spontaneous menses occurs in that timeframe. Daily use (Answer D) can suppress menstrual periods and prevent or decrease intermenstrual bleeding, so micronized daily progesterone is not the best step for this patient.

Medroxyprogesterone (Answer E) functions as a contraceptive and it can be a short-term strategy to control or stop intermenstrual or heavy bleeding, but it would not be a good long-term strategy because it leads to estrogen deficiency and bone loss with long-term use.

Educational Objective
Recommend a management strategy for oligomenorrhea in a woman with polycystic ovary syndrome when oral contraceptives are contraindicated.

UpToDate Topic Review(s)
Treatment of polycystic ovary syndrome in adults

Reference(s)

Legro RS, Arslanian SA, Ehrmann DA, et al; Endocrine Society. Diagnosis and treatment of polycystic ovary syndrome: an Endocrine Society clinical practice guideline. *J Clin Endocrinol Metab.* 2013;98(12):4565-4592. PMID: 24151290

Centers for Disease Control and Prevention. US Medical Eligibility Criteria (US MEC) for Contraceptive Use, 2016. Atlanta, GA. Centers for Disease Control, 2016. Available at: http://www.cdc.gov/reproductivehealth/unintendedpregnancy/usmec.htm. Accessed for verification March 2019

Kearon C, Akl EA, Comerota AJ, et al. Antithrombotic therapy for VTE disease: antithrombotic therapy and prevention of thrombosis, 9th ed: American College of Chest Physicians Evidence-Based Clinical Practice Guidelines. *Chest.* 2012;141(2 Suppl):e419S-e496S. PMID: 22315268

108
ANSWER: B) Decreased hepatic type 1 deiodinase activity

Several nonthyroidal illnesses or situations can have a profound effect on thyroid hormone metabolism and thyroid function tests. The classic situation is the impact of a serious illness on thyroid parameters, as occurs in hospitalized patients, particularly in the intensive care unit. During chronic illness, there is reduced *TRH* gene expression, reduced TSH secretion and decreased pulsatility, decreased type 1 deiodinase activity in the liver, increased type 3 deiodinase activity in the liver, and increased type 2 deiodinase activity in muscle. These changes are manifest as a low serum TSH concentration, very low serum T_3 concentrations, low serum T_4 concentrations, and increased reverse T_3 concentrations. The hypothalamic suppression is believed to be a response in order to generally reduce catabolism, with some debate as to whether it is an adaptive or maladaptive response. The decreased type 1 deiodinase in the liver and the increased type 3 deiodinase in the liver mediate the fall in T_3 and the rise in reverse T_3, respectively. The alterations in type 2 deiodinase activity may modulate the activity of T_3 at a local tissue level. For example, the increased type 2 deiodinase activity in muscle may ensure adequate thyroid hormone within skeletal muscle. The difficulty interpreting these complex changes in thyroid hormones, which are also affected by whether the illness is acute or chronic and whether the patient receives enteral or parenteral nutrition, has led to the adage that thyroid function should not be assessed in a hospitalized patient unless there is a high suspicion of a thyroid problem. Another situation with complex effects on thyroid hormone metabolism is the so-called polar T_3 syndrome in which the daily production of T_3 increases with chronic cold exposure. Cold adaption is believed to be aided by high rates of production of T_3 from T_4 by type 2 deiodinase activity in brown adipose tissue.

In anorexic patients with low body weight, profound alterations in thyroid hormones and TSH are observed. Serum T_3 levels are low, reverse T_3 levels are high, T_4 levels are low, and TSH levels are low. Thus, these changes are very similar to changes seen in nonthyroidal illness. Although reverse T_3 levels are helpful in understanding the underlying physiology, they are not needed as part of the routine clinical evaluation of such a patient. Animal studies of fasting show decreased thyrotropin-releasing hormone expression (not increased expression [Answer E]) in the hypothalamus, as is seen in critical illness. In studies of normal volunteers who are subjected to fasting, 24-hour blood sampling demonstrates decreased TSH pulse amplitude (not increased pulsatility [Answer D]). This is, again, a change similar to that seen in nonthyroidal illness. Changes in hepatic deiodinases also seem to be similar in hospitalized patients in the chronic phase of critical illness and in those with anorexia or those who are fasting. In both cases, hepatic type 3 deiodinase activity is increased (not decreased [Answer C]). However, hepatic type 1 deiodinase activity is indeed decreased (Answer B).

Kisspeptin is responsible for stimulating GnRH neurons and thus supporting normal ovulation and fertility. Kisspeptin levels do appear to be altered in both anorexia and critical illness, at least in some studies. However, kisspeptin (Answer A) does not appear to be involved in modulating thyroid function.

Although anorexia presents with many clinical features that are also seen with hypothyroidism, such as bradycardia, hypothermia, and delayed ankle reflexes, these features may actually be manifestations of attempts to conserve energy. Treatment with thyroid hormone is not beneficial and may lead to undesirable weight loss and loss of muscle mass. When anorexic patients are fed, there is generally an increase in T_3, a lowering of reverse T_3, and an increase in TSH, although initially there may not be much change in T_4. Restoration of normal body weight is believed to be the only way to restore normal thyroid economy.

Educational Objective
Explain the effect of anorexia and low body weight on thyroid physiology and thyroid function.

UpToDate Topic Review(s)
Anorexia nervosa: Endocrine complications and their management

Reference(s)

Boelen A, Wiersinga WM, Fliers E. Fasting-induced changes in the hypothalamus-pituitary-thyroid axis. *Thyroid.* 2008;18(2):123-129. PMID: 18225975

Leslie RD, Isaacs AJ, Gomez J, Raggatt PR, Bayliss R. Hypothalamo-pituitary-thyroid function in anorexia nervosa: influence of weight gain. *Br Med J.* 1978;2(6136):526-528. PMID: 698555

Van den Berghe G. Non-thyroidal illness in the ICU: a syndrome with different faces. *Thyroid.* 2014;24(10):1456-1465. PMID: 24845024

Warren MP. Endocrine manifestations of eating disorders. *J Clin Endocrinol Metab.* 2011;96(2):333-343. PMID: 21159848

109 ANSWER: A) No specific therapy

The dual epidemics of obesity and type 2 diabetes have raised concerns regarding increased incidence of cancer and cancer-related mortality. Increased rates of pancreatic, hepatic, endometrial, and breast cancer have been observed in patients with type 2 diabetes and obesity. Data on the association of type 1 diabetes with cancers has been less robust. Of interest to this patient, epidemiologic studies show a lower incidence of prostate cancer in patients with diabetes; however, there is an increased prostate cancer–related mortality rate.

Proposed mechanisms for increased cancer rates in this population are hyperglycemia, insulin resistance, hyperinsulinemia, and up-regulated inflammatory cascades. Both obesity and type 2 diabetes are independently associated with increased cancer incidence. Intentional weight loss reduces the risk of malignancies. In studies assessing cancer risk following bariatric surgery, a 24% to 78% reduction in cancer risk was noted in treatment groups compared with risk in placebo groups. In the Nurses Health Study, a 17% increased risk of breast cancer was seen in patients who also had diabetes, and this was independent of age and obesity.

Despite associations among cancer, type 2 diabetes, and obesity, there is no pharmacologic intervention that is recommended to reduce the risk of cancer (Answer A). The American Cancer Society recommends a healthy lifestyle for cancer prevention. This includes maintaining a lean body weight without being underweight and engaging in 150 minutes of moderate exercise or 75 minutes of intense exercise a week. A diet rich in fruits and vegetables and low in red meat and calorically dense foods is recommended.

Although observational studies have shown improved cancer-related outcomes (in certain cancers) with glucose-lowering medications, none have shown consistent findings. The most widely described is the possible role of metformin (Answer B). Epidemiologic studies show reduced incidence of pancreatic, hepatocellular, breast, lung, and colorectal cancer in patients treated with metformin. Metformin exerts its glucose-lowering effects by activating/phosphorylating AMP-activated protein kinase. This results in decreased gluconeogenesis and possibly increased apoptosis. Other analyses have not shown a similar reduction in cancer rates, and results from prospective trials are still pending. Therefore, the evidence is not conclusive.

Pioglitazone (Answer D) has been associated with bladder cancer. In the PROactive trial, there were more cases of bladder cancer in the pioglitazone treatment group than in the placebo group, and meta-analyses suggested a connection. However, subsequent cohort studies that followed patients for nearly 3 years did not show increased risk of bladder cancer with pioglitazone use. There are no data on decreased risk of cancer with pioglitazone.

In one study of glibenclamide, the overall cancer incidence was increased by 20% to 25%, although there are also no consistent findings that sulfonylureas (Answer C) increase or decrease cancer risk.

The ORIGIN trial (Outcome Reduction With Initial Glargine Intervention), which enrolled 12,000 patients to evaluate the role of insulin glargine on cardiovascular outcomes, showed no effect of insulin (Answer E) on cancer.

Educational Objective
Counsel patients with type 2 diabetes mellitus regarding possible therapeutic interventions to reduce cancer risk.

UpToDate Topic Review(s)
Overview of medical care in adults with diabetes mellitus

Reference(s)
Shlomai G, Neel B, LeRoith D, Gallagher EJ. Type 2 diabetes mellitus and cancer: the role of pharmacotherapy. *J Clin Oncol.* 2016;34(35):4261-4269. PMID: 27903154

Gallagher EJ, LeRoith D. Obesity and diabetes: the increased risk of cancer and cancer-related mortality. *Physiol Rev.* 2015;95(3):727-748. PMID: 26084689

110 ANSWER: D) Measure plasma GHRH

While full-blown forms of acromegaly are often easy to diagnose, milder forms are more difficult to differentiate from normal population variants. Serum IGF-1 is a GH-dependent protein that circulates as a heterotrimer, bound to IGFBP-3 and acid-labile subunit. This patient has had 2 documented mild elevations of IGF-1. He has some signs and symptoms of acromegaly (hypertension, large hands, snoring), but none of these findings is specific for the disease. By definition, 2.5% of the general population has a serum IGF-1 level that is either above or below 2 standard deviations of the mean value (method used to determine normal values). Therefore, IGF-1 itself, unless markedly elevated or associated with obvious clinical features, cannot diagnose acromegaly in this patient. The gold standard for the diagnosis of acromegaly is the oral glucose suppression test. Unfortunately, even this test has some limitations. These are caused by the impact of assay methods on the absolute GH concentrations. Despite the cutoff of 1 ng/mL that was suggested by the latest Endocrine Society practice guideline, most pituitary experts use a cutoff of 0.4 ng/mL as suggested by the Acromegaly Consensus Group that considered the use of modern, more specific GH assays. This patient has acromegaly, independent from which cutoff is used and also based on the fact that the GH concentration did not seem to change at all during the test.

Once acromegaly is diagnosed, a pituitary-dedicated MRI should be performed. Because of the frequent delay in diagnosis, MRI often reveals a macroadenoma. Less frequently, patients have microadenomas (<1 cm in diameter), and rarely is the adenoma so small that it cannot be detected on MRI after gadolinium administration. When MRI fails to show an obvious pituitary adenoma, a possible etiology is the presence of a GHRH-secreting neuroendocrine tumor elsewhere in the body. These tumors cause less than 1% of acromegaly cases and are metastatic in about 50% of affected persons. They are usually well-differentiated neuroendocrine tumors, mostly from pancreatic or bronchial origin. In these cases, the pituitary visualized on MRI can be either normal or diffusely enlarged. Measurement of a random plasma GHRH level (Answer D) is usually helpful, as it is almost invariably markedly elevated independent from the timing of the blood draw.

Repeating a GH-suppression test after stopping metoprolol (Answer A) is not useful, as this medication does not influence the GH response to oral glucose. Measurement of free IGF-1 (Answer C) is presently limited to research studies, and it has not been shown to be helpful in the diagnosis of mild acromegaly. Similarly, measurement of IGFBP-3 (Answer B) is not helpful in diagnosing acromegaly. Pursuing no further evaluation (Answer E) is wrong, as this patient may have a GHRH-secreting tumor requiring surgical removal.

This patient's GHRH level was normal, and he therefore most likely has a small GH-secreting adenoma that is currently below the detection ability of MRI.

Educational Objective
Diagnose acromegaly in a patient with normal findings on pituitary MRI.

Reference(s)

Schilbach K, Strasburger CJ, Bidlingmaier M. Biochemical investigations in diagnosis and follow up of acromegaly. *Pituitary*. 2017;20(1):33-45. PMID: 28168377

Katznelson L, Laws ER Jr, Melmed S, Molitch ME, Murad MH, Utz A, Wass JA; Endocrine Society. Acromegaly: an endocrine society clinical practice guideline. *J Clin Endocrinol Metab*. 2014;99(11):3933-3951. PMID: 25356808

Giustina A, Chanson P, Bronstein MD, et al; Acromegaly Consensus Group. A consensus on criteria for cure of acromegaly. *J Clin Endocrinol Metab*. 2010;95(7):3141-3148. PMID: 20410227

Borson-Chazot F, Garby L, Raverot G, Claustrat F, Raverot V, Sassolas G; GTE group. Acromegaly induced by ectopic secretion of GHRH: a review 30 years after GHRH discovery. *Ann Endocrinol (Paris)*. 2012;73(6):497-502. PMID: 23122576

111   ANSWER: B) Zoledronic acid

The patient described in this vignette has asymptomatic Paget disease of bone. His imaging studies are consistent with Paget disease involving his entire right hemipelvis (sclerosis on the radiograph and increased radionuclide uptake on the bone scan), and his bone-specific alkaline phosphatase level is markedly elevated (>5 times the upper normal limit). Paget disease affects both men and women, with a small male predominance in some studies. Its frequency increases with advancing age, with rates in the United States estimated to be approximately 2% to 3% among individuals older than 55 years. However, several issues may have led to an underestimation of the prevalence of Paget disease, including the fact that it is often asymptomatic. Paget disease can affect any bone in the body, but has a predilection for the skull, spine, pelvis, and long bones of the lower extremities. Both genetic and environmental causes, including the possible role of viral infection, are thought to contribute to the development of the disease. Some of the symptoms and complications related to Paget disease include bone pain, osteoarthritis of adjacent joints, "chalk-stick" fractures, hearing loss, paraplegia, increased cardiac output, hypercalcemia, and rarely, osteosarcoma. Indications to treat asymptomatic Paget disease of bone include serum alkaline phosphatase more than 2 to 4 times the upper normal limit, pagetic changes at sites where complications could occur (eg, skull, spine, weight-bearing bones, and pagetic bone abutting a joint), planned surgery at an active pagetic site, and hypercalcemia in association with immobilization in patients with polyostotic disease. Therefore, this patient meets criteria to treat. Recommending no treatment (Answer E) is incorrect.

The primary agents for the treatment of Paget disease of bone are bisphosphonates. With this patient's history of esophageal stricture, an oral bisphosphonate such as risedronate (Answer A) should be avoided, making zoledronic acid (Answer B), which is an intravenous bisphosphonate, the best treatment choice in this case. It is important to note that studies have demonstrated more rapid, more frequent, and more sustained disease control after a single intravenous infusion of zoledronic acid compared with 60 days of daily oral risedronate, as well as superior effects on quality of life, including pain relief.

Denosumab (Answer C), a fully human monoclonal antibody to the receptor activator of nuclear factor kappaB ligand (RANKL), is an agent currently approved for the treatment of osteoporosis, for the prevention of skeletal-related events in patients with multiple myeloma, for patients with bone metastases from solid tumors, and for the treatment of hypercalcemia of malignancy refractory to bisphosphonate therapy. Although denosumab is not currently approved for the treatment of Paget disease, there is some evidence that it may have clinical utility for this indication. While this would be off-label use, it may be an appealing option for patients with contraindications to bisphosphonates such as those with impaired kidney function.

Calcitonin (Answer D) is an antiresorptive agent that is less potent than bisphosphonates and is unlikely to result in sustained clinical remission. However, it is relatively safe and is approved in its subcutaneous formulation for the treatment of patients with Paget disease who are intolerant of bisphosphonates.

Educational Objective

Determine when treatment is indicated in a patient with Paget disease and recommend the most appropriate medication.

UpToDate Topic Review(s)
Treatment of Paget disease of bone

Reference(s)

Singer FR, Bone HG 3rd, Hosking DJ, et al; Endocrine Society. Paget's disease of bone: an Endocrine Society clinical practice guideline. *J Clin Endocrinol Metab.* 2014;99(12):4408-4422. PMID: 25406796

Reid IR, Sharma S, Kalluru R, Eagleton C. Treatment of Paget's disease of bone with denosumab: case report and literature review. *Calcif Tissue Int.* 2016;99(3):322-325. PMID: 27193832

Reid IR, Miller P, Lyles K, et al. Comparison of a single infusion of zoledronic acid with risedronate for Paget's disease. *N Engl J Med.* 2005;353(9):898-908. PMID: 16135834

Hosking D, Lyles K, Brown JP, et al. Long-term control of bone turnover in Paget's disease with zoledronic acid and risedronate. *J Bone Miner Res.* 2007;22(1):142-148. PMID: 17032148

Reid IR, Lyles K, Su G, et al. A single infusion of zoledronic acid produces sustained remissions in Paget disease: data to 6.5 years. *J Bone Miner Res.* 2011;26(9):2261-2270. PMID: 21638319

112 ANSWER: E) Copper

Roux-en-Y gastric bypass (RYGB) is a type of bariatric surgery with both restrictive and malabsorptive components. A 15- to 30-cc gastric pouch is created from the proximal stomach and it is anastomosed to the jejunum (Roux limb). The duodenum is then anastomosed to the jejunum 100 to 150 cm distal to the gastrojejunostomy. After RYGB, patients are started on a multivitamin with iron and calcium citrate, as they are at increased risk for micronutrient malabsorption. After RYGB, routine monitoring is recommended for iron, folic acid, 25-hydroxyvitamin D, and vitamin B_{12}. However, monitoring of copper, zinc, selenium, and thiamine is only recommended in patients with clinical findings of deficiencies of these micronutrients.

This patient presents with symptoms of zinc deficiency and his blood work confirms the diagnosis. Zinc is the second most prevalent trace element in the body. It participates in normal cell growth and differentiation, protects cells from free radical damage, and has a role in several enzymatic reactions. Cells with rapid turnover (ie, skin, gastrointestinal mucosa) are greatly affected in patients with zinc deficiency. Symptoms of zinc deficiency include alopecia, acrodermatitis, glossitis, diarrhea, poor wound healing, and hypogonadism in men. The recommended dietary allowance for adults is 8 mg daily for women and 11 mg daily for men. Red meat is the richest source of zinc, providing about 50% of dietary zinc.

After RYGB, zinc's absorption decreases because both the duodenum and proximal jejunum, main sites of zinc absorption, are bypassed and there is less hydrochloric acid, which is required for zinc absorption. Zinc is transported across the brush border membrane surface of cells in the small intestine via ZIP4. When zinc concentrations in these cells is very high—for example, when an individual is taking a supplemental dose of this trace element—a promoter for the metallothionein gene is activated and enhanced transcription of this gene occurs. This increases the level of thionein polypeptides, which bind to any available zinc and copper. The binding affinity of this protein is higher for copper than for zinc, so more copper is bound, which prevents copper from being transported across the basolateral membrane to plasma. Then these intestinal cells are sloughed off into the intestinal tract and excreted, which leads to low copper levels. The current recommendation is that when a patient is receiving zinc, it is important that they also receive supplemental copper (Answer E) to maintain the ratio of 1 mg of copper per 8 to 15 mg of zinc. This will decrease the risk of copper deficiency. Cobalamin (Answer A), iron (Answer B), folic acid (Answer C), and thiamine (Answer D) are not affected by zinc supplementation, so extra supplementation is not needed.

Copper deficiency mainly causes hematologic and neurologic clinical manifestations. Hematologic manifestations include anemia (microcytic, normocytic, or macrocytic), leukopenia, neutropenia, and pancytopenia. Neurologic manifestations include myelopathy presenting with sensory ataxia and a spastic gait, peripheral neuropathy, optic neuritis, and cognitive impairment. The hematologic manifestations of copper deficiency, in most cases, resolve promptly after copper supplementation; however, neurologic improvement is either slow, incomplete, or absent.

Educational Objective

After bariatric surgery, anticipate the risk of copper deficiency in the setting of zinc supplementation.

UpToDate Topic Review(s)

Bariatric surgery: Postoperative nutritional management

Reference(s)

Salle A, Demarsy D, Poirier AL, et al. Zinc deficiency: a frequent and underestimated complication after bariatric surgery. *Obes Surg.* 2010;20(12):1660-1670. PMID: 20706804

Shankar P, Boylan M, Sriram K. Micronutrient deficiencies after bariatric surgery. *Nutrition.* 2010;26(11-12):1031-1037. PMID: 20363593

Mahawar KK, Bhasker AG, Bindal V, et al. Zinc deficiency after gastric bypass for morbid obesity: a systematic review. *Obes Surg.* 2017;27(2):522-529. PMID: 27885534

Cousins RJ. Absorption, transport, and hepatic metabolism of copper and zinc: special reference to metallothionein and ceruloplasmin. *Physiol Rev.* 1985;65(2):238-309. PMID: 3885271

Kumar N. Copper deficiency myelopathy (human swayback). *Mayo Clin Proc.* 2006;81(10):1371-1384. PMID: 17036563

113 ANSWER: D) Administer insulin glargine + fixed-dose insulin aspart with meals and on a correctional scale

Hyperglycemia in the hospital setting is associated with increased complications, in-hospital mortality, and hospitalization costs. The latter is driven primarily by increased length of stay and increased 30-day readmissions. The American Diabetes Association recommends that insulin treatment be initiated for patients with glucose levels consistently greater than or equal to 180 mg/dL (≥10.0 mmol/L) with a glycemic target of 140 to 180 mg/dL (7.8-10.0 mmol/L) for most critically ill and noncritically ill patients. Given these guidelines, this patient's poor glycemic control while on his home regimen (hemoglobin A_{1c} = 8.4% [68 mmol/mol]) and the association of sulfonylureas with hypoglycemia make resuming metformin and glipizide (Answer A) an incorrect choice. Use of oral hypoglycemic agents is restricted by many inpatient pharmacies for the above reasons.

The aforementioned guidelines specifically discourage the sole use of correctional-scale insulin (Answer B). Basal insulin only (Answer E) or basal + correctional insulin (Answer C) is suggested for patients who are nothing-by-mouth status or who have poor oral intake. In this case, there is no indication of poor oral intake. Findings from the Basal Plus trial suggest no difference in glycemic control between a basal-bolus regimen (Answer D) and basal + correctional-only insulin. This trial did not report on hospital complications. However, findings from a randomized controlled trial comparing basal-bolus insulin with correctional-scale insulin showed that basal-bolus insulin improved glycemic control and reduced hospital complications in patients in a general surgery ward, lending support for administering insulin glargine + fixed-dose insulin aspart with meals and on a correctional scale as the best choice for glycemic management in this patient. Furthermore, this approach is consistent with the 2019 American Diabetes Association standards of clinical care guidelines.

The choice of insulin dose may be difficult in such cases and no studies have compared different dosing regimens. However, many authors have shared their approaches, and the Endocrine Society guidelines have specific suggestions for choice of insulin regimen. For patients similar to the one presented in this vignette (age <70 years and estimated glomerular filtration rate >60 mg/min per 1.73 m^2), a total daily dose of 0.4 units per kg is suggested, with 50% to be given as basal insulin and 50% to be given as bolus rapid-acting insulin analogue divided into equal doses before meals.

Educational Objective

Manage hyperglycemia in a hospitalized patient with diabetes mellitus.

UpToReview(s)

Management of diabetes mellitus in hospitalized patients

Reference(s)

Umpierrez G, Smiley D, Jacobs S, et al. Randomized study of basal-bolus insulin therapy in the inpatient management of patients with type 2 diabetes undergoing general surgery (RABBIT 2 Surgery). *Diabetes Care.* 2011;34(2):256-261. PMID: 21228246

Umpierrez GE, Hellman R, Korytowski MT, et al; Endocrine Society. Management of hyperglycemia in hospitalized patients in non-critical care setting: an Endocrine Society clinical practice guideline. *J Clin Endocrinol Metab.* 2012;97(1):16-38. PMID: 22223765

American Diabetes Association. 15. Diabetes care in the hospital: standards of medical care in diabetes-2019. *Diabetes Care.* 2019;42(Suppl 1):S173-S181. PMID: 30559241

Umpierrez GE, Smiley D, Hermayer K et al. Randomized study comparing a basal-bolus with a basal plus correction insulin regimen for the hospital management of medical and surgical patients with type 2 diabetes. *Diabetes Care.* 2013;36(8):2169-2174. PMID: 23435159

114 ANSWER: B) Germinoma

Although pituitary adenomas can present at any age, onset of hypopituitarism in adolescence or young adulthood merits consideration of other specific conditions such as craniopharyngioma (Answer A) and germinoma (germ-cell tumor) (Answer B).

This patient has normal secondary sexual characteristics, but has now developed widespread anterior pituitary dysfunction with resultant secondary amenorrhea, suggesting the presence of a lesion that developed after puberty. Bilateral inferior quadrantanopia points to a suprasellar lesion that is compressing the optic chiasm from above. The postcontrast sagittal MRI shows a complex heterogeneous mass in the region of the hypothalamus (*see image, white arrow*). However, the main clue to the nature of the underlying pathology is the presence of a second independent lesion in the region of the pineal gland (*see image, white arrowhead*). The co-occurrence of suprasellar and pineal lesions is highly suggestive of a germinoma. Note the suprasellar mass is distinct from the normal pituitary gland and demonstrates more heterogeneous gadolinium uptake.

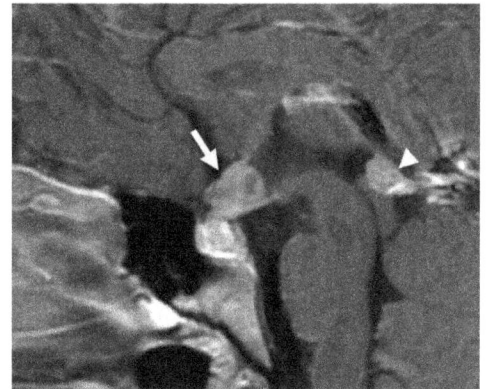

Germ-cell tumors may secrete hCG, which can be detected in the serum or cerebrospinal fluid. Therefore, following identification of a possible germinoma on clinical and radiologic grounds, further investigation would typically begin with measurement of serum (± cerebrospinal fluid) tumor markers. Surgery is generally held in reserve to provide histologic confirmation of the diagnosis, especially when there are normal serum and cerebrospinal fluid tumor markers. Germinomas tend to be very vascular, making complete resection extremely difficult to achieve. Fortunately, most germinomas respond well to chemotherapy and radiotherapy, with a greater than 85% overall 5-year survival. The extent of endocrine dysfunction varies, but panhypopituitarism can occur. Some patients present with profound thirst and polyuria due to diabetes insipidus.

In a patient of this age, the radiologic appearance of the sellar mass could be compatible with a craniopharyngioma (Answer A), which often presents with similar endocrine disruption and vision compromise. CT may reveal calcification within the lesion. However, although these tumors can be locally invasive, one would not expect to see a second lesion at a separate site within the CNS, as is clearly evident in this case.

Similarly, Rathke cleft cyst (Answer D) can exhibit a similar appearance, although its origin from the Rathke pouch at the junction of the anterior and posterior lobes of the pituitary gland is often apparent.

Suprasellar meningiomas (Answer E) typically come to medical attention due to compression of the optic pathways, but endocrine function is often surprisingly well preserved even with sizeable lesions. In addition, outside the context of an inherited tumor syndrome (eg, neurofibromatosis type 2 in which multiple tumors may be seen), they rarely present at this age.

For the reasons reviewed above, the radiologic findings are not consistent with a nonfunctioning pituitary adenoma (Answer C).

Educational Objective
Construct a differential diagnosis for a suprasellar mass in a young adult and identify typical radiologic features of a germinoma.

UpToDate Topic Review(s)
Intracranial germ cell tumors

Reference(s)

Osorio DS, Allen JC. Management of CNS germinoma. *CNS Oncology.* 2015;4(4):273-279. PMID: 26118663

Lian X, Hou X, Yan J, et al. Treatment outcomes of intracranial germinoma: a retrospective analysis of 170 patients from a single institution. *J Canc Res Clin Oncol.* 2019;145(3):709-715. PMID: 30209611

115 **ANSWER: D) Adjuvant mitotane monotherapy**

This patient had a complete resection of a high-grade stage III adrenocortical carcinoma and should be offered adjuvant therapy with mitotane (Answer D). Adrenocortical carcinoma is a rare and usually aggressive malignancy with few effective therapeutic options. The most effective therapy is surgical resection. Complete, and even incomplete, surgical resection can substantially improve prognosis. The addition of adjuvant medical therapies can further improve prognosis and overall survival. Thus, no further therapy (Answer A) is incorrect.

The most important step in treating patients with adrenocortical carcinoma is referral to an experienced tertiary care center. Experienced surgeons are most capable of achieving a complete resection via radical adrenalectomy and lymph node sampling, which translates to the best long-term outcomes. The pathology is then used to determine the grade and stage of the cancer (*see staging table*). In this patient's case, at least 2 of 10 lymph nodes have malignant cells. Therefore, even though the surgery may seem complete and there were no distant metastases, this patient's cancer is stage III. The grade of the tumor is determined by the Ki67 proliferation index, where less than 10% is considered low-grade and greater than 10% is considered high-grade. Thus, this patient has a high-grade stage III adrenocortical carcinoma and has not undergone a complete (R0) surgical resection.

Adjuvant mitotane therapy is recommended for high-grade stage I and II disease, as well as for all stage III and IV disease and instances when a complete surgical resection is not performed/possible. Mitotane is a derivative of the pesticide DDT and is used for its potential adrenolytic and/or adrenostatic properties. Patients on mitotane should be treated with glucocorticoids, as many will develop adrenal insufficiency. With higher levels of mitotane, patients often need supraphysiologic dosages of glucocorticoids because mitotane increases cortisol-binding globulin and accelerates glucocorticoid metabolism by activating P450 CYP3A4. In the largest retrospective cohort studies performed to date, adjuvant mitotane monotherapy following a complete surgical resection in stage III adrenocortical carcinoma increased progression-free survival and suggested a trend towards improved overall survival.

In some centers, adjuvant radiotherapy is also considered, particularly for stage III disease. Progression of disease while on mitotane (ie, development of advanced adrenocortical carcinoma) should trigger an intensification of therapy, which could include chemotherapy (etoposide, doxorubicin, cisplatin) (Answers B and E), radiotherapy, immunotherapy, and/or repeated surgery or radiofrequency ablation of metastases. There are insufficient data to support the efficacy of chemotherapy, radiotherapy, or immunotherapy as first-line adjuvant therapies; however, many centers do sometimes use these treatments as first-line on a case-by-case basis. Streptozotocin (Answer C) has been shown to be inferior to etoposide, doxorubicin, and cisplatin in a randomized controlled trial; however, it can be considered as an alternative chemotherapy when there is progression of disease on etoposide, doxorubicin, and cisplatin.

Stage	Description
I	T1, N0, M0 • Primary tumor ≤5 cm • Localized; no local invasion, negative lymph nodes, no distant metastases
II	T2, N0, M0 • Primary tumor >5 cm • Localized; no local invasion, negative lymph nodes, no distant metastases
III	T1-T2, N1, M0 T3-T4, N0-N1, M0 • Primary tumor infiltration into surrounding periadrenal tissue, invasion into adjacent organs, tumor thrombus in vena cava or renal vein, or positive lymph node involvement • No distant metastases
IV (advanced)	T1-T4, N0-N1, M1 • Distant metastases, regardless of other factors

Adapted from Else T, Kim A, Sabolch A, et al. Adrenocortical carcinoma. Endocr Rev. 2014;35(2):282-326.

Educational Objective
Make treatment recommendations on the basis of staging of adrenocortical carcinoma.

UpToDate Topic Review(s)
Treatment of adrenocortical carcinoma

Reference(s)

Fassnacht M, Dekkers OM, Else T, et al. European Society of Endocrinology Clinical Practice Guidelines on the management of adrenocortical carcinoma in adults, in collaboration with the European Network for the Study of Adrenal Tumors. *Eur J Endocrinol.* 2018;179(4):G1-G46. PMID: 30299884

Else T, Kim A, Sabolch A, et al. Adrenocortical carcinoma. *Endocr Rev.* 2014;35(2):282-326. PMID: 24423978

116 ANSWER: B) Discontinue both oral contraceptives and cabergoline

Cabergoline is the drug of choice to treat various forms of hyperprolactinemia. Although concerns were recently raised about the effects of cabergoline on heart valve anatomy and function, a significant risk of valvular disease was observed only in patients taking 3 mg daily, a dosage almost never used to treat hyperprolactinemia. Nevertheless, a small degree of worry remains about the long-term effects of low cabergoline dosages. Therefore, treatment cessation should be considered if possible. Cabergoline is a pregnancy category B drug (animal reproduction studies have failed to demonstrate a risk to the fetus, but there are no adequate and well-controlled studies in pregnant women). A seminal paper from Colao et al published in 2003 reported that 66.5% of patients with microprolactinomas or macroprolactinomas who had received cabergoline for longer than 2 years, and whose prolactin was well controlled by 0.5 mg of cabergoline weekly, maintained a normal prolactin level after cabergoline withdrawal. In a follow-up article, the same group identified a serum prolactin concentration of 5.4 ng/mL or less (≤0.2 nmol/L) and maximal residual tumor diameter of 3.1 mm or smaller on MRI as predictors of remission. When both features occurred, the chance of hyperprolactinemia recurrence was only 20%, while it was 90% if neither of the 2 features was present. The chance of recurrence was about 50% if only the prolactin criterion was met and 56% if only the tumor size criterion was met. A recent meta-analysis by Xia et al that included 1106 patients from 24 studies found an overall success rate of cabergoline withdrawal of 36.6% in patients on low-dosage maintenance therapy (0.5 mg weekly). In this particular patient (whose prolactin level is lower than 5.4 ng/mL with no residual tumor on MRI), the chance of remaining euprolactinemic after ceasing cabergoline is about 80%. In preparation for a pregnancy, it is reasonable to stop cabergoline and the oral contraceptive (Answer B) and to monitor prolactin and the patient's menstrual period pattern (Answer B).

All studies of cabergoline withdrawal have shown that when recurrence occurs, an increase in prolactin is observed before any evidence of tumor growth. Therefore, cabergoline withdrawal is safe and should be attempted, given the high chance of being successful in this case. While the occurrence of clinically significant growth of a residual adenoma during pregnancy would be low (given the recent MRI showing no visible adenoma), the patient should be informed of possible regrowth during pregnancy.

Continuing cabergoline at this point (Answer A) seems unnecessary, as the patient has a good chance of being cured and becoming pregnant while off the dopaminergic agent.

Because there are more safety data on bromocriptine than on cabergoline at the time of conception, some practitioners switch patients who desire pregnancy from cabergoline to bromocriptine (Answer C). While this may be a reasonable approach, there is a possibility that this patient may not need any dopaminergic medication at all.

The landmark 2004 Colao et al study enrolled patients who had been on cabergoline for a minimum of 2 years. Therefore, there is no need to treat for a minimum of 5 years (Answer D) before attempting withdrawal.

If her prolactinoma is cured, she should be able to conceive naturally, without assisted reproductive technologies (Answer E).

Educational Objective
Counsel patients with prolactinoma regarding cabergoline withdrawal.

UpToDate Topic Review(s)
Management of hyperprolactinemia

Reference(s)

Colao A, Di Sarno A, Cappabianca P, Di Somma C, Pivonello R, Lombardi G. Withdrawal of long-term cabergoline therapy for tumoral and nontumoral hyperprolactinemia. *N Engl J Med.* 2003;349(21):2023-2033. PMID: 14627787

Colao A, Di Sarno A, Guerra E, et al. Predictors of remission of hyperprolactinaemia after long-term withdrawal of cabergoline therapy. *Clin Endocrinol (Oxf).* 2007;67(3):426-433. PMID: 17573902

Xia MY, Lou XH, Lin SJ, Wu ZB. Optimal timing of dopamine agonist withdrawal in patients with hyperprolactinemia: a systematic review and meta-analysis. *Endocrine*. 2018;59(1):50-61. PMID: 29043560

Salvatori R. Dopamine agonist withdrawal in hyperprolactinemia: when and how. *Endocrine*. 2018;59(1):4-6. PMID: 29124662

117 ANSWER: E) Recommend testicular sperm extraction and intracytoplasmic sperm injection

Klinefelter syndrome (47,XXY) is a common cause of primary hypogonadism in men, with an estimated prevalence of 1 in 650 male births. Men with Klinefelter syndrome usually have small testicles and azoospermia, accounting for 10% of azoospermia cases. Sperm in ejaculate is uncommon, and, if present, is often associated with chromosomal mosaicism. Historically, men with Klinefelter syndrome and their partners were referred for fertility treatment with donor semen (Answer A). However, studies in the late 1990s reported that many men with Klinefelter syndrome and azoospermia actually harbor minor testicular foci with production of small numbers of spermatozoa. For men with Klinefelter syndrome and azoospermia, fertility is now possible with techniques such as microdissection testicular sperm extraction followed by intracytoplasmic sperm injection (Answer E). In experienced centers, sperm retrieval rates per testicular sperm extraction cycle are around 44%, with similar pregnancy and live birth rates (around 40%).

Of note, the risk of chromosomal abnormalities in offspring of men with Klinefelter syndrome does not appear to be increased, most likely because spermatozoa from men with Klinefelter syndrome originate in euploid germ cells where the extra X chromosome is lost. Preimplantation genetic diagnosis is therefore not currently recommended.

In contrast to the established benefits of testicular sperm extraction combined with intracytoplasmic sperm injection, the effect of treatments such as hCG (Answer C) or selective estrogen-receptor modulators (Answer B) on spermatogenesis is not well understood, and there are no clinical data demonstrating effectiveness. Likewise there is no rationale to reduce testosterone replacement. While testosterone treatment can suppress spermatogenesis, reducing or stopping testosterone treatment (Answer D) has no proven impact in men with defective spermatogenesis due to Klinefelter syndrome. Whether previous testosterone therapy affects sperm retrieval rates by testicular sperm extraction remains debated.

Educational Objective
Counsel men with Klinefelter syndrome regarding fertility issues.

UpToDate Topic Review(s)
Treatments for male infertility
Causes of primary hypogonadism in males

Reference(s)
Gravholt CH, Chang S, Wallentin M, Fedder J, Moore P, Skakkebæk A. Klinefelter syndrome: integrating genetics, neuropsychology, and endocrinology. *Endocr Rev*. 2018;39(4):389-423. PMID: 29438472

Corona G, Pizzocaro A, Lanfranco F, et al; Klinefelter ItaliaN Group (KING). Sperm recovery and ICSI outcomes in Klinefelter syndrome: a systematic review and meta-analysis. *Hum Reprod Update*. 2017;23(3):265-275. PMID: 28379559

118 ANSWER: E) Perform a urinalysis

This vignette highlights the difficulty in diagnosing diabetic ketoacidosis (DKA) when the serum bicarbonate level is normal. This patient also has a diagnosis of gastroparesis, which, at first glance, appears to be the cause of the nausea and vomiting. The astute clinician would note that the anion gap is 19 (normal is <12). Because this patient has type 1 diabetes, one should always consider DKA in the differential diagnosis of nausea and vomiting. He has a normal bicarbonate level because he is also volume contracted and has been losing chloride in the form of hydrochloric acid from emesis of gastric contents. This results in a coexisting metabolic alkalosis. A clue to the metabolic alkalosis is calculating the "delta-delta" of the anion gap, which is the relationship between the increase delta in the plasma anion gap and the decrease delta in the plasma bicarbonate concentration. For pure DKA, the ratio of these 2 changes approximates 1. A ratio higher or lower than 1 signifies a coexisting acid-base disorder. In the current vignette, the increase in the anion gap above normal is 7, and the decrease in bicarbonate is 0, affirming a coexisting disorder—metabolic alkalosis.

In this vignette, urinalysis (Answer E) is the easiest method to determine the presence or absence of ketones. Although not listed as an answer, measuring β-hydroxybutyrate would also confirm the presence of ketosis. Once this is confirmed, the patient can be treated for underlying DKA, which is the cause of his nausea and vomiting. Treatment of his nausea with parenteral antiemetics (Answer A) or discharging the patient and changing his diet to frequent small meals (Answer C) is incorrect because neither step addresses the cause of the nausea—DKA. Performing a cosyntropin-stimulation test to screen for adrenal insufficiency (Answer B) is not necessary, as that is not the underlying cause of his nausea and vomiting and does not explain the anion gap. Discharging the patient and changing the antiemetic to erythromycin (Answer D) is incorrect, as he should be admitted to the hospital and treated for DKA.

Educational Objective
Diagnose diabetic ketoacidosis on the basis of an elevated anion gap when the serum bicarbonate level is normal.

UpToDate Topic Review(s)
Diabetic ketoacidosis and hyperosmolar hyperglycemic state in adults: Clinical features, evaluation, and diagnosis

Reference(s)

Kamel KS, Halperin ML. Acid-base problems in diabetic ketoacidosis. *N Engl J Med.* 2015;372(20):1969-1970. PMID: 25970063

Kitabchi AE, Umpierrez GE, Miles JM, Fisher JN. Hyperglycemic crises in adult patients with diabetes. *Diabetes Care.* 2009;32(7):1335-1343. PMID: 19564476

119 ANSWER: C) Denosumab

The initial assessment of hypercalcemia must include measurement of PTH to determine whether the condition is PTH dependent or independent. Although primary hyperparathyroidism is the most common cause of hypercalcemia in outpatients, the most common cause of hypercalcemia in hospitalized patients is hypercalcemia of malignancy, as is the case in this particular patient. Hypercalcemia of malignancy occurs in up to 30% of patients with malignancy, with the most common associated cancers being lung, breast, urinary tract, and multiple myeloma. When present, hypercalcemia of malignancy is generally a poor prognostic sign with a mean survival of 2 to 3 months. As in this patient, common presenting symptoms include fatigue and mental confusion, as well as nausea, anorexia, bone pain, and polyuria. Most patients with hypercalcemia of malignancy have tumoral overproduction of PTHrP, a hormone that serves a physiologic role in embryologic development and mammary gland function. Overproduction of PTHrP in this setting increases osteoclastic bone resorption and renal reabsorption of calcium, often resulting in profound hypercalcemia. Less commonly, hypercalcemia of malignancy is due to localized osteolysis that is triggered by tumor cell secretion of osteoclast-activating cytokines in bone, or is due to tumor cell overproduction of calcitriol that enhances intestinal absorption and bone resorption of calcium.

Initial therapies for a patient with hypercalcemia of malignancy due to PTHrP are aggressive intravenous hydration, as affected patients are usually markedly hypovolemic because of polyuria and reduced oral intake, and correction of hypophosphatemia, if present, with oral phosphate. Although used historically in hypercalcemic patients to enhance renal calcium excretion, loop diuretics such as furosemide (Answer A) are not proven beneficial in this setting and may exacerbate electrolyte disturbances. Intravenous bisphosphonates such as pamidronate (Answer B) and zoledronic acid are first-line agents in patients with hypercalcemia of malignancy due to PTHrP, with onset of the calcium-lowering effect within 1 to 3 days. Sometimes hypercalcemia of malignancy, however, is refractory to bisphosphonates, as is the case with this patient. Therefore, use of the less potent bisphosphonate pamidronate is inappropriate for her.

Denosumab (Answer C), the monoclonal antibody to receptor-activated nuclear factor kappa-B ligand (RANKL), which is approved for the treatment of osteoporosis, is FDA approved to treat hypercalcemia of malignancy that is refractory to bisphosphonate therapy and is the appropriate choice for this patient. Denosumab is administered at a dosage of 120 mg subcutaneously on days 1, 8, and 15, with a maintenance dosage of 120 mg every 4 weeks. Treated patients are at a higher risk of hypocalcemia, particularly if more advanced renal dysfunction is present. As such, they should receive vitamin D supplementation to ensure an adequate 25-hydroxyvitamin D level (>30 ng/mL [>74.9 nmol/L]). As with parenteral bisphosphonates, patients treated with denosumab are at higher risk of osteonecrosis of the jaw (~1.8% incidence over 14 months), although this is generally less important given the poor prognosis in most patients.

Calcitonin (Answer D) has limited effectiveness in hypercalcemia of malignancy due to the markedly lower antiosteoclastic effect, as well as tachyphylaxis with continued use. Prednisone (Answer E) is beneficial in patients with hypercalcemia of malignancy who have elevated serum 1,25-dihydroxyvitamin D levels due to tumor overproduction, which is not present in this patient.

Educational Objective
Explain the role of denosumab in hypercalcemia refractory to conventional therapy in a patient with humoral hypercalcemia of malignancy.

UpToDate Topic Review(s)
Hypercalcemia of malignancy: Mechanisms

Reference(s)
Hu MI, Glezerman IG, Leboulleux S, et al. Denosumab for treatment of hypercalcemia of malignancy. *J Clin Endocrinol Metab.* 2014;99(9):3144-3152. PMID: 24915117

120 ANSWER: D) Fluoxetine

The patient described in this vignette has binge eating disorder (BED). Binge eating is characterized by 2 distinct features: 1) eating in a discrete period an amount of food that is larger than what most people would eat in a similar period under similar circumstances and 2) there is a sense of lack of control over eating during an episode. BED is characterized by recurrent episodes of binge eating that are associated with 3 or more of the following: 1) eating much more rapidly than normal, 2) eating until feeling uncomfortably full, 3) eating large amounts of food when not feeling physically hungry, 4) eating alone because of feeling embarrassed by how much one is eating, and 5) feeling disgusted with oneself, depressed, or very guilty afterward. Also, affected individuals have marked distress regarding binge eating and the episodes are not associated with inappropriate compensatory behavior as in bulimia nervosa. Episodes of binge eating in patients with BED occur at least once a week for 3 months. BED can be classified as mild, moderate, severe, or extreme depending on the number of binge-eating episodes per week. The lifetime prevalence of BED in adults is 2% for men and 3.5% for women. This disorder is more prevalent in individuals seeking weight-loss treatment than in the general population.

Treatment for BED includes psychotherapy such as cognitive behavioral therapy and pharmacotherapy. Antidepressants, anticonvulsant agents, stimulants, and weight-loss medications have been studied for the treatment of BED. Selective serotonin reuptake inhibitors have been the most frequently studied medications in this setting. When compared with placebo, fluoxetine is associated with a significant reduction in the frequency of binge eating. Both fluoxetine and sertraline have been shown to reduce the frequency of binges and to improve binge behavior to a similar degree as measured by the binge-eating scale. Among anticonvulsant medications, topiramate reduces the number of binge-eating days per week (-3.5 ± 1.9 vs -2.5 ± 2.1) and binge episodes per week (-5.0 ± 4.3 vs -3.4 ± 3.8) compared with placebo. Sixteen percent of patients on topiramate discontinued the study because of adverse effects compared with 8% in the placebo group.

Weight-loss medications studied in the treatment of BED include sibutramine, fenfluramine, and orlistat. The first 2 drugs have been withdrawn from the market in the United States. Orlistat has not shown reduction in binge eating compared with placebo, but it does help with weight loss. In the stimulant group, lisdexamfetamine has US FDA approval for treatment of moderate to severe BED. Lisdenxamfetamine is started at a dosage of 30 mg daily, and the dosage is increased by 20 mg increments up to 70 mg daily. A randomized placebo-controlled trial showed a greater percentage of participants achieving 4-week binge-eating cessation in the treatment group (50 mg/daily, 42.2% [$P = 0.1$] and 70 mg/daily, 50% [$P < .01$]) compared with the placebo group (21.3%).

In this vignette, it is important to recognize that the patient has mild BED and she would benefit from treatment of this condition first. Therefore, the best suggestion is to start fluoxetine (Answer D). The addition of a selective serotonin reuptake inhibitor to bupropion is generally well tolerated. Empagliflozin (an SGLT-2 inhibitor) (Answer A), phentermine (a sympathomimetic approved for short-term use) (Answer B), lorcaserin (a selective serotonin receptor agonist) (Answer C), and liraglutide (a GLP-1 receptor agonist) (Answer E) have not been studied for effectiveness in treating BED. Also, her type 2 diabetes is well controlled, so adding an SGLT-2 inhibitor or liraglutide is not indicated now.

Educational Objective
Diagnose binge eating disorder and recommend appropriate treatment.

UpToDate Topic Review(s)
Binge eating disorder in adults: Overview of treatment

Reference(s)

Hudson JI, Hiripi E, Pope HG Jr, Kessler RC. The prevalence and correlates of eating disorders in the National Comorbidity Survey Replication [published correction appears in *Biol Psychiatry*. 2012;72(2):164]. *Biol Psychiatry*. 2007;61(3):348-358. PMID: 16815322

Reas DL, Grilo CM. Pharmacological treatment of binge eating disorder: update review and synthesis. *Expert Opin Pharmacother*. 2015;16(10):1463-1478. PMID: 26044518

McElroy SL, Hudson JI, Capece JA, et al. Topiramate for the treatment of binge eating disorder associated with obesity: a placebo-controlled study. *Biol Psychiatry*. 2007;61(9):1039-1048. PMID: 17258690

McElroy SL, Hudson JI, Mitchell JE. Efficacy and safety of lisdexamfetamine for treatment of adults with moderate to severe binge-eating disorder: a randomized clinical trial. *JAMA. Psychiatry*. 2015;72(3):235-246. PMID: 25587645

ENDOCRINE SELF-ASSESSMENT PROGRAM 2020

Part III

This question-mapping index groups question topics according to the 8 umbrella sections of ESAP (Adrenal, Bone-Calcium, Diabetes, Lipids-Obesity, Pituitary, Reproduction [Female], Reproduction [Male], and Thyroid). Relevant **question numbers** follow each topic.

www.ingramcontent.com/pod-product-compliance
Lightning Source LLC
Chambersburg PA
CBHW050438200326
41458CB00014B/4983